PN Pharmacology for Nursing
REVIEW MODULE EDITION 7.0

Contributors

Norma Jean E. Henry, MSN/Ed, RN

Honey C. Holman, MSN, RN

Debborah Williams, MSN, RN

Kellie Wilford, MSN, RN

Marsha S. Barlow, MSN RN

Mary Jane Janowski, RN, MA

Peggy L. Leehy, MSN, RN

Terri Lemon, DNP, MSN, RN

Consultants

Tracey Bousquet, BSN, RN

Deb Johnson-Schuh, RN, MSN, CNE

LaKeisha Wheless, MSN, RN

Lisa Bass, MSN, RN, CRNI, CNE

Penny Fauber, RN, BSN, MS, PhD

Ronda Points, RN, MSN/Ed

Director of content review: Kristen Lawler

Director of development: Derek Prater

Project management: Nicole Burke

Coordination of content review: Norma Jean E. Henry, Honey C. Holman

Copy editing: Kelly Von Lunen, Bethany Phillips

Layout: Spring Lenox, Randi Hardy, Charves Hervey, Rachel Cohen

Illustrations: Randi Hardy

Online media: Morgan Smith, Ron Hanson, Nicole Lobdell, Brant Stacy

Cover design: Jason Buck

Interior book design: Spring Lenox

IMPORTANT NOTICE TO THE READER

User's Guide

Welcome to the Assessment Technologies Institute® PN Pharmacology for Nursing Review Module Edition 7.0. The mission of ATI's Content Mastery Series® Review Modules is to provide user-friendly compendiums of nursing knowledge that will:
- Help you locate important information quickly.
- Assist in your learning efforts.
- Provide exercises for applying your nursing knowledge.
- Facilitate your entry into the nursing profession as a newly licensed nurse.

This newest edition of the Review Modules has been redesigned to optimize your learning experience. We've fit more content into less space and have done so in a way that will make it even easier for you to find and understand the information you need.

ORGANIZATION

This Review Module is organized into units covering pharmacological principles (Unit 1) and medications affecting the body systems and physiological processes (Units 2 to 12). Chapters within these units conform to one of two organizing principles for presenting the content.
- Nursing concepts
- Medications

Nursing concepts chapters begin with an overview describing the central concept and its relevance to nursing. Subordinate themes are covered in outline form to demonstrate relationships and present the information in a clear, succinct manner.

Medications chapters include an overview describing a disorder or group of disorders. Medications used to treat these disorders are grouped according to classification. A specific medication can be selected as a prototype or example of the characteristics of medications in this classification. These sections include information about how the medication works, its therapeutic uses, and routes of administration. Next, you will find information about complications, contraindications, and medication and food interactions, as well as nursing interventions and client education to help prevent and/or manage these issues. Finally, the chapter includes information on nursing administration of the medication and evaluation of the medication's effectiveness.

ACTIVE LEARNING SCENARIOS AND APPLICATION EXERCISES

Each chapter includes opportunities for you to test your knowledge and to practice applying that knowledge. Active Learning Scenario exercises pose a nursing scenario and then direct you to use an ATI Active Learning Template (included at the back of this book) to record the important knowledge a nurse should apply to the scenario. An example is then provided to which you can compare your completed Active Learning Template. The Application Exercises include NCLEX-style questions, such as multiple-choice and multiple-select items, providing you with opportunities to practice answering the kinds of questions you might expect to see on ATI assessments or the NCLEX. After the Application Exercises, an answer key is provided, along with rationales.

NCLEX® CONNECTIONS

To prepare for the NCLEX-PN, it is important to understand how the content in this Review Module is connected to the NCLEX-PN test plan. You can find information on the detailed test plan at the National Council of State Boards of Nursing's website, www.ncsbn.org. When reviewing content in this Review Module, regularly ask yourself, "How does this content fit into the test plan, and what types of questions related to this content should I expect?"

To help you in this process, we've included NCLEX Connections at the beginning of each unit and with each question in the Application Exercises Answer Keys. The NCLEX Connections at the beginning of each unit point out areas of the detailed test plan that relate to the content within that unit. The NCLEX Connections attached to the Application Exercises Answer Keys demonstrate how each exercise fits within the detailed content outline. These NCLEX Connections will help you understand how the detailed content outline is organized, starting with major client needs categories and subcategories and followed by related content areas and tasks. The major client needs categories are:
- Safe and Effective Care Environment
  - Management of Care
  - Safety and Infection Control
- Health Promotion and Maintenance
- Psychosocial Integrity
- Physiological Integrity
  - Basic Care and Comfort
  - Pharmacological and Parenteral Therapies
  - Reduction of Risk Potential
  - Physiological Adaptation

An NCLEX Connection might, for example, alert you that content within a unit is related to:
- Pharmacological and Parenteral Therapies
  - Adverse Effects/Contraindications/Side Effects/ Interactions
    - Identify a contraindication to the administration of a medication to the client.

QSEN COMPETENCIES

As you use the Review Modules, you will note the integration of the Quality and Safety Education for Nurses (QSEN) competencies throughout the chapters. These competencies are integral components of the curriculum of many nursing programs in the United States and prepare you to provide safe, high-quality care as a newly licensed nurse. Icons appear to draw your attention to the six QSEN competencies.

Safety: The minimization of risk factors that could cause injury or harm while promoting quality care and maintaining a secure environment for clients, self, and others.

Patient-Centered Care: The provision of caring and compassionate, culturally sensitive care that addresses clients' physiological, psychological, sociological, spiritual, and cultural needs, preferences, and values.

Evidence-Based Practice: The use of current knowledge from research and other credible sources, on which to base clinical judgment and client care.

Informatics: The use of information technology as a communication and information-gathering tool that supports clinical decision-making and scientifically based nursing practice.

Quality Improvement: Care related and organizational processes that involve the development and implementation of a plan to improve health care services and better meet clients' needs.

Teamwork and Collaboration: The delivery of client care in partnership with multidisciplinary members of the health care team to achieve continuity of care and positive client outcomes.

ICONS

Icons are used throughout the Review Module to draw your attention to particular areas. Keep an eye out for these icons.

(N) This icon is used for NCLEX Connections.

(G) This icon indicates gerontological considerations, or knowledge specific to the care of older adult clients.

Qs This icon is used for content related to safety and is a QSEN competency. When you see this icon, take note of safety concerns or steps that nurses can take to ensure client safety and a safe environment.

QPCC This icon is a QSEN competency that indicates the importance of a holistic approach to providing care.

QEBP This icon, a QSEN competency, points out the integration of research into clinical practice.

QI This icon is a QSEN competency and highlights the use of information technology to support nursing practice.

QQI This icon is used to focus on the QSEN competency of integrating planning processes to meet clients' needs.

QTC This icon highlights the QSEN competency of care delivery using an interprofessional approach.

M◇ This icon appears at the top-right of pages and indicates availability of an online media supplement, such as a graphic, animation, or video. If you have an electronic copy of the Review Module, this icon will appear alongside clickable links to media supplements. If you have a hard copy version of the Review Module, visit www.atitesting.com for details on how to access these features.

FEEDBACK

ATI welcomes feedback regarding this Review Module. Please provide comments to comments@atitesting.com.

Table of Contents

NCLEX® Connections   1

UNIT 1

Pharmacological Principles

CHAPTER 1	Pharmacokinetics and Routes of Administration	3
CHAPTER 2	Safe Medication Administration and Error Reduction	11
CHAPTER 3	Dosage Calculation	17
CHAPTER 4	Intravenous Therapy	29
CHAPTER 5	Adverse Effects, Interactions, and Contraindications	35

NCLEX® Connections   41

UNIT 2

Medications Affecting the Nervous System

CHAPTER 6	Anxiety and Trauma- and Stressor-Related Disorders	43
CHAPTER 7	Depressive Disorders	49
CHAPTER 8	Bipolar Disorders	59
CHAPTER 9	Psychotic Disorders	65
CHAPTER 10	Medications for Children and Adolescents Who Have Mental Health Issues	73
CHAPTER 11	Substance Use Disorders	83
CHAPTER 12	Chronic Neurologic Disorders	89
CHAPTER 13	Eye and Ear Disorders	101
	Eye disorders	*101*
	Ear disorders	*104*
CHAPTER 14	Miscellaneous Central Nervous System Medications	109
CHAPTER 15	Sedative-Hypnotics	117

NCLEX® Connections 123

UNIT 3 *Medications Affecting the Respiratory System*

CHAPTER 16   Airflow Disorders   125

Bronchodilators   125

Anti-inflammatory agents   128

CHAPTER 17   Upper Respiratory Disorders   133

NCLEX® Connections 141

UNIT 4 *Medications Affecting the Cardiovascular System*

CHAPTER 18   Medications Affecting Urinary Output   143

CHAPTER 19   Medications Affecting Blood Pressure   151

CHAPTER 20   Cardiac Glycosides and Heart Failure   163

CHAPTER 21   Angina and Antilipemic Agents   169

Angina   169

Antilipemic agents   171

NCLEX® Connections 179

UNIT 5 *Medications Affecting the Hematologic System*

CHAPTER 22   Medications Affecting Coagulation   181

CHAPTER 23   Growth Factors   193

NCLEX® Connections   199

UNIT 6   *Medications Affecting the Gastrointestinal System and Nutrition*

CHAPTER 24   Peptic Ulcer Disease   201

CHAPTER 25   Gastrointestinal Disorders   207

CHAPTER 26   Vitamins, Minerals, and Supplements   217

NCLEX® Connections   227

UNIT 7   *Medications Affecting the Reproductive System*

CHAPTER 27   Medications Affecting the Reproductive Tract   229

NCLEX® Connections   239

UNIT 8   *Medications for Joint and Bone Conditions*

CHAPTER 28   Connective Tissue Disorders   241

CHAPTER 29   Bone Disorders   251

NCLEX® Connections   257

UNIT 9   *Medications for Pain and Inflammation*

CHAPTER 30   Nonopioid Analgesics   259

CHAPTER 31   Opioid Agonists and Antagonists   265

CHAPTER 32   Adjuvant Medications for Pain   271

CHAPTER 33   Miscellaneous Pain Medications   277

NCLEX® Connections   285

UNIT 10   *Medications Affecting the Endocrine System*

CHAPTER 34   Diabetes Mellitus   287

CHAPTER 35   Endocrine Disorders   295

NCLEX® Connections   305

UNIT 11   *Medications Affecting the Immune System*

CHAPTER 36   Immunizations   307

NCLEX® Connections   315

UNIT 12   *Medications for Infection*

CHAPTER 37   Principles of Antimicrobial Therapy   317

CHAPTER 38   Antibiotics Affecting the Bacterial Cell Wall   321

CHAPTER 39   Antibiotics Affecting Protein Synthesis   327

CHAPTER 40   Urinary Tract Infections   333

CHAPTER 41   Mycobacterial, Fungal, and Parasitic Infections   339

CHAPTER 42   Viral Infections, HIV, and AIDS   345

References   *353*

Active Learning Templates   *A1*

Basic Concept   A1

Diagnostic Procedure   A3

Growth and Development   A5

Medication   A7

Nursing Skill   A9

System Disorder   A11

Therapeutic Procedure   A13

ⓝ NCLEX® Connections

When reviewing the following chapters, keep in mind the relevant topics and tasks of the NCLEX outline, in particular:

Safety and Infection Control

ACCIDENT/ERROR/INJURY PREVENTION
Identify the client's allergies and intervene as appropriate.

Evaluate the appropriateness of a health care provider's order for the client.

REPORTING OF INCIDENT/EVENT/IRREGULAR OCCURRENCE/VARIANCE
Identify situations requiring completion of incident/event/irregular occurrence/variance report (medication administration error, client fall).

Acknowledge and document practice error (incident report).

Pharmacological Therapies

ADVERSE EFFECTS/CONTRAINDICATIONS/SIDE EFFECTS/ INTERACTIONS: Identify a contraindication to the administration of prescribed or over-the-counter medication to the client.

DOSAGE CALCULATIONS: Perform calculations needed for medication administration.

MEDICATION ADMINISTRATION
Follow the rights of medication administration.

Collect required client data prior to medication administration.

Calculate and monitor intravenous (IV) flow rate.

CHAPTER 1

CHAPTER 1 *Pharmacokinetics and Routes of Administration*

Pharmacokinetics refers to how medications travel through the body. Medications undergo a variety of biochemical processes that result in absorption, distribution, metabolism, and excretion.

PHASES OF PHARMACOKINETICS

ABSORPTION

Absorption is the transmission of medications from the location of administration (gastrointestinal [GI] tract, muscle, blood vessels, skin, mucous membranes, subcutaneous tissue) to the bloodstream. The most common routes of administration are enteral (through the GI tract) and parenteral (by injection). Each of these routes has a unique pattern of absorption.
- The rate of medication absorption determines how soon the medication will take effect.
- The amount of medication the body absorbs determines the intensity of its effects.
- The route of administration affects the rate and amount of absorption.

Oral

BARRIERS TO ABSORPTION: Medications must pass through the layer of epithelial cells that line the GI tract.

ABSORPTION PATTERN: Varies greatly due to the following.
- Stability and solubility of the medication
- GI pH and emptying time
- Presence of food in the stomach or intestines
- Other concurrent medications
- Forms of medications (enteric-coated pills, liquids)

Sublingual, buccal

BARRIERS TO ABSORPTION: Swallowing before dissolution allows gastric pH to inactivate the medication.

ABSORPTION PATTERN: Quick absorption systemically through highly vascular mucous membranes

Other mucous membranes (rectal, vaginal)

BARRIERS TO ABSORPTION: Presence of stool in the rectum or infectious material in the vagina limits tissue contact.

ABSORPTION PATTERN: Easy absorption with both local and systemic effects

Inhalation via mouth, nose

BARRIERS TO ABSORPTION: Inspiratory effort

ABSORPTION PATTERN: Rapid absorption through alveolar capillary networks

Intradermal, topical

BARRIERS TO ABSORPTION: Close proximity of epidermal cells

ABSORPTION PATTERN
- Slow, gradual absorption
- Effects primarily local but also systemic, especially with lipid-soluble medications passing through subcutaneous fatty tissue

Subcutaneous, intramuscular

BARRIERS TO ABSORPTION: There is no significant barrier. Capillary walls have large spaces between cells that medications easily pass through.

ABSORPTION PATTERN
- **Solubility of the medication in water:** Highly soluble medications have rapid absorption (10 to 30 min); poorly soluble medications have slow absorption.
- **Blood perfusion at the site of injection:** Sites with high blood perfusion have rapid absorption; sites with low blood perfusion have slow absorption.

Intravenous

BARRIERS TO ABSORPTION: None

ABSORPTION PATTERN
- **Immediate:** enters directly into the blood
- **Complete:** reaches the blood in its entirety

DISTRIBUTION

Distribution is the transportation of medications to sites of action by bodily fluids. Factors influencing distribution include the following.

Circulation: Conditions that inhibit blood flow or perfusion, such as peripheral vascular or cardiac disease, can delay medication distribution.

Permeability of the cell membrane: The medication must be able to pass through tissues and membranes to reach its target area. Medications that are lipid-soluble or have a transport system can cross the blood-brain barrier and the placenta.

Plasma protein binding: Medications compete for protein binding sites (primarily albumin) within the bloodstream. The ability of a medication to bind to a protein can affect how much of the medication will leave and travel to target tissues. Two medications can compete for the same binding sites, resulting in toxicity.

METABOLISM

Metabolism (biotransformation) changes medications into less active or inactive forms by the action of enzymes. This occurs primarily in the liver, but it also takes place in the kidneys, lungs, intestines, and blood.

FACTORS INFLUENCING THE RATE OF MEDICATION METABOLISM

- **Age:** Infants have a limited medication-metabolizing capacity. The aging process also can influence medication metabolism, but varies with the individual. In general, hepatic medication metabolism tends to decline with age. Older adults require smaller doses of medications due to the possibility of accumulation in the body. Ⓒ
- **Increase in some medication-metabolizing enzymes:** This can metabolize a particular medication sooner, requiring an increase in dosage of that medication to maintain a therapeutic level. It can also cause an increase in the metabolism of other concurrent-use medications.
- **First-pass effect:** The liver inactivates some medications on their first pass through the liver. Thus they require a nonenteral route (sublingual, IV) because of their high first-pass effect.
- **Similar metabolic pathways:** When the same pathway metabolizes two medications, it can alter the metabolism of one or both. In this way, the rate of metabolism can decrease for one or both of the medications, leading to medication accumulation.
- **Nutritional status:** Clients who are malnourished can be deficient in the factors necessary to produce specific medication-metabolizing enzymes, thus impairing medication metabolism.

OUTCOMES OF METABOLISM

- Increased renal excretion of medication
- Inactivation of medications
- Increased therapeutic effect
- Activation of prodrugs into active forms
- Decreased toxicity when active forms of medications become inactive forms
- Increased toxicity when inactive forms of medications become active forms

EXCRETION

Excretion is the elimination of medications from the body, primarily through the kidneys. Elimination also takes place through the liver, lungs, intestines, and exocrine glands (such as in breast milk). Kidney dysfunction can lead to an increase in the duration and intensity of a medication's response, so it is important to monitor BUN and creatinine levels.

MEDICATION RESPONSES

Medication dosing attempts to regulate medication responses to maintain plasma levels between the minimum effective concentration (MEC) and the toxic concentration. A plasma medication level is in the therapeutic range when it is effective and not toxic. Nurses use therapeutic levels of many medications to monitor clients' responses.

THERAPEUTIC INDEX

Medications with a high therapeutic index (TI) have a wide safety margin, so there is no need for routine serum medication-level monitoring. Medications with a low TI require close monitoring of serum medication levels.

- Nurses should consider the route of administration when monitoring for peak levels.
- For example, an oral medication can peak from 1 to 3 hr after administration. If the route is IV, the peak time might occur within 10 min. (Refer to a medication reference or a pharmacist for specific medication peak times.)
- For trough levels, obtain a blood sample immediately before the next medication dose, regardless of the route of administration.
- A plateau is a medication's concentration in plasma during a series of doses.

HALF-LIFE

Half-life (t½) refers to the time for the medication in the body to drop by 50%. Liver and kidney function affect half-life. It usually takes four half-lives to achieve a steady state of serum concentration (medication intake = medication metabolism and excretion).

SHORT HALF-LIFE

- Medications leave the body quickly (4 to 8 hr).
- Short-dosing interval or MEC drops between doses.

LONG HALF-LIFE

- Medications leave the body slowly (over more than 24 hr) with a greater risk for medication accumulation and toxicity.
- Medications can be given at longer intervals without loss of therapeutic effects.
- Medications take a longer time to reach a steady state.

PHARMACODYNAMICS

Pharmacodynamics describes the interactions between medications and target cells, body systems, and organs to produce effects. These interactions result in functional changes that are the mechanism of action of the medication. Medications interact with cells in one or two ways.

Agonists bind to or mimic the receptor activity that endogenous compounds regulate. For example, morphine is an agonist because it activates the receptors that produce analgesia, sedation, constipation, and other effects. (Receptors are the medication's target sites on or within the cells.)

Antagonists can block the usual receptor activity that endogenous compounds regulate or the receptor activity of other medications. For example, losartan (an angiotensin II receptor blocker) is an antagonist. It works by blocking angiotensin II receptors on blood vessels, which prevents vasoconstriction.

Partial agonists act as agonists and antagonists, with limited affinity to receptor sites. For example, nalbuphine acts as an antagonist at mu receptors and an agonist at kappa receptors, causing analgesia with minimal respiratory depression at low doses.

ROUTES OF ADMINISTRATION

ORAL OR ENTERAL

Tablets, capsules, liquids, suspensions, elixirs, lozenges

Most common route

NURSING ACTIONS
- Contraindications for oral medication administration include vomiting, decreased GI motility, absence of gag reflex, difficulty swallowing, and decreased level of consciousness.
- Have clients sit upright to facilitate swallowing.
- Administer irritating medications, such as analgesics, with small amounts of food.
- Do not mix with large amounts of food or beverages in case clients cannot consume the entire quantity.
- Avoid administration with interacting foods or beverages, such as grapefruit juice.
- In general, administer oral medications on an empty stomach (30 to 60 min before meals, 2 hr after meals).
- Follow the manufacturer's directions for crushing, cutting, and diluting medications. Break or cut scored tablets only. (See the Institute for Safe Medication Practices website, www.ismp.org).
- Make sure clients swallow enteric-coated or time-release medications whole.
- Use a liquid form of the medication to facilitate swallowing whenever possible.

ADVANTAGES
- Safe
- Inexpensive
- Easy and convenient

DISADVANTAGES
- Oral medications have highly variable absorption.
- Inactivation can occur in the GI tract or by first-pass effect.
- Clients must be cooperative and conscious.
- Contraindications include nausea and vomiting.

SUBLINGUAL AND BUCCAL

Directly enters the bloodstream and bypasses the liver

Sublingual: under the tongue

Buccal: between the cheek and the gum

CLIENT EDUCATION
- Keep the medication in place until complete absorption occurs.
- Do not eat or drink while the tablet is in place or until it has completely dissolved.

LIQUIDS, SUSPENSIONS, AND ELIXIRS

NURSING ACTIONS
- Follow directions for dilution and shaking.
- When administering the medication, pour it into a cup on flat surface. Make sure the base of the meniscus (lowest fluid line) is at the level of the dose.

TRANSDERMAL

Medication in a skin patch for absorption through the skin, producing systemic effects

CLIENT EDUCATION
- Apply patches as prescribed to ensure proper dosing.
- Wash the skin with soap and water, and dry it thoroughly before applying a new patch.
- Place the patch on a hairless area, and rotate sites daily to prevent skin irritation.

TOPICAL

- Painless
- Limited adverse effects

NURSING ACTIONS: Apply with a glove, tongue blade, or cotton-tipped applicator. Do not apply with a bare hand.

INSTILLATION (DROPS, OINTMENTS, SPRAYS)

Generally for eyes, ears, and nose

NURSING ACTIONS

- **Eyes**
  - Have clients sit upright or lie supine, tilt their head slightly, and look up at the ceiling.
  - Rest your dominant hand on the client's forehead, hold the dropper above the conjunctival sac about 1 to 2 cm, drop the medication into the center of the sac, avoid placing it directly on the cornea, and have the client close the eye gently. If they blink during instillation, repeat the procedure.
  - Apply gentle pressure with a finger and a clean facial tissue on the nasolacrimal duct for 30 to 60 seconds to prevent systemic absorption of the medication.
  - If instilling more than one medication in the same eye, wait at least 5 min between medications.
  - For eye ointment, apply a thin ribbon to the inner edge of the lower eyelid on the conjunctiva from the inner to the outer canthus.
- **Ears**
  - Have clients sit upright or lie on their side.
  - Straighten the ear canal by pulling the auricle upward and outward for adults or down and back for children. Hold the dropper 1 cm above the ear canal, instill the medication, and then gently apply pressure with a finger to the tragus of the ear, unless it is too painful.
  - Do not press a cotton ball deep into the ear canal. If necessary, gently place it into the outermost part of the ear canal.
  - Have clients remain in the side-lying position if possible for 2 to 3 min after instilling ear drops.
- **Nose**
  - Use medical aseptic technique when administering medications into the nose.
  - Have clients lie supine with their head positioned to allow the medication to enter the prescribed nasal passage.
  - Use the dominant hand to instill the drops, supporting the head with your nondominant hand.
  - Instruct clients to breathe through the mouth, stay in a supine position, and not blow their nose for 5 min after drop instillation.

INHALATION

Administered through metered-dose inhalers (MDI) or dry-powder inhalers (DPI)

MDI

CLIENT EDUCATION

- Remove the cap from the inhaler's mouthpiece.
- Shake the inhaler vigorously five or six times.
- Hold the inhaler with the mouthpiece at the bottom.
- Hold the inhaler with the thumb near the mouthpiece and the index and middle fingers at the top.
- Hold the inhaler about 2 to 4 cm (1 to 2 in) away from the front of the mouth or close the mouth around the mouthpiece of the inhaler with the opening pointing toward the back of the throat.
- Take a deep breath and then exhale.
- Tilt the head back slightly, press the inhaler, and, at the same time, begin a slow, deep inhalation breath. Continue to breathe in slowly and deeply for 3 to 5 seconds to facilitate delivery to the air passages.
- Hold the breath for 10 seconds to allow the medication to deposit in your airways.
- Take the inhaler out of the mouth and slowly exhale through pursed lips.
- Resume normal breathing.
- A spacer keeps the medication in the device longer, thereby increasing the amount of medication the device delivers to the lungs and decreasing the amount of medication in the oropharynx.
  - Remove the covers from the mouthpieces of the inhaler and of the spacer.
  - Insert the MDI into the end of the spacer.
  - Shake the inhaler five or six times.
  - Exhale completely, and then close the mouth around the spacer's mouthpiece. Continue as with an MDI.

DPI

CLIENT EDUCATION

- Do not shake the device.
- Take the cover off the mouthpiece.
- Follow the manufacturer's directions for preparing the medication, such as turning the wheel of the inhaler or loading a medication pellet.
- Exhale completely.
- Place the mouthpiece between the lips and take a deep inhalation breath through the mouth.
- Hold the breath for 5 to 10 seconds.
- Take the inhaler out of the mouth and slowly exhale through pursed lips.
- Resume normal breathing.
- If more than one puff is needed, wait the length of time the provider specifies before administering the second puff.
- Rinse the mouth out with water or brush teeth if using a corticosteroid inhaler to reduce the risk of fungal infections of the mouth.
- Remove the canister and rinse the inhaler, cap, and spacer once a day with warm running water and dry them completely before using the inhaler again.

NASOGASTRIC AND GASTROSTOMY TUBES

NURSING ACTIONS
- Verify proper tube placement.
- Use a syringe and allow the medication to flow in by gravity or push it in with the plunger of the syringe.
- To prevent clogging, flush the tubing before and after each medication with 15 to 30 mL warm sterile water.
- Flush with another 15 to 30 mL warm sterile water after instilling all the medications.

General guidelines
- Use liquid forms of medications. If not available, consider crushing medications if allowed.
- Do not administer sublingual medications through an NG tube. (Sublingual medications are given under the tongue.)
- Do not crush specifically prepared oral medications (extended/time-release, fluid-filled, enteric-coated).
- Administer each medication separately.
- Do not mix medications with enteral feedings.
- Completely dissolve crushed tablets and capsule contents in 15 to 30 mL sterile water prior to administration.

SUPPOSITORIES

NURSING ACTIONS
- Follow the manufacturer's directions for storage.
- Wear gloves for the procedure.
- Remove the wrapper, and lubricate the suppository if necessary.
- **Rectal suppositories (thin, bullet-shaped medication)**
  - Position clients in the left lateral or Sims' position.
  - Insert the suppository just beyond the internal sphincter.
  - Instruct clients to remain flat or in the left lateral position for at least 5 min after insertion to retain the suppository. Absorption times vary by medication.
- **Vaginal suppositories**
  - Position clients supine with knees bent and feet flat on the bed and close to their hips (modified lithotomy or dorsal recumbent position).
  - Use the applicator, if available.
  - Insert the suppository along the posterior wall of the vagina 7.5 to 10 cm (3 to 4 in).
  - Instruct clients to remain supine for at least 5 min after insertion to retain the suppository.
  - If using an applicator, wash it with soap and water. (If it is disposable, discard it.)

PARENTERAL

NURSING ACTIONS
- The vastus lateralis is best for infants 1 year and younger.
- The ventrogluteal site is preferable for IM injections and for injecting volumes greater than 2 mL.
- The deltoid site has a smaller muscle mass and can only accommodate up to 1 mL of fluid.
- Use a needle size and length indicated for the type of injection and the client's size. Syringe size should approximate the volume of medication.
- Use a tuberculin syringe for solution volumes less than 0.5 mL.
- Rotate injection sites to enhance medication absorption, and document each site.
- Do not use injection sites that are edematous, inflamed, or have moles, birthmarks, or scars.
- For IV administration, immediately monitor clients for therapeutic and adverse effects.
- Discard all sharps (broken ampule bottles, needles) in leak- and puncture-proof containers.

INTRADERMAL

NURSING ACTIONS
- Use for tuberculin testing or checking for medication or allergy sensitivities.
- Use small amounts of solution (0.01 to 0.1 mL) in a tuberculin syringe with a fine-gauge needle (25- to 27-gauge, ¼ to ⅝ inches long) in lightly pigmented, thin-skinned, hairless sites (inner surface of mid-forearm, scapular area of back) at 10° to 15° angle.
- Insert the needle with the bevel up. A small bleb should appear.
- Do not massage the site after injection.

SUBCUTANEOUS AND INTRAMUSCULAR

NURSING ACTIONS
- **Subcutaneous**
  - Use for small doses of nonirritating, water-soluble medications (insulin, heparin).
  - Use a 3/8- to 5/8-inch, 25- to 27-gauge needle or a 28- to 31-gauge insulin syringe. Inject no more than 1.5 mL of solution.
  - Select sites that have an adequate fat-pad size (abdomen, upper hips, lateral upper arms, thighs).
  - For average-size clients, pinch up the skin and inject at a 45° to 90° angle. For clients who are obese, use a 90° angle.
- **Intramuscular**
  - Use for irritating medications, solutions in oils, and aqueous suspensions.
  - The most common sites are ventrogluteal, dorsogluteal, deltoid, and vastus lateralis (pediatric).
  - Use a needle size 18- to 27-gauge (usually 22- to 25-gauge), 1- to 1.5-inch long, and inject at a 90° angle. Solution volume is usually 1 to 3 mL. Divide larger volumes into two syringes and use two sites.

ADVANTAGES

- Used for poorly soluble medications.
- Used for administering medications that have slow absorption for an extended period of time (depot preparations).

DISADVANTAGES

- There can be pain with the risk for local tissue damage and nerve damage.
- There is a risk for infection at the insertion site.

Z-TRACK

NURSING ACTIONS

- Use this technique for IM injections because it is less painful and it prevents medication from leaking back into subcutaneous tissue.
- Use for medications that cause visible or permanent skin stains, such as iron preparations, and those that are highly irritating to tissues.
- Pull the skin and underlying tissues about 2.5 cm (1 in) to the side and hold it there.
- Insert the needle at a 90° angle and inject the medication.
- Wait 10 seconds, and then release the tissue while withdrawing the needle.

INTRAVENOUS

NURSING ACTIONS

- Use for administering medications, fluid, and blood products.
- Vascular access devices can be for short-term use (catheters) or long-term use (infusion ports). Use 16-gauge devices for clients who have trauma, 18-gauge during surgery and for blood administration, and 22- to 24-gauge for children, older adults, and clients who have medical issues or are stable postoperatively.
- Peripheral veins in the arm or hand are preferable. Ask clients which site they prefer. For newborns, use veins in the head, lower legs, and feet. After administration, immediately monitor for therapeutic and adverse effects.

ADVANTAGES

- Onset is rapid, and absorption into the blood is immediate, which provides an immediate response.
- This route allows control over the precise amount of medication to administer.
- It allows for administration of large volumes of fluid.
- It dilutes irritating medications in free-flowing IV fluid.

DISADVANTAGES

- Absorption of the medication into the blood is immediate. This is potentially dangerous if giving the wrong dosage or the wrong medication.
- There is an increased risk for infection or embolism with IV injections.
- Poor circulation can inhibit the medication's distribution.

EPIDURAL

NURSING ACTIONS

- Clients receive IV opioid analgesia (morphine or fentanyl) via this route.
- The provider advances the catheter through the needle into the epidural space at the level of the fourth or fifth vertebra.
- The provider programs an infusion pump to administer the medication.

Application Exercises

1. A provider prescribes phenobarbital for a client who has a seizure disorder. The medication has a half-life of 36 hr. How many times per day should the nurse expect to administer this medication?

    A. One

    B. Two

    C. Three

    D. Four

2. A nurse is reviewing medication dosages and factors that influence medication metabolism. Which of the following factors should the nurse identify as a reason to administer lower medication dosages? (Select all that apply.)

    A. Increased renal excretion

    B. Increased medication-metabolizing enzymes

    C. Liver failure

    D. Peripheral vascular disease

    E. Concurrent use of medication the same pathway metabolizes

3. A nurse is preparing to administer eye drops to a client. Which of the following actions should the nurse take? (Select all that apply.)

    A. Have the client lie on her side.

    B. Ask the client to look up at the ceiling.

    C. Tell the client to blink when the drops enter her eye.

    D. Drop the medication into the center of the client's conjunctival sac.

    E. Instruct the client to close her eye gently after instillation.

4. A nurse is reinforcing discharge teaching with a client who has a new prescription for transdermal patches. Which of the following statements should the nurse identify as an indication that the client understands the instructions?

    A. "I will clean the site with an alcohol swab before I apply the patch."

    B. "I will rotate the application sites weekly."

    C. "I will apply the patch to an area of skin with no hair."

    D. "I will place the new patch on the site of the old patch."

5. A nurse reviewing a client's medical record notes a new prescription for verifying the trough level of the client's medication. Which of the following actions should the nurse take?

    A. Obtain a blood specimen immediately prior to administering the next dose of medication.

    B. Verify that the client has been taking the medication for 24 hr before obtaining a blood specimen.

    C. Ask the client to provide a urine specimen after the next dose of medication.

    D. Administer the medication, and obtain a blood specimen 30 min later.

PRACTICE Active Learning Scenario

A nurse is showing a client how to use a metered-dose inhaler (MDI) with a spacer. What should the nurse include in the instructions? Use the ATI Active Learning Template: Therapeutic Procedure to complete this item.

INDICATIONS: Identify the medication absorption pattern and a barrier to absorption.

CLIENT EDUCATION: Describe the steps to follow when using an MDI with a spacer.

Application Exercises Key

1. A. **CORRECT:** Medications with long half-lives remain at their therapeutic levels between doses for long periods of time. The nurse should expect to administer this medication once a day.

    B. A medication the nurse administers twice a day would have a shorter half-life. An example is vancomycin.

    C. A medication the nurse administers three times a day would have a shorter half-life. An example is zidovudine.

    D. A medication the nurse administers four times a day would have a shorter half-life. An example is ibuprofen.

    (N) *NCLEX® Connection: Pharmacological Therapies, Medication Administration*

2. A. Increased renal excretion decreases the concentration of the medication, requiring an increased dosage.

    B. Increased medication-metabolizing enzymes decrease the concentration of the medication, requiring an increased dosage.

    C. **CORRECT:** Liver failure decreases metabolism and thus increases the concentration of a medication. This requires decreasing the dosage.

    D. Peripheral vascular disease impairs distribution, requiring an increased dosage.

    E. **CORRECT:** When one pathway metabolizes two medications, the medications compete for metabolism, thereby increasing the concentration of one or both medications. This requires decreasing the dosage of one or both medications.

    (N) *NCLEX® Connection: Pharmacological Therapies, Expected Actions/Outcomes*

3. A. The client should be sitting or in a supine position to facilitate the instillation of eye drops.

    B. **CORRECT:** The client should look upward to keep the drops from falling onto her cornea.

    C. The client should not blink so that she doesn't eject the eye drops. If she does blink, the nurse should repeat the instillation.

    D. **CORRECT:** The nurse should drop the medication into the center of the conjunctival sac to promote distribution.

    E. **CORRECT:** The client should close her eye gently to promote distribution of the medication.

    (N) *NCLEX® Connection: Pharmacological Therapies, Medication Administration*

4. A. The client should wash his skin with soap and water and dry it thoroughly before applying a transdermal patch.

    B. The client should rotate application sites daily to prevent skin irritation.

    C. **CORRECT:** The client should apply the patch to a hairless area of skin to promote absorption of the medication.

    D. The client should rotate application sites daily to prevent skin irritation.

    (N) *NCLEX® Connection: Pharmacological Therapies, Medication Administration*

5. A. **CORRECT:** To verify trough levels of a medication, the nurse should obtain a blood specimen immediately before administering the next dose of medication.

    B. The length of time the client has been taking the medication does not affect trough levels.

    C. Trough levels are from serum, not urine.

    D. Trough levels reflect the least concentration of the medication in the client's blood. It will be higher after administration of the medication.

    (N) *NCLEX® Connection: Pharmacological Therapies, Expected Actions/Outcomes*

PRACTICE Answer

Using the ATI Active Learning Template: Therapeutic Procedure

INDICATIONS
- Medication absorption pattern: Rapid absorption through the alveolar capillary network. A spacer keeps the medication in the device longer, thereby increasing the amount of medication the device delivers to the lungs and decreasing the amount of medication in the oropharynx.
- Barrier to absorption: Inadequate respiratory effort

CLIENT EDUCATION
- Remove the covers from the mouthpieces of the inhaler and of the spacer.
- Insert the MDI into the end of the spacer.
- Shake the inhaler five or six times.
- Exhale completely, and then close your mouth around the spacer's mouthpiece.
- Take a deep breath and then exhale.
- Tilt your head back slightly, press the inhaler, and, at the same time, begin a slow, deep inhalation breath. Continue to breathe in slowly and deeply for 3 to 5 seconds to facilitate delivery to the air passages.
- Hold your breath for 10 seconds to allow the medication to deposit in your airways.
- Take the mouthpiece out of your mouth and slowly exhale through pursed lips.
- Resume normal breathing.

(N) *NCLEX® Connection: Pharmacological and Parenteral Therapies, Medication Administration*

UNIT 1 PHARMACOLOGICAL PRINCIPLES

CHAPTER 2 # Safe Medication Administration and Error Reduction

Providers who may legally write prescriptions in the United States include physicians, advanced practice nurses, dentists, and physician assistants. These providers are responsible for obtaining clients' medical history, performing a physical examination, diagnosing, prescribing medications, monitoring responses to therapy, and modifying prescriptions as necessary.

NURSE RESPONSIBILITIES

- Having knowledge of federal, state (nurse practice acts), and local laws and facility policies that govern the prescribing, dispensing, and administration of medications
- Preparing, administering, and evaluating responses to medications
- Developing and maintaining an up-to-date knowledge base of medications they administer
  - Uses
  - Mechanisms of action
  - Routes of administration
  - Safe dosage ranges
  - Adverse effects
  - Precautions
  - Contraindications
  - Interactions
- Maintaining acceptable practice and skills competencies
- Determining the accuracy of medication prescriptions
- Reporting all medication errors
- Safeguarding and storing medications
- Following legal mandates when administering controlled substances **Qs**
- Calculating medication doses accurately
- Understanding the responsibilities of other members of the health care team regarding medications

2.1 Essential knowledge prior to medication administration

Medication category/class

Medications have a pharmacological action, therapeutic use, body system target, chemical makeup, and classification for use during pregnancy.

For example, lisinopril is an ACE inhibitor (pharmacological action) and an antihypertensive (therapeutic use).

Mechanism of action

This is how medications produce their therapeutic effect.

For example, glipizide is an oral hypoglycemic agent that lowers blood glucose levels primarily by stimulating pancreatic islet cells to release insulin.

Therapeutic effect

This is the expected effect (physiological response) for which the nurse administers a medication to a specific client. One medication can have more than one therapeutic effect.

For example, one client receives acetaminophen to lower fever, whereas another client receives it to relieve pain.

Side effects

These are expected and predictable effects that result at therapeutic dosages.

For example, morphine for pain relief usually results in constipation.

Adverse effects

These are undesirable, inadvertent, unexpected, and potentially dangerous responses to a medication. Some are immediate, whereas others take weeks or months to develop.

For example, the antibiotic gentamicin can cause hearing loss.

Toxic effects

Medications can have specific risks and manifestations of toxicity. They develop after taking a medication for a long time or when toxic amounts build up due to faulty metabolism or excretion.

For example, nurses monitor clients taking digoxin for dysrhythmias, a manifestation of cardiotoxicity. Hypokalemia places these clients at greater risk for digoxin toxicity.

Medication interactions

Medications can interact with each other, resulting in beneficial or harmful effects.

For example, giving the beta-blocker atenolol concurrently with the calcium channel blocker nifedipine helps prevent reflex tachycardia.

An example of an undesirable interaction is the result of giving omeprazole (a proton pump inhibitor) concurrently with phenytoin (an anticonvulsant). This can increase the serum level of phenytoin.

Obtain a complete medication history, and be knowledgeable of clinically significant interactions.

Be aware that medications can also interact beneficially or harmfully with food and with herbal and dietary supplements.

Precautions/ Contraindications

These are conditions (diseases, age, pregnancy, lactation) that make it risky or completely unsafe for clients to take specific medications.

For example, tetracyclines can stain developing teeth. Therefore, children younger than 8 years should not take these medications. Another example is that myasthenia gravis is a contraindication for fentanyl, an opioid analgesic.

Some medications require caution with some conditions.

For example, the kidneys excrete vancomycin without changing it. Therefore, administering this medication to clients who have kidney impairment requires caution.

Preparation, dosage, administration

It is important to know any specific considerations for preparation, safe dosages, dosage calculations, and how to administer the medication.

For example, morphine is available in many formulations. Oral doses of morphine are generally higher than parenteral doses due to extensive first-pass effect. Clients who have chronic severe pain, such as with cancer, generally take oral doses of morphine.

Nursing implications

Know how to monitor therapeutic effects and side effects, prevent and treat adverse effects, provide comfort, and instruct clients about the safe use of medications.

MEDICATION CATEGORY AND CLASSIFICATION

NOMENCLATURE

The chemical name is the name of the medication that reflects its chemical composition and molecular structure (isobutylphenyl propanoic acid).

The generic name is the official or nonproprietary name the United States Adopted Names Council gives a medication. Each medication has only one generic name (ibuprofen).

The trade name is the brand or proprietary name the company that manufactures the medication gives it. One medication can have multiple trade names (Advil, Motrin).

CONSIDERATIONS

Nurses administer prescription medications under the supervision of providers. Some medications can be habit-forming, or have potential harmful effects and require more stringent supervision. Qs

Uncontrolled substances require monitoring by a provider, but do not generally pose risks of abuse and addiction. Antibiotics are uncontrolled prescription medications.

Controlled substances have a potential for abuse and dependence and have a schedule classification. Heroin is Schedule I and has no medical use in the U.S. Medications Schedules II through V have legitimate applications. Each subsequent level has a decreasing risk of abuse and dependence. For example, morphine is a Schedule II medication that has a greater risk for abuse and dependence than phenobarbital, which is Schedule IV.

- New medications in development undergo the rigorous testing procedures of the U.S. Food and Drug Administration (FDA) to determine both effectiveness and safety before approval. However, new medications can have unidentified or unreported adverse effects. Nurses observing these can report them at www.fda.gov/medwatch.
- The FDA's Pregnancy Risk Categories (A, B, C, D, X) classify medications according to their potential harm during pregnancy, with Category A being the safest and Category X the most dangerous. Teratogenesis from unsafe medications is most likely to occur during the first trimester. Before administering any medication to a client who is or could be pregnant, determine whether it is safe for use during pregnancy.

MEDICATION PRESCRIPTIONS

Each facility has written policies for medication prescriptions, including which providers may write, receive, and transcribe medication prescriptions. Qtc

Types of medication prescriptions

Routine or standard prescriptions
- These prescriptions identify medications nurses give on a regular schedule with or without a termination date or a specific number of doses. Without a termination date, the prescription remains in effect until the provider discontinues it or discharges the client.
- Providers must represcribe some medications (opioids, antibiotics) within a specific amount of time or they will automatically discontinue.

Single or one-time prescriptions are for administration once at a specific time or as soon as possible. These prescriptions are common for preoperative or preprocedural medications. For example, a one-time prescription instructs the nurse to administer lorazepam 2 mg IM at 0700.

Stat prescriptions are only for administration once and immediately, typically in emergencies when a client's condition changes suddenly. For example, a stat prescription instructs the nurse to administer diphenhydramine 50 mg IM stat.

PRN prescriptions specify at what dosage, what frequency, and under what conditions a nurse may administer the medication. The nurse uses clinical judgment to determine the client's need for the medication. For example, a PRN (*pro re nata*) prescription instructs the nurse to administer tramadol 50 mg PO every 4 hr PRN for back pain. When administering PRN medications, the nurse documents findings that demonstrate the client's need for the medication and the time of administration.

Standing prescriptions: Providers write standing prescriptions for specific circumstances or for specific units. For example, a critical care unit has standing prescriptions for treating clients who have asystole. Another example is a heparin protocol.

Components of a medication prescription

- Client's full name
- Date and time of the prescription
- Name of the medication (generic or brand)
- Strength and dosage of the medication
- Route of administration
- Time and frequency of administration: exact times, intervals, or number of times per day (according to the facility's policy or the specific qualities of the medication)
- Quantity to dispense and the number of refills
- Signature of the prescribing provider

Communicating medication prescriptions

Origin of medication prescriptions: Providers or nurses who take verbal or telephone prescriptions from a provider write medication prescriptions on the client's medical record. When the nurse writes a medication prescription on the client's medical record, the facility's policy specifies how much time the provider has to sign the prescription. Nurses transcribe medication prescriptions onto the medication administration record (MAR).

Taking a telephone prescription
- If possible, have a second nurse listen on an extension or on a speaker in a private area (to ensure confidentiality).
- Make sure that the prescription is complete and correct by reading back to the provider the client's name, medication name, dosage, time of administration, frequency, and route.
- To ensure correct spelling, use aids such as "B as in boy." State numbers separately, such as "one, five" for 15.
- Remind the provider to verify the prescription and sign it within the amount of time the facility's policy specifies.
- Enter the prescription in the client's health record.

Medication reconciliation

The Joint Commission requires policies and procedures for medication reconciliation. Nurses compile a list of each client's current medications, including all medications with their dosages and frequency. They compare the list with new medication prescriptions and reconcile it with the provider to resolve any discrepancies. This process should take place at admission, when transferring clients between units or facilities, and at discharge.

DATA COLLECTION PRIOR TO MEDICATION THERAPY

Nurses obtain the following information before initiating medication therapy, and update it as necessary.

Health history

- Age
- Health problems and current reason for seeking care
- All medications currently taken (prescription and nonprescription): name, dose, route, and frequency of each
- Any adverse or side effects possibly from medication therapy, as well as therapeutic effects
- Use of herbal or natural products for medicinal purposes
- Use of caffeine, tobacco, alcohol, or other substances
- Clients' understanding of the purpose of the medications along with the client's beliefs, feelings, and concerns Qᴘᴄᴄ
- All medication and food allergies

Physical examination

A systematic physical examination provides a baseline for evaluating the therapeutic effects of medication therapy and for detecting possible side and adverse effects.

RIGHTS OF SAFE MEDICATION ADMINISTRATION

Right client

Verify clients' identification before each medication administration. The Joint Commission requires two client identifiers.
- Acceptable identifiers include the client's name, assigned identification number, telephone number, birth date, or another person-specific identifier, such as a photo identification card.
- Check identification bands for name and identification number.
- Check for allergies by asking clients, looking for an allergy bracelet or medal, and reviewing the MAR.
- Use barcode scanners to identify clients. Qι

Right medication

Correctly interpret medication prescriptions, verifying completeness and clarity.
- Read medication labels and compare them with the MAR three times.
  - Before removing the container
  - When removing the amount of medication from the container
  - In the presence of the client before administering the medication
- Leave unit-dose medication in its package until administration.
- When using automated medication dispensing systems, perform the same checks and adapt as necessary. Qι

Right dose

- Use a unit-dose system to help prevent errors. If not available, calculate the correct medication dose.
- Check a drug reference to make sure the dose is within the expected range.
- When performing medication calculations or conversions, have another nurse check the dosage calculation.
- Prepare medication dosages using standard measurement devices (graduated cups, syringes). Some medication dosages (such as some cytotoxic medications) require a second verifier or witness. Automated medication dispensing systems use a machine to control the dispensing of medications.

Right time

Administer medication on time to maintain a consistent therapeutic blood level.
- It is generally acceptable to administer the medication 30 min before or after the scheduled time. Refer to the drug reference or the facility's policy for exceptions.
- Give priority to time-critical medications that must act at specific times (preoperatively).

Right route

The most common routes of administration are oral, topical, subcutaneous, IM, and IV. Additional routes include sublingual, buccal, intradermal, transdermal, epidural, inhalation, nasal, ophthalmic, otic, rectal, vaginal, intraosseous, and via enteral tubes.

- Select the correct preparation for the route prescribed (otic vs. ophthalmic topical ointment or drops).
- Always use different syringes for enteral and parenteral medication administration.
- Know the scope of practice for the PN outlined in the state nurse practice act regarding specific classifications of medications and routes of administration. This can vary by state.
- Know how to administer medication safely and correctly.

Right documentation

- Immediately record the medication, dose, route, time, and any pertinent information, including the client's response to the medication. Document the medication after administration, not before.
- For some medications, in particular those to alleviate pain, evaluate the client's response and document it later, perhaps after 30 min.

Right client education

- Inform clients about the medication: its purpose, what to expect, how to take it, and what to report.
- To individualize client education, determine what the client already knows, needs to know, and wants to know about the medication. Qᴾᶜᶜ

Right to refuse

- Respect clients' right to refuse any medication.
- Explain the consequences, inform the provider, and document the refusal.

Right data collection

Collect any essential data before and after administering any medication. For example, measure apical heart rate before giving digoxin.

Right evaluation

Follow up with clients to verify therapeutic effects as well as side and adverse effects.

MEDICATION ERROR PREVENTION

COMMON MEDICATION ERRORS

- Wrong medication or IV fluid
- Incorrect dose or IV rate
- Wrong client, route, or time
- Administration of an allergy-inducing medication
- Omission of a dose or administration of extra doses
- Incorrect discontinuation of a medication or IV fluid
- Inaccurate prescribing
- Inadvertently giving a medication that has a similar name

USING THE NURSING PROCESS TO PREVENT MEDICATION ERRORS Qₛ

Data collection

- Be knowledgeable about medications before administering them. Use recommended resources.
  - Providers (nurses, physicians, pharmacists)
  - Poison control centers
  - Sales representatives from drug companies
  - Nursing pharmacology textbooks and medication handbooks
  - *Physicians' Desk Reference*
  - Professional journals
  - Professional websites
- Obtain information about diagnoses and conditions that affect medication administration (ability to swallow; allergies; heart, liver, and kidney disorders).
  - Identify allergies.
  - Obtain necessary preadministration data (heart rate, blood pressure, serum levels) to determine the appropriateness of the medication and to obtain baseline data for evaluating the effectiveness of medications.
  - Omit or delay doses as necessary due to clients' status.
- Determine whether the prescription is complete, including the name of the client, date and time, name of the medication, dosage, route of administration, times of administration or frequency, and signature of the prescribing provider.
- Interpret the medication prescription accurately. The Institute for Safe Medication Practices (ISMP) is a nonprofit organization working to educate health care providers and consumers about safe medication practices. The ISMP and the FDA identify the most common medical abbreviations that result in misinterpretation, mistakes, and injury. For a complete list, go to www.ismp.org.
  - **Error-Prone Abbreviation List:** Abbreviations that have caused a high number of medication errors
  - **Confused Medication Name List:** Sound-alike and look-alike medication names
  - **High-Alert Medication List:** Medications that, if a nurse administers them in error, have a high risk for resulting in significant harm to clients. Strategies to prevent errors include limiting access; using auxiliary labels and automated alerts; standardizing the prescription, preparation, and administration; and using automated or independent double checks.
- Question the provider if the prescription is unclear or seems incorrect for the client. Refuse to administer a medication if it seems unsafe, and notify the charge nurse or supervisor.
- Providers usually make dosage changes gradually. Question them about abrupt and excessive changes.

Planning

- Identify client outcomes for medication administration.
- Set priorities (which medications to give first or before specific treatments or procedures).

Implementation

- Avoid distractions during medication preparation (poor lighting, ringing phones). Interruptions can increase the risk of error.
- Prepare medications for one client at a time.
- Check the labels for the medication's name and concentration. Read labels carefully. Measure doses accurately, and double-check dosages of high-alert medications (insulin, heparin) with a colleague. Check the medication's expiration date.
- Doses are usually one to two tablets or one single-dose vial. Question multiple tablets or vials for a single dose.
- Follow the rights of medication administration consistently and carefully. Take the MAR to the bedside.
- Do not administer medications that someone else prepared.
- Reinforce teaching about medications and the importance of proper identification before medication administration.
- Encourage clients to voice concerns if a dosage or medication seems incorrect.
- Omit or delay a dose when clients question the size of a dose or the appearance of a medication.
- Follow correct procedures for all routes of administration.
- Communicate clearly both verbally and in writing.
- Use verbal prescriptions only for emergencies, and follow the facility's protocol for telephone prescriptions. Nursing students may **not** accept verbal or telephone orders.
- Follow all laws and regulations for preparing and administering controlled substances. Keep them in a secure area. Have another nurse witness the discarding of controlled substances.
- Do not leave medications at the bedside. Some facilities' policies allow exceptions, such as for topical medications.
- Follow the principles of client and family education for medications.

Evaluation

- Evaluate, document, and report clients' responses to medications.
- Use knowledge of the therapeutic effect and common side and adverse effects of medications to compare expected outcomes with actual findings.
- Identify, document, and report side and adverse effects.
- Report all errors, and implement corrective measures immediately.
  - Complete an incident report within the time frame the facility specifies, usually 24 hr. This report should include the following. Qଠ
    - Client identification
    - Name and dose of the medication
    - Time and place of the incident
    - Accurate and objective account of the event
    - Who was notified
    - What actions were taken
    - Signature of the person who completed the report
  - Do not reference or include this report in the client's medical record.
  - Medication errors relate to systems, procedures, product design, or practice patterns. Report all errors to help the facility's risk managers determine how errors occur and what changes to make to avoid similar errors in the future.

Application Exercises

1. A nurse is preparing a client's medications. Which of the following actions should the nurse take in following legal practice guidelines? (Select all that apply.)

    A. Maintain skill competency.

    B. Determine the dosage.

    C. Monitor for adverse effects.

    D. Safeguard medications.

    E. Identify the client's diagnosis.

2. A nurse reviewing a client's health record notes a new prescription for lisinopril 10 mg PO once every day. The nurse should identify this as which of the following types of prescription?

    A. Single

    B. Stat

    C. Routine

    D. Standing

3. A nurse is reviewing a new prescription for prochlorperazine 25 mg PR PRN for nausea and vomiting for a client who has postoperative nausea and vomiting. The nurse should clarify which of the following parts of the prescription with the provider?

    A. Medication

    B. Dosage

    C. Route

    D. Frequency

4. A nurse is collecting data from a client before preparing to administer medications. Which of the following data should the nurse be sure to collect? (Select all that apply.)

    A. Use of herbal teas

    B. Daily fluid intake

    C. Current health status

    D. Previous surgical history

    E. Food allergies

5. A newly hired nurse asks another nurse about the procedure for accepting a telephone prescription. Which of the following statements should the nurse identify as indicating understanding of the process?

    A. "A second nurse enters the prescription into the client's medical record."

    B. "Another nurse should listen to the phone call."

    C. "The provider can clarify the prescription when he signs the health record."

    D. "I should omit the read-back if this is a one-time prescription."

Application Exercises Key

1. A. **CORRECT:** Maintaining skill competency and using correct administration techniques are legal responsibilities of the nurse.

   B. A nurse should verify that the prescribed dosage is within the expected range, but determining the medication's dosage is the provider's responsibility.

   C. **CORRECT:** A nurse is legally responsible for monitoring for side and adverse effects of medications.

   D. **CORRECT:** Safeguarding of medications, such as controlled substances, is a legal responsibility of the nurse.

   E. A nurse should know about a client's diagnosis, but identifying a diagnosis is the provider's responsibility.

   (N) NCLEX® Connection: Pharmacological Therapies, Expected Actions/Outcomes

2. A. A single or one-time prescription is for administration once at a specific time or as soon as possible.

   B. A stat prescription is only for administration once and immediately.

   C. **CORRECT:** A routine or standard prescription identifies medications to give on a regular schedule with or without a termination date or a specific number of doses. The nurse will administer this medication every day until the provider discontinues it.

   D. Providers write standing prescriptions for specific circumstances or for specific units.

   (N) NCLEX® Connection: Safety and Infection Control, Accident/Error/Injury Prevention

3. A. This prescription includes the medication's generic name, prochlorperazine.

   B. This prescription includes the medication's dosage of 25 mg.

   C. This prescription includes the medication's route, which is rectal (PR).

   D. **CORRECT:** Though the medication is prescribed PRN, the prescription does not include the time or frequency of medication administration. The nurse must clarify this with the prescribing provider.

   (N) NCLEX® Connection: Safety and Infection Control, Accident/Error/Injury Prevention

4. A. **CORRECT:** The nurse should inquire about the client's use of herbal products, which often contain caffeine, prior to medication administration because caffeine can affect medication biotransformation.

   B. Daily fluid intake is important for ensuring adequate hydration, but it is not part of essential data collection prior to medication administration.

   C. **CORRECT:** The nurse should review the client's current health status because new prescriptions can cause alterations in current health status.

   D. Surgical history is important for determining risks or alterations in the client's health status, but it is not part of essential data collection prior to medication administration.

   E. **CORRECT:** The nurse should inquire about food allergies during essential data collection to identify any potential reactions or interactions.

   (N) NCLEX® Connection: Safety and Infection Control, Accident/Error/Injury Prevention

5. A. The nurse who accepts the telephone prescription should enter it into the client's medical record to prevent errors in translation.

   B. **CORRECT:** A second nurse should listen to a telephone prescription to prevent errors in communication.

   C. The nurse should verify that the prescription is complete and accurate at the time she takes it by reading it back to the prescribing provider.

   D. A telephone prescription includes reading back all types of medication prescriptions.

   (N) NCLEX® Connection: Safety and Infection Control, Accident/Error/Injury Prevention

A nurse is reviewing information about preventing medication errors. What should the nurse apply about using the nursing process to prevent medication errors? Use the ATI Active Learning Template: Basic Concept to complete this item.

NURSING INTERVENTIONS: Using the nursing process to prevent medication errors, list the following.

- Three data collection actions
- One planning action
- Four implementation actions
- Three evaluation actions

PRACTICE Answer

Using the ATI Active Learning Template: Basic Concept

NURSING INTERVENTIONS

Data collection
- Be knowledgeable about the medication to administer. Use recommended resources.
- Obtain information about medical diagnoses and conditions that affect medication administration.
- Determine whether the medication prescription is complete.
- Interpret the medication prescription accurately.
- Question the provider if the prescription is unclear or seems incorrect for the client.
- Question the provider about abrupt and excessive changes in dosage.

Planning
- Identify clients' outcomes for medication administration.
- Set priorities (which medications to give first or before specific treatments or procedures).

Implementation
- Avoid distractions and interruptions during medication preparation.
- Prepare medications for one client at a time.
- Check labels for the medication's name and concentration.
- Question multiple tablets or vials for a single dose.
- Follow the rights of medication administration consistently and carefully.
- Do not administer medications that someone else prepared.
- Encourage clients to voice concerns if a medication or dosage seems incorrect.
- Follow correct procedures for all routes of administration.
- Communicate clearly both verbally and in writing.
- Use verbal prescriptions only for emergencies, and follow the facility's protocol for telephone prescriptions.
- Follow all laws and regulations for preparing and administering controlled substances.
- Do not leave medications at the bedside.
- Follow the principles of client and family education for medications.

Evaluation
- Evaluate, document, and report clients' responses to medications.
- Use knowledge of the therapeutic effect and common side and adverse effects of medications to compare expected outcomes with actual findings.
- Identify, document, and report side and adverse effects.
- Report all errors, and implement corrective measures immediately.

(N) NCLEX® Connection: Safety and Infection Control, Reporting of Incident/Event/Irregular Occurrence Variance

UNIT 1   PHARMACOLOGICAL PRINCIPLES

CHAPTER 3   *Dosage Calculation*

Basic medication dose conversion and calculation skills are essential for providing safe nursing care.

Nurses are responsible for administering the correct amount of medication by calculating the precise amount of medication to give. Nurses can use three different methods for dosage calculation: ratio and proportion, formula (desired over have), and dimensional analysis.

TYPES OF CALCULATIONS

- Solid oral medication
- Liquid oral medication
- Injectable medication
- Correct doses by weight
- IV infusion rates

STANDARD CONVERSION FACTORS

Weight
- 1 mg = 1,000 mcg
- 1 g = 1,000 mg
- 1 kg = 1,000 g
- 1 lb = 16 oz
- 1 kg = 2.2 lb
- 1 gr = 60 mg

Volume
- 1 oz = 30 mL
- 1 L = 1,000 mL
- 1 tsp = 5 mL
- 1 tbsp = 15 mL
- 1 tbsp = 3 tsp

GENERAL ROUNDING GUIDELINES

ROUNDING UP: If the number to the right is equal to or greater than 5, round up by adding 1 to the number on the left.

ROUNDING DOWN: If the number to the right is less than 5, round down by dropping the number, leaving the number to the left as is.

For dosages less than 1.0: Round to the nearest hundredth.
- For example (rounding up): 0.746 mL = 0.75 mL. The calculated dose is 0.746 mL. Look at the number in the thousandths place (6). Six is greater than 5. To round to hundredths, add 1 to the 4 in the hundredths place and drop the 6. The rounded dose is 0.75 mL.
- Or (rounding down): 0.743 mL = 0.74 mL. The calculated dose is 0.743 mL. Look at the number in the thousandths place (3). Three is less than 5. To round to the hundredth, drop the 3 and leave the 4 as is. The rounded dose is 0.74 mL.

For dosages greater than 1.0: Round to the nearest tenth.
- For example (rounding up): 1.38 = 1.4. The calculated dose is 1.38 mg. Look at the number in the hundredths place (8). Eight is greater than 5. To round to the tenth, add 1 to the 3 in the tenth place and drop the 8. The rounded dose is 1.4 mg.
- Or (rounding down): 1.34 mL = 1.3 mL. The calculated dose is 1.34 mL. Look at the number in the hundredths place (4). Four is less than 5. To round to the tenth, drop the 4 and leave the 3 as is. The rounded dose is 1.3 mL.

Solid dosage

Example: A nurse is preparing to administer phenytoin 0.2 g PO every 12 hr. Available is phenytoin 100 mg/capsule. How many capsules should the nurse administer per dose? (Round the answer to the nearest whole number.)

USING RATIO AND PROPORTION

STEP 1: What is the unit of measurement the nurse should calculate?

capsules

STEP 2: What is the dose the nurse should administer? Dose to administer = Desired

0.2 g

STEP 3: What is the dose available? Dose available = Have

100 mg

STEP 4: Should the nurse convert the units of measurement? Yes (g ≠ mg)

1 g = 1,000 mg (1 × 1,000)

0.2 g = 200 mg (0.2 × 1,000)

STEP 5: What is the quantity of the dose available? = Quantity

1 capsule

STEP 6: Set up the equation and solve for X.

$$\frac{Have}{Quantity} = \frac{Desired}{X}$$

$$\frac{100 \text{ mg}}{1 \text{ capsule}} = \frac{200 \text{ mg}}{X \text{ capsule}}$$

X = 2

STEP 7: Round, if necessary.

STEP 8: Re-evaluate to determine whether the amount to administer makes sense. If there are 100 mg/capsule and the prescription reads 0.2 g (200 mg), it makes sense to administer 2 capsules. The nurse should administer phenytoin 2 capsules PO every 12 hr.

USING DESIRED OVER HAVE

STEP 1: What is the unit of measurement the nurse should calculate?

capsules

STEP 2: What is the dose the nurse should administer? Dose to administer = Desired

0.2 g

STEP 3: What is the dose available? Dose available = Have

100 mg

STEP 4: Should the nurse convert the units of measurement? Yes (g ≠ mg)

1 g = 1,000 mg (1 × 1,000)

0.2 g = 200 mg (0.2 × 1,000)

STEP 5: What is the quantity of the dose available? = Quantity

1 capsule

STEP 6: Set up the equation and solve for X.

$$\frac{Desired \times Quantity}{Have} = X$$

$$\frac{200 \text{ mg} \times 1 \text{ capsule}}{100 \text{ mg}} = X \text{ capsule}$$

$$X = 2$$

STEP 7: Round, if necessary.

STEP 8: Re-evaluate to determine whether the amount to administer makes sense. If there are 100 mg/capsule and the prescription reads 0.2 g (200 mg), it makes sense to administer 2 capsules. The nurse should administer phenytoin 2 capsules PO every 12 hr.

USING DIMENSIONAL ANALYSIS

STEP 1: What is the unit of measurement the nurse should calculate?

capsules

STEP 2: What is the quantity of the dose available? = Quantity

1 capsule

STEP 3: What is the dose available? Dose available = Have

100 mg

STEP 4: What is the dose the nurse should administer? Dose to administer = Desired

0.2 g

STEP 5: Should the nurse convert the units of measurement? Yes (g ≠ mg)

1,000 mg = 1 g

0.2 g = 200 mg (0.2 × 100)

STEP 6: Set up the equation and solve for X.

$$X = \frac{Quantity}{Have} \times \frac{Conversion \ (Have)}{Conversion \ (Desired)} \times Desired$$

$$X \text{ capsule} = \frac{1 \text{ capsule}}{100 \text{ mg}} \times \frac{1,000 \text{ mg}}{1 \text{ g}} \times 0.2 \text{ g}$$

$$X = 2$$

STEP 7: Round, if necessary.

STEP 8: Re-evaluate to determine whether the amount to administer makes sense. If there are 100 mg/capsule and the prescription reads 0.2 g (200 mg), it makes sense to administer 2 capsules. The nurse should administer phenytoin 2 capsules PO every 12 hr.

Liquid dosage

Example: A nurse is preparing to administer amoxicillin 0.25 g PO every 8 hr. Available is amoxicillin oral suspension 250 mg/5 mL. How many mL should the nurse administer per dose? (Round the answer to the nearest whole number.)

USING RATIO AND PROPORTION

STEP 1: What is the unit of measurement the nurse should calculate?

mL

STEP 2: What is the dose the nurse should administer? Dose to administer = Desired

0.25 g

STEP 3: What is the dose available? Dose available = Have

250 mg

STEP 4: Should the nurse convert the units of measurement? Yes (g ≠ mg)

1 g = 1,000 mg (1 × 1,000)

0.25 g = 250 mg (0.25 × 1,000)

STEP 5: What is the quantity of the dose available? = Quantity

5 mL

STEP 6: Set up the equation and solve for X.

$$\frac{Have}{Quantity} = \frac{Desired}{X}$$

$$\frac{250 \text{ mg}}{5 \text{ mL}} = \frac{250 \text{ mg}}{X \text{ mL}}$$

$$X = 5$$

STEP 7: Round, if necessary.

STEP 8: Re-evaluate to determine whether the amount to administer makes sense. If there are 250 mg/5 mL and the prescription reads 0.25 g (250 mg), it makes sense to administer 5 mL. The nurse should administer amoxicillin 5 mL PO every 8 hr.

USING DESIRED OVER HAVE

STEP 1: What is the unit of measurement the nurse should calculate?

mL

STEP 2: What is the dose the nurse should administer? Dose to administer = Desired

0.25 g

STEP 3: What is the dose available? Dose available = Have

250 mg

STEP 4: Should the nurse convert the units of measurement? Yes (g ≠ mg)

1 g = 1,000 mg (1 × 1,000)

0.25 g = 250 mg (0.25 × 1,000)

STEP 5: What is the quantity of the dose available? = Quantity

5 mL

STEP 6: Set up the equation and solve for X.

$$\frac{Desired \times Quantity}{Have} = X$$

$$\frac{250\ mg \times 5\ mL}{250\ mg} = X\ mL$$

$$5 = X$$

STEP 7: Round, if necessary.

STEP 8: Re-evaluate to determine whether the amount to administer makes sense. If there are 250 mg/5 mL and the prescription reads 0.25 g (250 mg), it makes sense to administer 5 mL. The nurse should administer amoxicillin 5 mL PO every 8 hr.

USING DIMENSIONAL ANALYSIS

STEP 1: What is the unit of measurement the nurse should calculate?

mL

STEP 2: What is the quantity of the dose available? = Quantity

5 mL

STEP 3: What is the dose available? Dose available = Have

250 mg

STEP 4: What is the dose the nurse should administer? Dose to administer = Desired

0.25 g

STEP 5: Should the nurse convert the units of measurement? Yes (g ≠ mg)

1,000 mg = 1 g

0.25 g = 250 mg (0.25 × 1,000)

STEP 6: Set up the equation and solve for X.

$$X = \frac{Quantity}{Have} \times \frac{Conversion\ (Have)}{Conversion\ (Desired)} \times Desired$$

$$X\ mL = \frac{5\ mL}{250\ mg} \times \frac{1,000\ mg}{1\ g} \times 0.25\ g$$

$$X = 5$$

STEP 7: Round, if necessary.

STEP 8: Re-evaluate to determine whether the amount to administer makes sense. If there are 250 mg/5 mL and the prescription reads 0.25 g (250 mg), it makes sense to administer 5 mL. The nurse should administer amoxicillin 5 mL PO every 8 hr.

Injectable dosage

Example: A nurse is preparing to administer heparin 8,000 units subcutaneously every 8 hr. Available is heparin injection 10,000 units/mL. How many mL should the nurse administer per dose? (Round the answer to the nearest tenth. Use a leading zero if it applies. Do not use a trailing zero.)

USING RATIO AND PROPORTION

STEP 1: What is the unit of measurement the nurse should calculate?

mL

STEP 2: What is the dose the nurse should administer? Dose to administer = Desired

8,000 units

STEP 3: What is the dose available? Dose available = Have

10,000 units

STEP 4: Should the nurse convert the units of measurement? No

STEP 5: What is the quantity of the dose available? = Quantity

1 mL

STEP 6: Set up the equation and solve for X.

$$\frac{Have}{Quantity} = \frac{Desired}{X}$$

$$\frac{10,000\ units}{1\ mL} = \frac{8,000\ units}{X\ mL}$$

$$X = 0.8$$

STEP 7: Round, if necessary.

STEP 8: Re-evaluate to determine whether the amount to administer makes sense. If there are 10,000 units/mL and the prescription reads 8,000 units, it makes sense to administer 0.8 mL. The nurse should administer heparin injection 0.8 mL subcutaneously every 8 hr.

USING DESIRED OVER HAVE

STEP 1: What is the unit of measurement the nurse should calculate?

mL

STEP 2: What is the dose the nurse should administer? Dose to administer = Desired

8,000 units

STEP 3: What is the dose available? Dose available = Have

10,000 units

STEP 4: Should the nurse convert the units of measurement? No

STEP 5: What is the quantity of the dose available? = Quantity

1 mL

STEP 6: Set up an equation and solve for X.

$$\frac{Desired \times Quantity}{Have} = X$$

$$\frac{8,000 \text{ units} \times 1 \text{ mL}}{10,000 \text{ units}} = X \text{ mL}$$

$$0.8 = X$$

STEP 7: Round, if necessary.

STEP 8: Re-evaluate to determine whether the amount to administer makes sense. If there are 10,000 units/mL and the prescription reads 8,000 units, it makes sense to administer 0.8 mL. The nurse should administer heparin injection 0.8 mL subcutaneously every 8 hr.

USING DIMENSIONAL ANALYSIS

STEP 1: What is the unit of measurement the nurse should calculate?

mL

STEP 2: What is the quantity of the dose available? = Quantity

1 mL

STEP 3: What is the dose available? Dose available = Have

10,000 units

STEP 4: What is the dose the nurse should administer? Dose to administer = Desired

8,000 units

STEP 5: Should the nurse convert the units of measurement? No

STEP 6: Set up an equation and solve for X.

$$X = \frac{Quantity}{Have} \times \frac{Conversion \ (Have)}{Conversion \ (Desired)} \times Desired$$

$$X \text{ mL} = \frac{1 \text{ mL}}{10,000 \text{ units}} \times 8,000 \text{ units}$$

$$X = 0.8$$

STEP 7: Round, if necessary.

STEP 8: Re-evaluate to determine whether the amount to administer makes sense. If there are 10,000 units/mL and the prescription reads 8,000 units, it makes sense to administer 0.8 mL. The nurse should administer heparin injection 0.8 mL subcutaneously every 8 hr.

Dosages by weight

Example: A nurse is preparing to administer cefixime 8 mg/kg/day PO to divide equally every 12 hr to a toddler who weighs 22 lb. Available is cefixime suspension 100 mg/5 mL. How many mL should the nurse administer per dose? (Round the answer to the nearest whole number.)

STEP 1: What is the unit of measurement the nurse should calculate?

kg

STEP 2: Set up an equation and solve for X.

$$\frac{2.2 \text{ lb}}{1 \text{ kg}} = \frac{client's \ weight \ in \ lb}{X \text{ kg}}$$

$$\frac{2.2 \text{ lb}}{1 \text{ kg}} = \frac{22 \text{ lb}}{X \text{ kg}}$$

$$X = 10$$

STEP 3: Round, if necessary.

STEP 4: Re-evaluate to determine whether the equivalent makes sense. If 1 kg = 2.2 lb, it makes sense that 22 lb = 10 kg.

STEP 5: What is the unit of measurement the nurse should calculate?

mg

STEP 6: Set up an equation and solve for X.

$$mg \times kg/day = X$$

$$\frac{8 \text{ mg} \times 10 \text{ kg}}{1 \text{ day}} = 80 \text{ mg}$$

STEP 7: Round, if necessary.

STEP 8: Re-evaluate to determine whether the amount makes sense. If the prescription reads 8 mg/kg/day to divide equally every 12 hr and the toddler weighs 10 kg, it makes sense to give 80 mg/day, or 40 mg every 12 hr.

USING RATIO AND PROPORTION

STEP 9: What is the unit of measurement the nurse should calculate?

mL

STEP 10: What is the dose the nurse should administer? Dose to administer = Desired

40 mg (half of 80 mg/day for every 12 hr dosing)

STEP 11: What is the dose available? Dose available = Have

100 mg

STEP 12: Should the nurse convert the units of measurement? No

STEP 13: What is the quantity of the dose available? = Quantity

5 mL

STEP 14: Set up the equation and solve for X.

$$\frac{Have}{Quantity} = \frac{Desired}{X}$$

$$\frac{100 \text{ mg}}{5 \text{ mL}} = \frac{40 \text{ mg}}{X \text{ mL}}$$

$$X = 2$$

STEP 15: Round, if necessary.

STEP 16: Re-evaluate to determine whether the amount to give makes sense. If there are 100 mg/5 mL and the prescription reads 40 mg, it makes sense to give 2 mL. The nurse should administer cefixime suspension 2 mL PO every 12 hr.

USING DESIRED OVER HAVE

STEP 9: What is the unit of measurement the nurse should calculate?

mL

STEP 10: What is the dose the nurse should administer? Dose to administer = Desired

40 mg (half of 80 mg/day for every 12 hr dosing)

STEP 11: What is the dose available? Dose available = Have

100 mg

STEP 12: Should the nurse convert the units of measurement? No

STEP 13: What is the quantity of the dose available? = Quantity

5 mL

STEP 14: Set up an equation and solve for X.

$$\frac{Desired \times Quantity}{Have} = X$$

$$\frac{40 \text{ mg} \times 5 \text{ mL}}{100 \text{ mg}} = X \text{ mL}$$

$$2 = X$$

STEP 15: Round, if necessary.

STEP 16: Re-evaluate to determine whether the amount to give makes sense. If there are 100 mg/5 mL and the prescription reads 40 mg, it makes sense to give 2 mL. The nurse should administer cefixime suspension 2 mL PO every 12 hr.

USING DIMENSIONAL ANALYSIS

STEP 9: What is the unit of measurement the nurse should calculate?

mL

STEP 10: What is the quantity of the dose available? = Quantity

5 mL

STEP 11: What is the dose available? Dose available = Have

100 mg

STEP 12: What is the dose the nurse should administer? Dose to administer = Desired

40 mg (half of 80 mg/day for every 12 hr dosing)

STEP 13: Should the nurse convert the units of measurement? No

STEP 14: Set up an equation and solve for X.

$$X = \frac{Quantity}{Have} \times \frac{Conversion\ (Have)}{Conversion\ (Desired)} \times Desired$$

$$X \text{ mL} = \frac{5 \text{ mL}}{100 \text{ mg}} \times 40 \text{ mg}$$

$$X = 2$$

STEP 15: Round, if necessary.

STEP 16: Re-evaluate to determine whether the amount to give makes sense. If there are 100 mg/5 mL and the prescription reads 40 mg, it makes sense to give 2 mL. The nurse should administer cefixime suspension 2 mL PO every 12 hr.

IV flow rates

Nurses calculate IV flow rates for large-volume continuous IV infusions and intermittent IV bolus infusions using electronic infusion pumps (mL/hr) and manual IV tubing (gtt/min).

! The nurse should know the scope of practice for the LPN outlined in the state Nurse Practice Act regarding administration of IV fluids and medications. This can vary from state to state.

IV INFUSIONS WITH ELECTRONIC INFUSION PUMPS

Infusion pumps control an accurate rate of fluid infusion. Infusion pumps deliver a specific amount of fluid during a specific amount of time. For example, an infusion pump can deliver 150 mL in 1 hr or 50 mL in 20 min.

Example: A nurse is preparing to administer dextrose 5% in water (D_5W) 500 mL IV to infuse over 4 hr. The nurse should set the IV infusion pump to deliver how many mL/hr? (Round the answer to the nearest whole number.)

STEP 1: What is the unit of measurement the nurse should calculate?

mL/hr

STEP 2: What is the volume the nurse should infuse?

500 mL

STEP 3: What is the total infusion time?

4 hr

STEP 4: Should the nurse convert the units of measurement? No

STEP 5: Set up the equation and solve for X.

$$\frac{Volume \text{ (mL)}}{Time \text{ (hr)}} = X \text{ mL/hr}$$

$$\frac{500 \text{ mL}}{4 \text{ hr}} = X \text{ mL/hr}$$

125 = X

STEP 6: Round, if necessary.

STEP 7: Re-evaluate to determine whether the IV flow rate makes sense. If the prescription reads 500 mL to infuse over 4 hr, it makes sense to administer 125 mL/hr. The nurse should set the IV pump to deliver D_5W 500 mL IV at 125 mL/hr.

Example: A nurse is preparing to administer cefotaxime 1 g intermittent IV bolus over 45 min. Available is cefotaxime 1 g in 100 mL 0.9% sodium chloride (0.9% NaCl). The nurse should set the IV infusion pump to deliver how many mL/hr? (Round the answer to the nearest whole number.)

STEP 1: What is the unit of measurement the nurse should calculate?

mL/hr

STEP 2: Should the nurse convert the units of measurement? Yes (min ≠ hr) Yes (g ≠ mL)

$$\frac{60 \text{ min}}{45 \text{ min}} = \frac{1 \text{ hr}}{X \text{ hr}} \qquad \frac{100 \text{ mL}}{1 \text{ g}} = \frac{X \text{ mL}}{1 \text{ g}}$$

$X = 0.75$ $\qquad\qquad\qquad\qquad X = 100$

STEP 3: What is the total infusion time?

45 min

STEP 4: What is the volume the nurse should infuse?

100 mL

STEP 5: Set up an equation and solve for X.

$$\frac{Volume \text{ (mL)}}{Time \text{ (hr)}} = X \text{ mL/hr}$$

$$\frac{100 \text{ mL}}{0.75 \text{ hr}} = X \text{ mL/hr}$$

133.3333 = X

STEP 6: Round, if necessary.

133.3333 = 133

STEP 7: Re-evaluate to determine whether the IV flow rate makes sense. If the prescription reads 100 mL to infuse over 45 min (0.75 hr), it makes sense to administer 133 mL/hr. The nurse should set the IV pump to deliver cefotaxime 1 g in 100 mL of 0.9% NaCl IV at 133 mL/hr.

MANUAL IV INFUSIONS

If an electronic infusion pump is not available, regulate the IV flow rate using the roller clamp on the IV tubing. When setting the flow rate, count the number of drops that fall into the drip chamber over 1 min. Then calculate the flow rate using the drop factor on the manufacturer's package containing the administration set. The drop factor is the number of drops per milliliter of solution.

> Example: A nurse is preparing to administer lactated Ringer's (LR) 1,500 mL IV to infuse over 10 hr. The drop factor of the manual IV tubing is 15 gtt/mL. The nurse should adjust the manual IV infusion to deliver how many gtt/min? (Round the answer to the nearest whole number.)

USING RATIO AND PROPORTION AND DESIRED OVER HAVE

STEP 1: What is the unit of measurement the nurse should calculate?

gtt/min

STEP 2: What is the quantity of the drop factor that is available?

15 gtt/mL

STEP 3: What is the volume the nurse should infuse?

1,500 mL

STEP 4: What is the total infusion time?

10 hr

STEP 5: Should the nurse convert the units of measurement? No (mL = mL) Yes (hr ≠ min)

$$\frac{1 \text{ hr}}{60 \text{ min}} = \frac{10 \text{ hr}}{X \text{ min}}$$

$X = 600$ min

STEP 6: Set up the equation and solve for X.

$$\frac{Volume \text{ (mL)}}{Time \text{ (min)}} \times Drop\ factor \text{ (gtt/mL)} = X$$

$$\frac{1,500 \text{ mL}}{600 \text{ min}} \times 15 \text{ gtt/mL} = X \text{ gtt/min}$$

$37.5 = X$

STEP 7: Round, if necessary.

$37.5 = 38$

STEP 8: Re-evaluate to determine whether the IV flow rate makes sense. If the prescription reads 1,500 mL to infuse over 10 hr (600 min), it makes sense to administer 38 gtt/min. The nurse should adjust the manual IV infusion to deliver LR 1,500 mL IV at 38 gtt/min.

USING DIMENSIONAL ANALYSIS

STEP 1: What is the unit of measurement the nurse should calculate?

gtt/min

STEP 2: What is the quantity of the drop factor that is available?

15 gtt/mL

STEP 3: What is the total infusion time?

10 hr

STEP 4: What is the volume the nurse should infuse?

1,500 mL

STEP 5: Should the nurse convert the units of measurement? No (mL = mL) Yes (hr ≠ min)

$$\frac{1 \text{ hr}}{60 \text{ min}} = \frac{10 \text{ hr}}{X \text{ min}}$$

$X = 600$ min

STEP 6: Set up the equation and solve for X.

$$X = \frac{Quantity}{1 \text{ mL}} \times \frac{Conversion\ (Have)}{Conversion\ (Desired)} \times \frac{Volume}{Time}$$

$$X \text{ gtt/min} = \frac{15 \text{ gtt}}{1 \text{ mL}} \times \frac{1 \text{ hr}}{60 \text{ min}} \times \frac{1,500 \text{ mL}}{10 \text{ hr}}$$

$X = 37.5$

STEP 7: Round, if necessary.

$37.5 = 38$

STEP 8: Re-evaluate to determine whether the IV flow rate makes sense. If the prescription reads 1,500 mL to infuse over 10 hr (600 min), it makes sense to administer 38 gtt/min. The nurse should adjust the manual IV infusion to deliver LR 1,500 mL IV at 38 gtt/min.

> Example: A nurse is preparing to administer ranitidine 150 mg by intermittent IV bolus. Available is ranitidine 150 mg in 100 mL of 0.9% sodium chloride (0.9% NaCl) to infuse over 30 min. The drop factor of the manual IV tubing is 10 gtt/mL. The nurse should adjust the manual IV infusion to deliver how many gtt/min? (Round the answer to the nearest whole number.)

USING RATIO AND PROPORTION AND DESIRED OVER HAVE

STEP 1: What is the unit of measurement the nurse should calculate?

gtt/min

STEP 2: Should the nurse convert the units of measurement? Yes (mg ≠ mL)

$$\frac{150 \text{ mg}}{100 \text{ mL}} = \frac{150 \text{ mg}}{X \text{ mL}}$$

X = 100

STEP 3: What is the total infusion time?

30 min

STEP 4: What is the quantity of the drop factor that is available?

10 gtt/mL

STEP 5: What is the volume the nurse should infuse?

100 mL

STEP 6: Set up an equation and solve for X.

$$\frac{Volume \text{ (mL)}}{Time \text{ (min)}} \times Drop\ factor \text{ (gtt/mL)} = X$$

$$\frac{100 \text{ mL}}{30 \text{ min}} \times 10 \text{ gtt/mL} = X \text{ gtt/min}$$

33.3333 = X

STEP 7: Round, if necessary.

33.3333 = 33

STEP 8: Re-evaluate to determine whether the IV flow rate makes sense. If the amount prescribed is 100 mL to infuse over 30 min, it makes sense to administer 33 gtt/min. The nurse should adjust the manual IV infusion to deliver ranitidine 150 mg in 100 mL of 0.9% NaCl IV at 33 gtt/min.

USING DIMENSIONAL ANALYSIS

STEP 1: What is the unit of measurement to calculate?

gtt/min

STEP 2: What is the quantity of the drop factor that is available?

10 gtt/mL

STEP 3: What is the total infusion time?

30 min

STEP 4: Should the nurse convert the units of measurement? Yes (mg ≠ mL)

$$\frac{150 \text{ mg}}{100 \text{ mL}} = \frac{150 \text{ mg}}{X \text{ mL}}$$

X = 100

STEP 5: What is the volume the nurse should infuse?

100 mL

STEP 6: Set up an equation and solve for X.

$$X = \frac{Quantity}{1 \text{ mL}} \times \frac{Conversion\ (Have)}{Conversion\ (Desired)} \times \frac{Volume}{Time}$$

$$X \text{ gtt/min} = \frac{10 \text{ gtt}}{1 \text{ mL}} \times \frac{100 \text{ mL}}{30 \text{ min}}$$

X = 33.3333

STEP 7: Round, if necessary.

33.3333 = 33

STEP 8: Re-evaluate to determine whether the IV flow rate makes sense. If the amount prescribed is 100 mL to infuse over 30 min, it makes sense to administer 33 gtt/min. The nurse should adjust the manual IV infusion to deliver ranitidine 150 mg in 100 mL of 0.9% NaCl IV at 33 gtt/min.

Application Exercises

1. A nurse is preparing to administer vancomycin 1 g by intermittent IV bolus. Available is vancomycin 1 g in 100 mL of dextrose 5% in water (D₅W) to infuse over 45 min. The drop factor of the manual IV tubing is 10 gtt/mL. The nurse should adjust the manual IV infusion to deliver how many gtt/min? (Round the answer to the nearest whole number. Do not use a trailing zero.)

2. A nurse is preparing to administer clindamycin 200 mg by intermittent IV bolus. Available is clindamycin injection 200 mg in 100 mL 0.9% sodium chloride (0.9% NaCl) to infuse over 30 min. The nurse should set the IV pump to deliver how many mL/hr? (Round the answer to the nearest whole number. Do not use a trailing zero.)

3. A nurse is preparing to administer furosemide 80 mg PO daily. Available is furosemide oral solution 10 mg/1 mL. How many mL should the nurse administer? (Round the answer to the nearest whole number. Do not use a trailing zero.)

4. A nurse is preparing to administer haloperidol 2 mg PO every 12 hr. Available is haloperidol 1 mg/tablet. How many tablets should the nurse administer? (Round the answer to the nearest whole number. Do not use a trailing zero.)

5. A nurse is preparing to administer amoxicillin 20 mg/kg/day PO to divide equally every 12 hr to a preschooler who weighs 44 lb. Available is amoxicillin suspension 250 mg/5 mL. How many mL should the nurse administer per dose? (Round the answer to the nearest whole number. Do not use a trailing zero.)

6. A nurse is preparing to administer heparin 15,000 units subcutaneously every 12 hr. Available is heparin injection 20,000 units/mL. How many mL should the nurse administer per dose? (Round the answer to the nearest tenth. Use a leading zero if it applies. Do not use a trailing zero.)

7. A nurse is preparing to administer acetaminophen 650 mg PO every 6 hr PRN for pain. Available is acetaminophen liquid 500 mg/5 mL. How many mL should the nurse administer per dose? (Round the answer to the nearest tenth. Use a leading zero if it applies. Do not use a trailing zero.)

8. A nurse is preparing to administer dextrose 5% in water (D₅W) 750 mL IV to infuse over 6 hr. The nurse should set the IV pump to deliver how many mL/hr? (Round the answer to the nearest whole number. Do not use a trailing zero.)

Application Exercises Key

1. **22** gtt/min

Using Ratio and Proportion and Desired Over Have

STEP 1: What is the unit of measurement the nurse should calculate?   gtt/min

STEP 2: Should the nurse convert the units of measurement?   Yes

$$\frac{1\,g}{100\,mL} \times \frac{1\,g}{X\,mL} = 100\,mL$$

STEP 3: What is the total infusion time?   45 min

STEP 4: What is the volume the nurse should infuse?   100 mL

STEP 5: What is the quantity of the drop factor that is available?   10 gtt/mL

STEP 6: Set up an equation and solve for X.

$$\frac{Volume\,(mL)}{Time\,(min)} \times Drop\,factor\,(gtt/mL) = X$$

$$\frac{100\,mL}{45\,min} \times 10\,gtt/mL = X\,gtt/mL$$

$$22.2222 = X$$

STEP 7: Round, if necessary.   22.2222 = 22

STEP 8: Re-evaluate to determine whether the IV flow rate makes sense. If the amount prescribed is 100 mL to infuse over 45 min, it makes sense to administer 22 gtt/min. The nurse should adjust the manual IV infusion to deliver vancomycin 1 g in 100 mL of D$_5$W IV at 22 gtt/min.

Using Dimensional Analysis

STEP 1: What is the unit of measurement to calculate?   gtt/min

STEP 2: What is the quantity of the drop factor that is available?   10 gtt/mL

STEP 3: What is the total infusion time?   45 min

STEP 4: Should the nurse convert the units of measurement?   Yes

$$\frac{1\,g}{100\,mL} \times \frac{1\,g}{X\,mL} = 100\,mL$$

STEP 5: What is the volume the nurse should infuse?   100 mL

STEP 6: Set up an equation and solve for X.

$$X = \frac{Quantity}{1\,mL} \times \frac{Conversion\,(Have)}{Conversion\,(Desired)} \times \frac{Volume}{Time}$$

$$X\,gtt/min = \frac{10\,gtt}{1\,mL} \times \frac{100\,mL}{45\,min}$$

$$X = 22.2222$$

STEP 7: Round, if necessary.   22.2222 = 22

STEP 8: Re-evaluate to determine whether the IV flow rate makes sense. If the amount prescribed is 100 mL to infuse over 45 min, it makes sense to administer 22 gtt/min. The nurse should adjust the manual IV infusion to deliver vancomycin 1 g in 100 mL of D$_5$W IV at 22 gtt/min.

Ⓝ *NCLEX® Connection: Pharmacological Therapies, Medication Administration*

---

2. **200** mL/hr

STEP 1: What is the unit of measurement the nurse should calculate?   mL/hr

STEP 2: Should the nurse convert the units of measurement?   Yes (mg ≠ mL)   Yes (min ≠ hr)

$$\frac{60\,min}{30\,min} = \frac{1\,hr}{X\,hr} \quad \frac{200\,mg}{100\,mg} = \frac{200\,mg}{X\,mL}$$

$$X = 0.5 \qquad X = 100$$

STEP 3: What is the volume the nurse should infuse?   100 mL

STEP 4: What is the total infusion time?   30 min

STEP 5: Set up an equation and solve for X.

$$\frac{Volume\,(mL)}{Time\,(hr)} = X\,mL/hr \qquad \frac{100\,mL}{0.5\,hr} = X\,mL/hr$$

$$200 = X$$

STEP 6: Round, if necessary.

STEP 7: Re-evaluate to determine whether the IV flow rate makes sense. If the prescription reads 100 mL to infuse over 30 min (0.5 hr), it makes sense to administer 200 mL/hr. The nurse should set the IV pump to deliver clindamycin 200 mg in 100 mL of 0.9% NaCl IV at 200 mL/hr.

Ⓝ *NCLEX® Connection: Pharmacological Therapies, Medication Administration*

---

3. **8** mL

Using Ratio and Proportion

STEP 1: What is the unit of measurement the nurse should calculate?   mL

STEP 2: What is the dose the nurse should administer? Dose to administer = Desired = 80 mg

STEP 3: What is the dose available? Dose available = Have = 10 mg

STEP 4: Should the nurse convert the units of measurement?   No

STEP 5: What is the quantity of the dose available? = Quantity = 1 mL

STEP 6: Set up the equation and solve for X.

$$\frac{Have}{Quantity} = \frac{Desired}{X} \quad \frac{10\,mg}{1\,mL} \times \frac{80\,mg}{X\,mL}$$

$$X = 8$$

STEP 7: Round, if necessary.

STEP 8: Re-evaluate to determine whether the amount to administer makes sense. If there are 10 mg/1 mL and the prescription reads 80 mg, it makes sense to administer 8 mL. The nurse should administer furosemide 8 mL PO daily.

Using Desired Over Have

STEP 1: What is the unit of measurement the nurse should calculate?   mL

STEP 2: What is the dose the nurse should administer? Dose to administer = Desired = 80 mg

STEP 3: What is the dose available? Dose available = Have = 10 mg

STEP 4: Should the nurse convert the units of measurement? No

STEP 5: What is the quantity of the dose available? = Quantity = 1 mL

STEP 6: Set up the equation and solve for X.

$$\frac{Desired \times Quantity}{Have} = X \quad \frac{80\,mg \times 1\,mL}{10\,mg} = X\,mL$$

$$8 = X$$

STEP 7: Round, if necessary.

STEP 8: Re-evaluate to determine whether the amount to administer makes sense. If there are 10 mg/1 mL and the prescription reads 80 mg, it makes sense to administer 8 mL. The nurse should administer furosemide 8 mL PO daily.

Using Dimensional Analysis

STEP 1: What is the unit of measurement the nurse should calculate?   mL

STEP 2: What is the quantity of the dose available? = Quantity = 1 mL

STEP 3: What is the dose available? Dose available = Have = 10 mg

STEP 4: What is the dose the nurse should administer? Dose to administer = Desired = 80 mg

STEP 5: Should the nurse convert the units of measurement?   No

STEP 6: Set up the equation and solve for X.

$$X = \frac{Quantity}{Have} \times \frac{Conversion\,(Have)}{Conversion\,(Desired)} \times Desired$$

$$X\,mL = \frac{1\,mL}{10\,mg} \times 80$$

$$X = 8$$

STEP 7: Round, if necessary.

STEP 8: Re-evaluate to determine whether the amount to administer makes sense. If there are 10 mg/1 mL and the prescription reads 80 mg, it makes sense to administer 8 mL. The nurse should administer furosemide 8 mL PO daily.

Ⓝ *NCLEX® Connection: Pharmacological Therapies, Dosage Calculations*

4. **2** tablets

Using Ratio and Proportion

STEP 1: What is the unit of measurement the nurse should calculate? tablet

STEP 2: What is the dose the nurse should administer? Dose to administer = Desired = 2 mg

STEP 3: What is the dose available? Dose available = Have = 1 mg

STEP 4: Should the nurse convert the units of measurement? No

STEP 5: What is the quantity of the dose available? = Quantity = 1 tablet

STEP 6: Set up the equation and solve for X.

$$\frac{Have}{Quantity} = \frac{Desired}{X} \qquad \frac{1\ mg}{1\ tablet} \times \frac{2\ mg}{X\ tablets}$$

$$X = 2$$

STEP 7: Round, if necessary.

STEP 8: Re-evaluate to determine whether the amount to administer makes sense. If there is 1 mg/tablet and the prescription reads 2 mg, it makes sense to administer 2 tablets. The nurse should administer haloperidol 2 tablets every 12 hr.

Using Desired Over Have

STEP 1: What is the unit of measurement the nurse should calculate? tablet

STEP 2: What is the dose the nurse should administer? Dose to administer = Desired = 2 mg

STEP 3: What is the dose available? Dose available = Have = 1 mg

STEP 4: Should the nurse convert the units of measurement? No

STEP 5: What is the quantity of the dose available? = Quantity = 1 tablet

STEP 6: Set up the equation and solve for X.

$$\frac{Desired \times Quantity}{Have} = X$$

$$\frac{2\ mg \times 1\ tablet}{1\ mg} = X\ tablets$$

$$2 = X$$

STEP 7: Round, if necessary.

STEP 8: Re-evaluate to determine whether the amount to administer makes sense. If there is 1 mg/tablet and the prescription reads 2 mg, it makes sense to administer 2 tablets. The nurse should administer haloperidol 2 tablets every 12 hr.

Using Dimensional Analysis

STEP 1: What is the unit of measurement the nurse should calculate? tablets

STEP 2: What is the quantity of the dose available? = Quantity = 1 tablet

STEP 3: What is the dose available? Dose available = Have = 1 mg

STEP 4: What is the dose the nurse should administer? Dose to administer = Desired = 2 mg

STEP 5: Should the nurse convert the units of measurement? No

STEP 6: Set up the equation and solve for X.

$$X = \frac{Quantity}{Have} \times \frac{Conversion\ (Have)}{Conversion\ (Desired)} \times Desired$$

$$X\ tablets = \frac{1\ tablet}{1\ mg} \times 2\ mg$$

$$X = 2$$

STEP 7: Round, if necessary.

STEP 8: Re-evaluate to determine whether the amount to administer makes sense. If there is 1 mg/tablet and the prescription reads 2 mg, it makes sense to administer 2 tablets. The nurse should administer haloperidol 2 tablets every 12 hr.

Ⓝ *NCLEX® Connection: Pharmacological Therapies, Dosage Calculations*

---

5. **4** mL

STEP 1: What is the unit of measurement the nurse should calculate? kg

STEP 2: Set up an equation and solve for X.

$$\frac{2.2\ lb}{1\ kg} = \frac{client's\ weight\ in\ lb}{X\ kg} \qquad \frac{2.2\ lb}{1\ kg} \times \frac{44\ lb}{X\ kg}$$

$$X = 20$$

STEP 3: Round, if necessary.

STEP 4: Re-evaluate to determine whether the equivalent makes sense. If 1 kg = 2.2 lb, it makes sense that 44 lb = 20 kg.

STEP 5: What is the unit of measurement the nurse should calculate? mg

STEP 6: Set up an equation and solve for X. **mg × kg/day = X**

$$\frac{20\ mg \times 20\ kg}{1\ day} = 400\ mg/day$$

STEP 7: Round, if necessary.

STEP 8: Re-evaluate to determine whether the amount makes sense. If the prescription reads 20 mg/kg/day to divide equally every 12 hr and the preschooler weighs 20 kg, it makes sense to give 400 mg/day, or 200 mg every 12 hr.

Using Ratio and Proportion

STEP 9: What is the unit of measurement the nurse should calculate? mL

STEP 10: What is the dose the nurse should administer? Dose to administer = Desired = 200 mg

STEP 11: What is the dose available? Dose available = Have = 250 mg

STEP 12: Should the nurse convert the units of measurement? No

STEP 13: What is the quantity of the dose available? = Quantity = 5 mL

STEP 14: Set up the equation and solve for X.

$$\frac{Have}{Quantity} = \frac{Desired}{X} \qquad \frac{250\ mg}{5\ mL} \times \frac{200\ mg}{X\ mL}$$

$$X = 4$$

STEP 15: Round, if necessary.

STEP 16: Re-evaluate to determine whether the amount to give makes sense. If there are 250 mg/5 mL and the prescription reads 200 mg, it makes sense to give 4 mL. The nurse should administer amoxicillin suspension 4 mL PO every 12 hr.

Ⓝ *NCLEX® Connection: Pharmacological Therapies, Dosage Calculations*

Using Desired Over Have

STEP 9: What is the unit of measurement the nurse should calculate? mL

STEP 10: What is the dose the nurse should administer? Dose to administer = Desired 200 mg

STEP 11: What is the dose available? Dose available = Have = 250 mg

STEP 12: Should the nurse convert the units of measurement? No

STEP 13: What is the quantity of the dose available? = Quantity = 5 mL

STEP 14: Set up an equation and solve for X.

$$\frac{Desired \times Quantity}{Have} = X \qquad \frac{200\ mg \times 5\ mL}{250\ mg} = X\ mL$$

$$4 = X$$

STEP 15: Round, if necessary.

STEP 16: Re-evaluate to determine whether the amount to give makes sense. If there are 250 mg/5 mL and the prescription reads 200 mg, it makes sense to give 4 mL. The nurse should administer amoxicillin suspension 4 mL PO every 12 hr.

Using Dimensional Analysis

STEP 9: What is the unit of measurement the nurse should calculate? mL

STEP 10: What is the quantity of the dose available? = Quantity = 5 mL

STEP 11: What is the dose available? Dose available = Have = 250 mg

STEP 12: What is the dose the nurse should administer? Dose to administer = Desired = 200 mg

STEP 13: Should the nurse convert the units of measurement? No

STEP 14: Set up an equation and solve for X.

$$X = \frac{Quantity}{Have} \times \frac{Conversion\ (Have)}{Conversion\ (Desired)} \times Desired$$

$$X\ mL = \frac{5\ mL}{250\ mg} \times 200\ mg$$

$$X = 4$$

STEP 15: Round, if necessary.

STEP 16: Re-evaluate to determine whether the amount to give makes sense. If there are 250 mg/5 mL and the prescription reads 200 mg, it makes sense to give 4 mL. The nurse should administer amoxicillin suspension 4 mL PO every 12 hr.

6. **0.8** mL

<table>
<tr><td>Using Ratio and Proportion</td><td>Using Desired Over Have</td><td>Using Dimensional Analysis</td></tr>
</table>

Using Ratio and Proportion

STEP 1: What is the unit of measurement the nurse should calculate? mL

STEP 2: What is the dose the nurse should administer? Dose to administer = Desired = 15,000 units

STEP 3: What is the dose available? Dose available = Have = 20,000 units

STEP 4: Should the nurse convert the units of measurement? No

STEP 5: What is the quantity of the dose available? = Quantity = 1 mL

STEP 6: Set up the equation and solve for X.

$$\frac{Have}{Quantity} = \frac{Desired}{X}$$

$$\frac{20,000\ units}{1\ mL} \times \frac{15,000\ units}{X\ mL}$$

$X = 0.75$

STEP 7: Round, if necessary. 0.75 = 0.8

STEP 8: Re-evaluate to determine whether the amount to administer makes sense. If there are 20,000 units/mL and the prescription reads 15,000 units, it makes sense to administer 0.8 mL. The nurse should administer heparin injection 0.8 mL subcutaneously every 12 hr.

Using Desired Over Have

STEP 1: What is the unit of measurement the nurse should calculate? mL

STEP 2: What is the dose the nurse should administer? Dose to administer = Desired = 15,000 units

STEP 3: What is the dose available? Dose available = Have = 20,000 units

STEP 4: Should the nurse convert the units of measurement? No

STEP 5: What is the quantity of the dose available? = Quantity = 1 mL

STEP 6: Set up an equation and solve for X.

$$\frac{Desired \times Quantity}{Have} = X$$

$$\frac{15,000\ units \times 1\ mL}{20,000\ units} = X\ mL$$

$0.75 = X$

STEP 7: Round, if necessary. 0.75 = 0.8

STEP 8: Re-evaluate to determine whether the amount to administer makes sense. If there are 10,000 units/mL and the prescription reads 8,000 units, it makes sense to administer 0.8 mL. The nurse should administer heparin injection 0.8 mL subcutaneously every 12 hr.

Using Dimensional Analysis

STEP 1: What is the unit of measurement the nurse should calculate? mL

STEP 2: What is the quantity of the dose available? = Quantity = 1 mL

STEP 3: What is the dose available? Dose available = Have = 20,000 units

STEP 4: What is the dose the nurse should administer? Dose to administer = Desired = 15,000 units

STEP 5: Should the nurse convert the units of measurement? No

STEP 6: Set up an equation and solve for X.

$$X = \frac{Quantity}{Have} \times \frac{Conversion\ (Have)}{Conversion\ (Desired)} \times Desired$$

$$X\ mL = \frac{1\ mL}{20,000\ units} \times 15,000\ units$$

$X = 0.75$

STEP 7: Round, if necessary. 0.75 = 0.8

STEP 8: Re-evaluate to determine whether the amount to administer makes sense. If there are 10,000 units/mL and the prescription reads 8,000 units, it makes sense to administer 0.8 mL. The nurse should administer heparin injection 0.8 mL subcutaneously every 12 hr.

(N) *NCLEX® Connection: Pharmacological Therapies, Dosage Calculations*

---

7. **6.5** mL

Using Ratio and Proportion

STEP 1: What is the unit of measurement the nurse should calculate? mL

STEP 2: What is the dose the nurse should administer? Dose to administer = Desired = 650 mg

STEP 3: What is the dose available? Dose available = Have = 500 mg

STEP 4: Should the nurse convert the units of measurement? No

STEP 5: What is the quantity of the dose available? = Quantity = 5 mL

STEP 6: Set up the equation and solve for X.

$$\frac{Have}{Quantity} = \frac{Desired}{X}$$

$$\frac{500\ mg}{5\ mL} \times \frac{650\ mg}{X\ mL}$$

$X = 6.5$

STEP 7: Round, if necessary.

STEP 8: Re-evaluate to determine whether the amount to administer makes sense. If there are 500 mg/5 mL and the prescription reads 650 mg, it makes sense to administer 6.5 mL. The nurse should administer acetaminophen liquid 6.5 mL PO every 6 hr PRN for pain.

Using Desired Over Have

STEP 1: What is the unit of measurement the nurse should calculate? mL

STEP 2: What is the dose the nurse should administer? Dose to administer = Desired = 650 mg

STEP 3: What is the dose available? Dose available = Have = 500 mg

STEP 4: Should the nurse convert the units of measurement? No

STEP 5: What is the quantity of the dose available? = Quantity = 5 mL

STEP 6: Set up the equation and solve for X.

$$\frac{Desired \times Quantity}{Have} = X$$

$$\frac{650\ mg \times 5\ mL}{500\ mg} = X\ mL$$

$6.5 = X$

STEP 7: Round, if necessary.

STEP 8: Re-evaluate to determine whether the amount to administer makes sense. If there are 500 mg/5 mL and the prescription reads 650 mg, it makes sense to administer 6.5 mL. The nurse should administer acetaminophen liquid 6.5 mL PO every 6 hr PRN for pain.

Using Dimensional Analysis

STEP 1: What is the unit of measurement the nurse should calculate? mL

STEP 2: What is the quantity of the dose available? = Quantity = 5 mL

STEP 3: What is the dose available? Dose available = Have = 500 mg

STEP 4: What is the dose the nurse should administer? Dose to administer = Desired = 650 mg

STEP 5: Should the nurse convert the units of measurement? No

STEP 6: Set up the equation and solve for X.

$$X = \frac{Quantity}{Have} \times \frac{Conversion\ (Have)}{Conversion\ (Desired)} \times Desired$$

$$X\ mL = \frac{5\ mL}{500\ mg} \times 650\ mg$$

$X = 6.5$

STEP 7: Round, if necessary.

STEP 8: Re-evaluate to determine whether the amount to administer makes sense. If there are 500 mg/5 mL and the prescription reads 650 mg, it makes sense to administer 6.5 mL. The nurse should administer acetaminophen liquid 6.5 mL PO every 6 hr PRN for pain.

(N) *NCLEX® Connection: Pharmacological Therapies, Dosage Calculations*

---

8. **125** mL/hr

STEP 1: What is the unit of measurement the nurse should calculate? mL/hr

STEP 2: What is the volume the nurse should infuse? 750 mL

STEP 3: What is the total infusion time? 6 hr

STEP 4: Should the nurse convert the units of measurement? No

STEP 5: Set up the equation and solve for X.

$$\frac{Volume\ (mL)}{Time\ (hr)} = X\ mL/hr \quad \frac{750\ mL}{6\ hr} = X\ mL/hr$$

$125 = X$

STEP 6: Round, if necessary.

STEP 7: Re-evaluate to determine whether the IV flow rate makes sense. If the prescription reads 750 mL to infuse over 6 hr, it makes sense to administer 125 mL/hr. The nurse should set the IV pump to deliver D$_5$W 750 mL IV at 125 mL/hr.

(N) *NCLEX® Connection: Pharmacological Therapies, Medication Administration*

CHAPTER 4

CHAPTER 4 *Intravenous Therapy*

Intravenous therapy involves administering fluids via an IV catheter to administer medications; supplement fluid intake; or give fluid replacement, electrolytes, or nutrients.

Nurses administer large- and small-volume IV infusions on a continuous basis.

Nurses or pharmacists mix IV medication in a specific volume of fluid to give as a continuous or intermittent IV infusion. Nurses also administer medications as an IV bolus, giving the medication in a small amount of solution, concentrated or diluted, and injecting it over a short time (1 to 2 min or longer, depending on the medication).

The nurse should know the scope of practice for the PN outlined in the state nurse practice act regarding administration of IV fluids and medications. This can vary from state to state.

DESCRIPTION OF PROCEDURE

The provider prescribes the type of IV fluid, the volume to infuse, and either the rate at which to infuse the IV fluid or the total amount of time it should take to infuse the fluid. The nurse regulates the IV infusion, either with an IV pump or manually, to be sure to deliver the right amount.

Nurses administer large-volume IV infusions on a continuous basis, such as 0.9% sodium chloride IV to infuse at 100 mL/hr or dextrose 5% in water 500 mL to infuse IV over 3 hr.

A fluid bolus is a large amount of IV fluid to give in a short time, usually less than 1 hr. It rapidly replaces fluid loss from dehydration, shock, hemorrhage, burns, or trauma.

A large-gauge IV catheter (18-gauge or larger) is essential for maintaining the rapid rate necessary to give a fluid bolus to an adult.

ADVANTAGES

- Rapid effects
- Precise amounts
- Less discomfort after initial insertion than repeated IM or subcutaneous injections
- Constant therapeutic blood levels
- Less irritation to subcutaneous and muscle tissue than IM or subcutaneous injections
- Optimal route for irritant medications

DISADVANTAGES

- Circulatory fluid overload is possible if the infusion is large or too rapid.
- Immediate absorption leaves little time to correct errors.
- IV fluid administration can irritate the lining of the vein.
- Failure to maintain surgical asepsis can lead to local and systemic infection.
- IV fluid administration is costly and inconvenient.
- Embolism is a risk of IV infusion.

WAYS TO ADMINISTER IV MEDICATIONS

Give the medication the pharmacist mixed in a large volume of fluid (500 to 1,000 mL) as a continuous IV infusion, such as potassium chloride and vitamins.

Deliver the medication in premixed solution bags from the medication's manufacturer.

Administer volume-controlled infusions.
- Give some medications, such as antibiotics, intermittently in a small amount of solution (25 to 250 mL) through a continuous IV fluid system or with saline or heparin lock systems.
- Infuse the medications for short periods of time and on a schedule.
- Use a secondary ("piggyback") IV bag or bottle or tandem setup, a volume-control administration set, or a mini-infusion pump.

Give an IV bolus dose.
- Inject the medications in small amounts of solution, concentrated or diluted, over a short time (1 to 2 min or longer, depending on the medication).
- Administer medications directly into the peripheral IV or access port to achieve an immediate medication level in the bloodstream, such as with pain medication.
- Prepare medications in the correct concentration and at a safe rate (amount of medication per minute).
- Use extreme caution and observe for adverse reactions or complications (redness, burning, swelling, increasing pain) that indicate phlebitis, infiltration, or extravasation.

TYPES OF IV ACCESS

Peripheral vein via a catheter

Jugular or subclavian vein via a central venous access device through venipuncture (such as a peripherally inserted central catheter [PICC]) or by surgical intervention with implantation of access ports for long-term use

CONSIDERATIONS

PREPROCEDURE

EQUIPMENT
- Correct size catheter
  - 16-gauge for clients who have trauma, rapid fluid volume
  - 18- to 20-gauge for clients who are having surgery, rapid blood administration
  - 22- to 24-gauge for other clients (adults)
- Tubing
- Infusion pump
- Clean gloves
- Scissors or electric shaver for hair removal

NURSING ACTIONS
- Check the prescription (solution, rate).
- Check for allergies to latex, tape, or iodine.
- Follow the rights of medication administration (including compatibilities of all IV solutions).
- Perform hand hygiene.
- Examine the IV solution for clarity, leaks, and expiration date.
- Prime the tubing.
- Don clean gloves before catheter insertion.
- Examine extremities and veins.
- Clip hair at and around the insertion site with scissors or shave it with an electric shaver.
- Place the client in a comfortable position.
- Identify the client and explain the procedure.

INTRAPROCEDURE

NURSING ACTIONS
- **Select the vein by choosing**
  - Distal veins first on the nondominant hand
  - A site that is not painful or bruised and will not interfere with activity
  - A vein that is resilient and has a soft, bouncy feeling
- **Document in the medical record**
  - Date and time of insertion
  - Insertion site and appearance
  - Catheter size
  - Type of dressing
  - IV fluid and rate
  - Number, locations, and status of previously attempted catheterizations
  - The client's response

> Sample documentation: 1/16/20XX, 1423, Inserted 22-gauge IV catheter into right wrist cephalic vein (one attempt); applied sterile occlusive dressing. Lactated Ringer's infusing at 100 mL/hr per infusion pump without redness or edema at the site. Tolerated without complications. L. Turner, RN

- Be sure to document thoroughly and accurately throughout the client's course of IV therapy.

POSTPROCEDURE

NURSING ACTIONS: Maintain patency of the IV access device.
- Do not stop a continuous infusion or allow blood to back up into the catheter. Clots can form at the tip of the needle or catheter and can lodge against the vein's wall, blocking the flow of fluid.
- Make sure the IV insertion site's dressing is not too tight.
- Flush intermittent IV catheters with the solution the facility specifies after every medication administration or every 8 to 12 hr when not in use.
- Monitor the site and infusion rate at least every hour.

CLIENT EDUCATION
- Do not manipulate the flow rate device, change settings on the IV pump, or lie on the tubing.
- Report pain at the insertion site, sudden difficulty with breathing, or blood in the tubing.
- Avoid manipulating the tubing or infusion site and report nearly empty solution containers.

GUIDELINES FOR SAFE IV MEDICATION ADMINISTRATION
- Use an infusion pump to administer medications that can cause serious adverse reactions, such as potassium chloride. Never administer them by IV bolus. Double-check the dose of potassium prescribed and the correct dilution or amount of fluid.
- Add medications to a new IV fluid container, not to an IV container that is already hanging.
- Never administer IV medications through tubing that is infusing blood, blood products, or parenteral nutrition solutions.
- Verify the compatibility of medications with IV solutions before infusing a medication through tubing that is infusing an IV solution.

Needlestick prevention
- Be familiar with IV insertion equipment.
- Do not use needles when needleless systems are available.
- Use protective safety devices when available.
- Dispose of needles immediately in designated puncture-resistant receptacles.
- Do not break, bend, or recap needles.

Specific considerations

Older adult clients, clients who are taking anticoagulants, and clients who have fragile veins ⊚

- Avoid tourniquets. Use a blood pressure cuff to help visualize (but not overdistend) the veins to help prevent hematoma formation.
- Do not slap the extremity to visualize veins.
- Instruct the client to hold the hand below the level of the heart to help distend and thus visualize the veins.
- Avoid using the back of the client's hand.
- Avoid rigorous friction while cleaning the site.

Edema in extremities

- Apply digital pressure over the selected vein to displace edema.
- Apply pressure with an alcohol pad.
- Cannulate the vein quickly.

Obese clients: Use anatomical landmarks to find veins.

Preventing IV infusion–related infections ⓠ

- Use standard precautions.
- Perform hand hygiene before and after handling IV systems.
- Change IV sites according to facility policy (usually every 72 hr).
- Replace continuous and intermittent infusion tubing according to facility policy (usually every 24 or 48 hr).
- Remove catheters as soon as there is no need for them.
- Replace catheters when suspecting any break in surgical aseptic technique, such as during emergency insertions.
- Use a sterile needle or catheter for each insertion attempt.
- Avoid writing on IV bags with pens or markers, because ink could seep through the bag and contaminate the solution.
- Replace the tubing immediately for potential or actual contamination.
- Do not allow fluids to hang for more than 24 hr unless it is a closed system (pressure bags for hemodynamic monitoring).
- Wipe all ports with alcohol or an antiseptic swab before connecting IV lines or inserting a syringe to prevent the introduction of micro-organisms into the system.
- Never disconnect tubing for convenience or to reposition the client.
- Do not allow ports to remain open to air.

COMPLICATIONS

Complications require notification of the provider and complete documentation. Use new tubing and catheters for restarting IV infusions after detecting complications.

Infiltration (infiltration of a nonvesicant solution)

FINDINGS: Pallor, local swelling at the site, decreased skin temperature around the site, damp dressings, slowed infusion

TREATMENT
- Stop the infusion and remove the catheter.
- Elevate the extremity.
- Encourage active range of motion.
- Apply a cold or warm compress depending on the type of solution that infiltrated the tissue.
- Check with the provider to determine whether the client still needs IV therapy. If so, restart the infusion proximal to the site or in another extremity.

PREVENTION
- Carefully select the site and catheter.
- Secure the catheter.

Extravasation (infiltration of a vesicant or tissue-damaging medication)

FINDINGS: Pain, burning, redness, swelling

TREATMENT
- Stop the infusion and notify the provider.
- Follow the facility's protocol, which can include infusing an antidote through the catheter before removal.

PREVENTION
- Closely monitor the IV site and dressing.
- Always use an infusion pump.

Hematoma

FINDINGS: Ecchymosis at the site

TREATMENT
- Do not apply alcohol.
- Apply pressure after IV catheter removal.
- Use a warm compress and elevation after bleeding stops.

PREVENTION
- Minimize tourniquet time.
- Remove the tourniquet before starting the IV infusion.
- Maintain pressure after IV catheter removal.

Catheter embolus

FINDINGS
- Missing catheter tip after discontinuation
- Severe pain at the site with migration; no manifestations if no migration
  - Decreasing blood pressure
  - Cyanosis in nail beds
  - Weak, rapid pulse

TREATMENT
- Place a tourniquet high on the extremity to limit venous flow.
- Prepare for removal under x-ray or via surgery to remove catheter fragments.
- Save the catheter after removal to determine the cause.

PREVENTION: Do not reinsert the stylet needle into the catheter.

Phlebitis/thrombophlebitis

FINDINGS
- Edema, erythema
- Throbbing, burning, or pain at the site
- Increased skin temperature
- Red line up the arm with a palpable band at the vein site
- Slowed infusion

TREATMENT
- Promptly discontinue the infusion and remove the catheter.
- Elevate the extremity.
- Apply a cold compress to minimize the flow of blood, then apply a warm compress to increase circulation.
- Check with the provider to determine whether the client still needs IV therapy. If so, restart the infusion proximal to the site or in another extremity.
- Obtain a specimen for culture at the site and prepare the catheter for culture if drainage is present.

PREVENTION
- Rotate sites at least every 72 hr according to facility policy.
- Monitor IV sites using a phlebitis scale.
- Avoid the lower extremities.
- Use hand hygiene.
- Use surgical aseptic technique.

Cellulitis

FINDINGS: Pain, warmth, edema, induration, red streaking, fever, chills, malaise

TREATMENT
- Promptly discontinue the infusion and remove the catheter.
- Elevate the extremity.
- Apply warm compresses three to four times per day.
- Obtain a specimen for culture at the site and prepare the catheter for culture if drainage is present.
- Administer antibiotics, analgesics, and antipyretics.

PREVENTION
- Rotate sites at least every 72 hr according to facility policy.
- Avoid the lower extremities.
- Use hand hygiene.
- Use surgical aseptic technique.

Fluid overload

FINDINGS
- Distended neck veins
- Increased blood pressure
- Tachycardia
- Shortness of breath
- Crackles in the lungs
- Edema
- Additional findings varying with the IV solution

TREATMENT
- Slow the IV rate or stop the infusion.
- Raise the head of the bed.
- Monitor vital signs and oxygen saturation.
- Adjust the rate after correcting fluid overload.
- Anticipate administering diuretics.

PREVENTION
- Use an infusion pump.
- Monitor I&O.

Application Exercises

1. A nurse is observing a client's IV infusion site. Which of the following findings should the nurse identify as indications of phlebitis? (Select all that apply.)

   A. Pallor

   B. Dampness

   C. Erythema

   D. Coolness

   E. Pain

2. A nurse manager is reviewing the facility's policies for IV therapy with the members of the team. The nurse manager should remind the team that which of the following techniques helps minimize the risk of catheter embolism?

   A. Performing hand hygiene before and after IV insertion

   B. Rotating IV sites at least every 72 hr

   C. Minimizing tourniquet time

   D. Avoiding reinserting the needle into an IV catheter

3. A nurse is preparing to initiate IV therapy for an older adult client. Which of the following actions should the nurse plan to take?

   A. Use a disposable razor to remove excess hair on the extremity.

   B. Select the back of the client's hand to insert the IV catheter.

   C. Distend the veins by using a blood pressure cuff.

   D. Direct the client to raise his arm above his heart.

4. A nurse is inspecting a client's IV catheter insertion site and notes a hematoma. Which of the following actions should the nurse take? (Select all that apply.)

   A. Stop the infusion.

   B. Apply alcohol to the insertion site.

   C. Apply warm compresses to the insertion site.

   D. Elevate the client's arm.

   E. Obtain a specimen for culture at the insertion site.

PRACTICE Active Learning Scenario

A nurse on a medical-surgical unit is providing care for a group of clients who are receiving IV therapy. The nurse is observing the clients for complications. Use the ATI Active Learning Template: Nursing Skill to complete this item.

INDICATIONS: Identify three indications for IV therapy.

POTENTIAL COMPLICATIONS: Identify four potential complications of IV therapy.

Application Exercises Key

1. A. Pallor at the insertion site is a manifestation of infiltration.

   B. Dampness at the insertion site indicates fluid leakage, which is a typical finding with infiltration.

   C. **CORRECT:** Erythema and warmth at the insertion site are manifestations of phlebitis.

   D. Coolness at the insertion site is a manifestation of infiltration.

   E. **CORRECT:** Pain and burning at the insertion site are manifestations of phlebitis.

   Ⓝ *NCLEX® Connection: Pharmacological Therapies, Expected Actions/Outcomes*

2. A. The nurse manager should remind the members of the team to perform hand hygiene to prevent infection, but this technique does not reduce the risk of catheter embolism.

   B. The nurse manager should remind the members of the team to rotate IV sites at least every 72 hr to help prevent phlebitis, but this technique does not minimize the risk of catheter embolism.

   C. The nurse manager should remind the members of the team to minimize tourniquet time to prevent hematoma formation, but this technique does not reduce the risk of catheter embolism.

   D. **CORRECT:** The nurse manager should remind the members of the team to avoid reinserting the stylet needle into an IV catheter. This action can result in severing the end of the catheter and consequently cause a catheter embolism.

   Ⓝ *NCLEX® Connection: Pharmacological Therapies, Medication Administration*

3. A. The nurse should remove excess hair by clipping it with scissors. Shaving with a disposable razor can cause skin damage that can lead to infection.

   B. In most instances, the nurse inserts the IV catheter into a distal site, such as the back of the client's hand. However, when inserting an IV catheter for an older adult, the nurse should select a site on the arm because older adults typically have fragile veins in the back of their hands.

   C. **CORRECT:** The nurse should distend the veins using a blood pressure cuff to reduce overfilling of the vein, which can result in a hematoma.

   D. The nurse should direct the client to hold his arm below the level of his heart to distend the vein.

   Ⓝ *NCLEX® Connection: Pharmacological Therapies, Expected Actions/Outcomes*

4. A. Hematoma formation is generally the result of an injury to blood vessels on insertion of an IV catheter. It does not affect the patency of the line or cause further injury unless the hematoma is expanding, so it is not necessary to stop the infusion. However, it is necessary to stop the bleeding if it is expanding.

   B. The nurse should not apply alcohol to the insertion site because it can be uncomfortable for the client and can increase capillary bleeding.

   C. **CORRECT:** Warm compresses can help promote healing of a hematoma.

   D. **CORRECT:** Elevation of the arm helps reduce edema, which can cause pressure and pain and additional bleeding in the area of the hematoma.

   E. A hematoma is not a result of infection, nor does it increase the risk for infection. Cultures are unnecessary.

   Ⓝ *NCLEX® Connection: Pharmacological Therapies, Adverse Effects/ Contraindications/Side Effects/Interactions*

PRACTICE Answer

Using the ATI Active Learning Template: Nursing Skill

INDICATIONS
- To administer medications
- To supplement fluid intake
- To replace electrolytes and nutrients

POTENTIAL COMPLICATIONS
- Infiltration
- Extravasation
- Cellulitis
- Fluid overload
- Catheter embolus
- Hematoma
- Phlebitis, thrombophlebitis

Ⓝ *NCLEX® Connection: Pharmacological and Parenteral Therapies, Parenteral/ Intravenous Therapies*

CHAPTER 5

CHAPTER 5 *Adverse Effects, Interactions, and Contraindications*

To ensure safe medication administration and prevent errors, nurses must know why a provider prescribes a medication and its intended therapeutic effect. They must also be aware of potential side or adverse effects, interactions, contraindications, and precautions.

Every medication has the potential to cause side and adverse effects. Side effects, such as drowsiness, occur when clients receive the therapeutic dose of a medication, such as an antihistamine. It is not usually necessary to stop taking the medication, although there are some nondrowsy formulations of some antihistamines the client might prefer. Adverse effects are undesirable, inadvertent, unexpected, and sometimes severe responses to the medication (anaphylaxis, cardiac dysrhythmias, hemorrhage). Providers immediately discontinue medications that cause severe adverse effects and can report them to the FDA via its voluntary MedWatch program.

Medications are chemicals that affect the body. When clients receive more than one medication, there is a potential for an interaction. Medications can also interact with foods, herbal medicines, and unconventional remedies.

Contraindications and precautions of specific medications refer to conditions clients have that make it unsafe or potentially harmful to receive these medications.

Responses to medications differ due to multiple factors (age, sex, disease processes, ethnicity, genetic variations).

ADVERSE MEDICATION EFFECTS

Central nervous system

Effects can result from central nervous system (CNS) stimulation (excitement) or CNS depression

NURSING ACTIONS
- If CNS stimulation is likely, clients can be at risk for seizures and therefore require precautions.
- If CNS depression is likely, advise clients not to drive or participate in other activities that can be dangerous. Qs

Anticholinergic

- Effects are a result of muscarinic receptor blockade.
- Most are in eyes, smooth muscle, exocrine glands, and the heart.

CLIENT EDUCATION: How to manage these effects to minimize danger and discomfort.

> For example, relieve dry mouth by sipping on liquids; manage photophobia by wearing sunglasses; and minimize urinary retention by urinating before taking the medication.

Cardiovascular

- Effects involve blood vessels and the heart.
- Antihypertensives can cause orthostatic hypotension.

CLIENT EDUCATION: If manifestations of orthostatic hypotension (lightheadedness, dizziness) occur, sit or lie down. Minimize orthostatic hypotension by changing position slowly.

Gastrointestinal (GI)

- Effects result from local irritation of the GI tract.
- Stimulation of the vomiting center also results in adverse effects.

NURSING ACTIONS
- NSAIDs can cause GI upset. Advise clients to take these medications with food or milk.
- Opioid analgesics slow peristalsis and can cause nausea and sedation. Advise clients taking opioids about methods to avoid constipation and GI irritation, and promote safety.

Hematologic

- Effects are relatively common and potentially life-threatening with some groups of medications.
- Bone marrow depression/suppression results from anticancer medications and hemorrhagic disorders from anticoagulants and thrombolytics.

CLIENT EDUCATION: Notify the provider if bleeding occurs (bruising, discolored urine and stool, petechiae, bleeding gums). Clients taking anticoagulants should avoid some herbal supplements, including ginkgo biloba, ginseng, and St. John's wort.

TOXICITY

- Toxicity is an adverse medication effect that is severe and can be life-threatening.
- Excessive dosing can cause toxicity, but it also can occur at therapeutic dose levels.

Hepatotoxicity

- Many medications can cause liver damage.
- Because the metabolism of most medications takes place in the liver, this organ is particularly vulnerable to medication-induced injury.
- Damage to liver cells can impair the metabolism of many medications, causing them to accumulate in the body and produce adverse effects.
- Many medications can alter liver function test results with no obvious manifestations of liver dysfunction.
- Combining two or more medications that are hepatotoxic increases the risk for liver damage.
- Clients who start taking a hepatotoxic medication require liver function tests then and periodically thereafter.
- Liver damage can result from an acetaminophen overdose. There is a greater risk of liver damage with chronic alcohol use. The antidote acetylcysteine can help minimize liver damage.

NURSING ACTIONS: Monitor clients for, and instruct them to watch for, manifestations of hepatotoxicity (nausea, vomiting, jaundice, dark urine, abdominal discomfort, anorexia).

Nephrotoxicity

- Kidney damage can occur with a number of medications, but it is primarily the result of some antimicrobial agents and NSAIDs, such as naproxen.
- Damage to the kidneys can interfere with medication excretion, leading to medication accumulation and adverse effects.
- The glomerular filtration rate of the kidneys decreases with advanced age, making older adults at increased risk for nephrotoxicity. Ⓒ

NURSING ACTIONS: Aminoglycosides, such as gentamicin (an antibiotic that treats serious infections aerobic bacilli cause), injure cells in the renal tubules of the kidney. Monitor serum creatinine and BUN, as well as peak and trough medication levels, for clients taking nephrotoxic medications.

ALLERGIC REACTION

- An allergic reaction is an immune response to a medication or other allergen.
- Previous exposure to the medication has resulted in the formation of antibodies.
- The intensity of allergic reactions can range from mild itching to severe rash to anaphylaxis.

NURSING ACTIONS
- Treat mild rashes and hives with diphenhydramine.
- Before administering any medications, obtain a complete medication history.

Anaphylactic reaction

Anaphylaxis is a life-threatening, immediate allergic reaction that causes respiratory distress, severe bronchospasm, laryngeal edema, a quick drop in blood pressure, and cardiovascular collapse.

NURSING ACTIONS: Treat anaphylaxis with epinephrine, bronchodilators, and antihistamines. Provide respiratory support, and inform the provider.

EXTRAPYRAMIDAL SYMPTOMS (EPSs)

- EPSs are movement disorders that include involuntary fine-motor tremors, rigidity, uncontrollable restlessness, and acute dystonias (spastic movements or muscle rigidity affecting the head, neck, eyes, face, tongue, back, and limbs).
- EPSs can occur within a few hours or take months to develop.
- EPSs are most often associated with medications affecting the CNS, such as those that treat mental health disorders.
- Anticholinergic medication can help minimize most EPSs.

IMMUNOSUPPRESSION

- Immunosuppression is a decreased or absent immune response.
- Immunosuppressant medications, such as glucocorticoids, can mask the usual manifestations of infection, such as fever.

NURSING ACTIONS: Monitor clients taking an immunosuppressant, such as a glucocorticoid, for delayed wound healing and subtle manifestations of infection, such as a sore throat.

CLIENT EDUCATION: Clients who take immunosuppressants should avoid contact with anyone who has a communicable disease.

INTERACTIONS

MEDICATION-MEDICATION INTERACTIONS

Increased therapeutic effects

Providers prescribe some medications for clients to take together to potentiate their action and increase therapeutic effects. Examples include taking two different medications to treat hypertension, or taking an opioid analgesic (such as oxycodone) along with an NSAID (such as ibuprofen).

CLIENTS EDUCATION: Clients who have asthma should use albuterol (a beta₂ adrenergic agonist) via inhaler and triamcinolone (a glucocorticoid) via inhaler to increase the absorption of triamcinolone.

Increased adverse effects

Clients can take two medications that have the same side or adverse effect. Taking these medications together can potentiate these effects. Diazepam and hydrocodone both have CNS depressant effects. Taking these medications together increases the risk for CNS depression.

Decreased therapeutic effects

One medication can increase the metabolism or block the effects of a second medication and therefore decrease the serum level and effectiveness of the second medication.

> For example, phenytoin increases hepatic medication-metabolizing enzymes that affect warfarin and thereby decreases the serum level and the effect of warfarin.

Decreased side/adverse effects

One medication can counteract the side or adverse effects of another medication.

> For example, ondansetron, an antiemetic, helps counteract the adverse effects of nausea and vomiting for clients receiving chemotherapy.

Increased serum levels, leading to toxicity

One medication can decrease the metabolism of a second medication and therefore increase the serum level of the second medication. This can lead to toxicity.

> For example, fluconazole inhibits hepatic medication-metabolizing enzymes that affect aripiprazole and thereby increases serum levels of this medication.

Over-the-counter (OTC) medication interactions

- Ingredients in OTC medications and herbal supplements can interact with other OTC or prescription medications.
  - Inactive ingredients, such as dyes, alcohol, and preservatives, can cause adverse reactions.
  - The potential for overdose exists because of the use of several preparations (including prescription and OTC medications and herbal supplements) with similar ingredients.
- Interactions between some prescription and OTC medications can interfere with their therapeutic effects.

NURSING ACTIONS
- Obtain a complete medication history.
- Instruct clients to follow the manufacturer's recommendation for dosage.

CLIENT EDUCATION
- Use caution and check with the provider before taking any OTC preparations such as antacids, laxatives, decongestants, herbal supplements, or cough syrups. For example, antacids can interfere with the absorption of ranitidine and other medications.
- Take antacids 1 hr apart from other medications.

MEDICATION-FOOD INTERACTIONS

Food can alter medication absorption or contain substances that react with some medications.

EXAMPLES
- Consuming foods that contain tyramine while taking monoamine oxidase inhibitors (MAOIs) can lead to a hypertensive crisis. Clients taking MAOIs should be aware of foods containing tyramine (aged cheese [cheddar, blue cheese], processed meats [salami, sausages]), and avoid them.
- Vitamin K can decrease the therapeutic effects of warfarin and place clients at risk for developing blood clots. Clients taking warfarin should include a consistent amount of vitamin K in their diet.
- Tetracycline can interact with a chelating agent (such as in milk) and form an insoluble, unabsorbable compound. Instruct clients not to take tetracycline within 2 hr of consuming dairy products.
- Grapefruit juice seems to act by inhibiting medication metabolism in the intestines, thus increasing the amount of medication available for absorption. This increases the medication's therapeutic effects and/or adverse reactions. Instruct clients to not drink grapefruit juice if they are taking a medication that interacts with grapefruit juice. QEBP
- Food often decreases the rate of medication absorption. For example, wheat bran and rolled oats can decrease the absorption of digoxin.
- Some foods increase the rate of absorption of some medications. For example, a high-calorie meal more than doubles the absorption of saquinavir, a medication that treats HIV infection.

CONTRAINDICATIONS AND PRECAUTIONS

- Some conditions and disorders can be contraindications for receiving a specific medication. For example, an allergy to penicillin is a contraindication for receiving any of the penicillins.
- Nurses and providers should take precautions for clients who are at increased risk for adverse reactions to a medication.

> Morphine depresses respiratory function, so clients who have asthma or any impairment in respiratory function require caution when receiving this medication.

CATEGORIES

The U.S. Food and Drug Administration places medications in categories according to the risk they pose to a fetus.

CATEGORY A: There is no evidence of risk to the fetus during pregnancy according to the results of adequate and well-controlled studies. Levothyroxine is a category A medication.

CATEGORY B: There is no evidence of risk to animal fetuses according to the results of studies, but there are no adequate and well-controlled studies of pregnant women. Insulin is a category B medication.

CATEGORY C: Studies have demonstrated adverse effects on animal fetuses. There are no adequate and well-controlled studies of pregnant women, but the potential benefits might warrant the use of the medication during pregnancy. Gabapentin is a category C medication.

CATEGORY D: Studies have demonstrated adverse effects on human fetuses according to the results of data from investigational or marketing experience, but the potential benefits might warrant the use of the medication during pregnancy. Lorazepam is a category D medication.

CATEGORY X: Studies have demonstrated adverse effects on animal and human fetuses according to the results of studies and data from investigational or marketing experience. Pregnancy is a contraindication for the use of the medication because the risks outweigh the potential benefits. Warfarin is a category X medication.

Application Exercises

1. A nurse in a clinic is caring for a group of clients. The nurse should contact the provider about a potential contraindication for a medication for which of the following clients? (Select all that apply.)

   A. A client at 8 weeks of gestation who takes levothyroxine to treat hypothyroidism

   B. A client who uses albuterol via inhaler and triamcinolone via inhaler to treat asthma

   C. A client who has chronic liver disease and is taking acetaminophen

   D. A client who is about to begin chemotherapy to treat ovarian cancer and has a new prescription for ondansetron

   E. A client who has a prosthetic heart valve, takes warfarin, and reports a possible pregnancy

2. A nurse is preparing to administer an IM dose of penicillin to a client who has a new prescription. The client states she took penicillin 3 years ago and developed a rash. Which of the following actions should the nurse take?

   A. Administer the prescribed dose.

   B. Withhold the medication.

   C. Ask the provider to change the prescription to an oral form.

   D. Administer an oral antihistamine at the same time.

3. A nurse is reinforcing discharge instructions for a client who has a new prescription for an antihypertensive medication. Which of the following statements should the nurse make?

   A. "Avoid foods that contain tyramine while taking this medication."

   B. "You should check your blood pressure every 8 hours while taking this medication."

   C. "The doctor will increase your medication dosage if you develop tachycardia."

   D. "Change positions slowly when you move from sitting to standing while taking this medication."

4. A nurse is reviewing a client's health record and notes that the client experiences permanent extrapyramidal effects from a medication taken previously. The nurse should identify that the medication affected which of the following of the client's systems?

   A. Cardiovascular

   B. Immune

   C. Central nervous

   D. Gastrointestinal

5. A nurse is caring for a client who is taking oral oxycodone. The client reports also taking ibuprofen in therapeutic doses three times a day. The nurse should identify that an interaction between these two medications can cause which of the following findings?

   A. A decrease in serum levels of ibuprofen, possibly leading to a need for increased doses of this medication

   B. A decrease in serum levels of oxycodone, possibly leading to a need for increased doses of this medication

   C. An increase in the expected therapeutic effect of both medications

   D. An increase in the expected adverse effects of both medications

PRACTICE Active Learning Scenario

A nurse is contributing to the plan of care for an older adult client who is receiving gentamicin IV bolus twice daily. The client has a history of musculoskeletal pain and takes naproxen daily for relief. What information should the nurse offer to include in the client's plan of care? Use the ATI Active Learning Template: Medication to complete this item.

THERAPEUTIC USES: Describe the use of gentamicin.

COMPLICATIONS: Describe two adverse effects.

NURSING INTERVENTIONS
- Describe two laboratory findings to monitor.
- Describe two nursing actions.

Application Exercises Key

1. A. Levothyroxine is a pregnancy category A medication. Pregnancy is not a contraindication for taking levothyroxine.

   B. Using albuterol (a beta₂ adrenergic agonist) via inhaler and triamcinolone (a glucocorticoid) via inhaler, increases the absorption of triamcinolone, which is a desirable effect.

   C. **CORRECT:** A liver disorder is a contraindication for taking acetaminophen due to the risk for toxicity. The nurse should notify the provider, who can prescribe a medication that does not contain acetaminophen.

   D. Ondansetron, an antiemetic, helps counteract the adverse effects of nausea and vomiting for clients receiving chemotherapy.

   E. **CORRECT:** Warfarin is a pregnancy category X medication, which can cause severe birth defects in the fetus. The nurse should notify the provider about the possibility of pregnancy.

   Ⓝ *NCLEX® Connection: Pharmacological Therapies, Adverse Effects/ Contraindications/Side Effects/Interactions*

2. A. Administering the penicillin IM in the dosage prescribed could cause a severe reaction.

   B. **CORRECT:** The nurse should withhold the medication and notify the provider of the client's previous reaction to penicillin so that the provider can prescribe a nonpenicillin antibiotic. Allergic reactions to penicillin can range from mild reactions to severe anaphylaxis.

   C. Administering penicillin orally rather than IM would not prevent an allergic reaction.

   D. Giving the penicillin along with an oral antihistamine might have some effectiveness if the client's reaction is mild, but it will not prevent a severe anaphylactic reaction.

   Ⓝ *NCLEX® Connection: Safety and Infection Control, Accident/Error/ Injury Prevention*

3. A. Foods that contain tyramine can cause a hypertensive crisis in clients taking monoamine oxidase inhibitors (MAOIs), but this is not a precaution for clients taking antihypertensive medication.

   B. Clients should check their blood pressure daily when taking an antihypertensive medication, but every 8 hr is unnecessary.

   C. Tachycardia is an adverse effect that would not warrant an increase in a dose of medication.

   D. **CORRECT:** Orthostatic hypotension is a common adverse effect of antihypertensive medications. The client should move slowly to a sitting or standing position and should sit or lie down if lightheadedness or dizziness occurs.

   Ⓝ *NCLEX® Connection: Pharmacological Therapies, Expected Actions/Outcomes*

4. A. Medications affecting the cardiovascular system generally do not cause extrapyramidal effects. However, they can cause neurological effects, such as dizziness, fatigue, and confusion.

   B. Medications affecting the immune system generally do not cause extrapyramidal effects, but they can cause neurological effects.

   C. **CORRECT:** Extrapyramidal effects are movement disorders that a number of central nervous system medications, such as conventional antipsychotic medications, can cause.

   D. Medications affecting the gastrointestinal system generally do not cause extrapyramidal effects, but they can cause neurological effects.

   Ⓝ *NCLEX® Connection: Pharmacological Therapies, Expected Actions/Outcomes*

5. A. Oxycodone and ibuprofen work by different mechanisms and are not antagonistic, so taking them together should not cause a decrease in serum levels of ibuprofen.

   B. Oxycodone and ibuprofen work by different mechanisms and are not antagonistic, so taking them together should not cause a decrease in serum levels of oxycodone.

   C. **CORRECT:** These medications work together to increase the pain-relieving effects of both medications. Oxycodone is an opioid analgesic, and ibuprofen is an NSAID. They work by different mechanisms, but the client is likely to have better pain relief when taking them together.

   D. Oxycodone and ibuprofen work by different mechanisms, so taking them together should not increase their adverse effects.

   Ⓝ *NCLEX® Connection: Pharmacological Therapies, Adverse Effects/ Contraindications/Side Effects/Interactions*

PRACTICE Answer

Using the ATI Active Learning Template: Medication

THERAPEUTIC USES: Gentamicin is a narrow-spectrum aminoglycoside antibiotic that treats serious infections aerobic bacilli cause.

COMPLICATIONS
- Gentamicin can injure cells of the proximal renal tubules.
- Naproxen and other NSAIDs can cause impaired kidney function.
- The glomerular filtration rate of the kidneys decreases with advanced age, making this client at increased risk for nephrotoxicity.

NURSING INTERVENTIONS
- Laboratory findings to monitor
  - BUN
  - Serum creatinine
  - Peak and trough levels of gentamicin
  - Specific gravity of urine
  - Urinalysis
- Nursing actions
  - Monitor intake and output.
  - Notify the provider of low urinary output.
  - Ensure adequate hydration for the client, and monitor for fluid overload.

Ⓝ *NCLEX® Connection: Pharmacological and Parenteral Therapies, Adverse Effects/ Contraindications/Side Effects Interactions*

ⓝ *NCLEX® Connections*

When reviewing the following chapters, keep in mind the relevant topics and tasks of the NCLEX outline, in particular:

Psychosocial Integrity

CHEMICAL AND OTHER DEPENDENCIES: Plan and provide care to client experiencing substance-related withdrawal or toxicity (nicotine, opioid, sedative).

Pharmacological Therapies

ADVERSE EFFECTS/CONTRAINDICATIONS/SIDE EFFECTS/ INTERACTIONS: Monitor the client for actual and potential adverse effects of medications (prescribed, over-the-counter, herbal supplements).

EXPECTED ACTIONS/OUTCOMES: Evaluate the client's response to medications (adverse reactions, interactions, therapeutic effects).

MEDICATION ADMINISTRATION
Administer medication by the oral route.

Administer a subcutaneous, intradermal, or intramuscular medication.

Administer medication by ear, eye, nose, inhalation, rectum, vagina, or skin route.

CHAPTER 6

Anxiety and Trauma- and Stressor-Related Disorders

Anxiety disorders include generalized anxiety disorder, panic disorder, obsessive-compulsive disorder, social anxiety disorder, and post-traumatic stress disorder. Persistent anxiety can become disabling and can require intervention with therapy, biofeedback, relaxation techniques, and the use of medications. Psychological manifestations of anxiety disorders can include fear and apprehension. Physical manifestations can include palpitations, tachycardia, and shortness of breath.

Sedative hypnotic anxiolytics: Benzodiazepines

SELECT PROTOTYPE MEDICATION: Alprazolam

OTHER MEDICATIONS
- Diazepam
- Lorazepam
- Chlordiazepoxide
- Clorazepate
- Oxazepam
- Clonazepam

PURPOSE

EXPECTED PHARMACOLOGICAL ACTION

Benzodiazepines enhance the inhibitory effects of gamma-aminobutyric acid (GABA) in the central nervous system (CNS). Relief from anxiety occurs rapidly following administration.

6.1 Medications at a glance

Major medications used to treat anxiety disorders

Benzodiazepine sedative hypnotic anxiolytics, such as lorazepam, alprazolam, and diazepam

Atypical anxiolytic/nonbarbiturate anxiolytics, such as buspirone

SELECTED ANTIDEPRESSANTS
- **Selective serotonin reuptake inhibitors (SSRIs):** paroxetine, sertraline, fluoxetine, citalopram, escitalopram, fluvoxamine
- **Serotonin-norepinephrine reuptake inhibitors (SNRIs):** venlafaxine, duloxetine

OTHER ANTIDEPRESSANTS: Tricyclic antidepressants (TCAs): amitriptyline, imipramine, clomipramine

Other medications used less frequently
- Monoamine oxidase inhibitor (MAOI): phenelzine
- Mirtazapine
- Trazodone
- Antihistamines, such as hydroxyzine pamoate and hydroxyzine hydrochloride
- Beta blockers, such as propranolol
- Alpha blockers, such as prazosin
- Anticonvulsants, such as gabapentin

In addition to anxiety disorders, some of these medications are used to treat adjustment disorders, dissociative disorders, and depressive disorders.

THERAPEUTIC USES

Generalized anxiety disorder (GAD) and panic disorder

OTHER USES FOR BENZODIAZEPINES
- Trauma- and stressor-related disorders: Acute stress disorder and post-traumatic stress disorder (PTSD)
- Hyperarousal manifestations of dissociative disorders
- Seizure disorders
- Insomnia
- Muscle spasm
- Alcohol withdrawal (for prevention and treatment of acute manifestations)
- Induction of anesthesia
- Amnesic prior to surgery or procedures

COMPLICATIONS

CNS depression

Sedation, lightheadedness, ataxia, decreased cognitive function

CLIENT EDUCATION
- Observe for CNS depression. Notify the provider if effects occur.
- Avoid activities that require alertness (driving, operating heavy equipment/machinery).
- Avoid alcohol and other antianxiety medications due to potentiated depressant effects, such as severe respiratory depression.

Anterograde amnesia

Difficulty recalling events that occur after dosing

CLIENT EDUCATION: Observe for manifestations. Notify the provider if effects occur.

Toxicity

Acute toxicity

Oral toxicity: drowsiness, lethargy, confusion

IV toxicity: can lead to respiratory depression, severe hypotension, or cardiac/respiratory arrest
Benzodiazepines for IV use include
- Diazepam
- Lorazepam

NURSING ACTIONS
- For oral toxicity, gastric lavage is used, followed by administration of activated charcoal or saline cathartics.
- Assist the RN or provider with IV administration of flumazenil for benzodiazepine overdose/toxicity to counteract sedation and reverse adverse effects.
- Monitor vital signs, maintain patent airway, and assist with providing fluids to maintain blood pressure.
- Have resuscitation equipment available.

Paradoxical response

Insomnia, excitation, euphoria, anxiety, rage

CLIENT EDUCATION: Watch for manifestations. Notify the RN and provider if these occur.

Withdrawal effects

Anxiety, insomnia, diaphoresis, tremors, lightheadedness, delirium, hypertension, muscle twitching, seizures

CLIENT EDUCATION
- Withdrawal effects are not common with short-term use.
- Clients who have been taking benzodiazepines regularly and in high doses should taper the dose over several weeks.

CONTRAINDICATIONS/PRECAUTIONS

- Benzodiazepines are mostly Pregnancy Risk Category D medications, with some being Category X. Both categories are avoided in clients who are pregnant or breastfeeding.
- Benzodiazepines are classified under Schedule IV of the Controlled Substances Act.
- Benzodiazepines are contraindicated in clients who have sleep apnea, respiratory depression, or glaucoma.
- Use benzodiazepines cautiously in older adult clients and those who have liver disease or a history of mental illness or a substance use disorder.
- Benzodiazepines are generally used short-term due to the risk for dependence. Qs

INTERACTIONS

CNS depressants (alcohol, barbiturates, opioids) can result in respiratory depression. Anticonvulsants and antihistamines can cause increased CNS depression.
CLIENT EDUCATION
- Avoid alcohol and other substances that cause CNS depression.
- Avoid activities that require alertness (driving, operating heavy equipment/machinery).

Grapefruit can reduce metabolism.
CLIENT EDUCATION: Avoid consuming grapefruit or products that contain grapefruit.

High-fat meals can reduce absorption.
CLIENT EDUCATION: Do not take with fatty foods.

NURSING ADMINISTRATION

- Advise clients to take the medication as prescribed and to avoid abrupt discontinuation of treatment to prevent withdrawal manifestations. Do not change the dosage or frequency without prior approval of the prescriber.
- When discontinuing benzodiazepines that have been taken regularly for long periods and in higher doses, taper the dose over several weeks. QEBP
- Administer the medication with meals or snacks if gastrointestinal upset occurs.
- Administer the medication at bedtime if possible due to sedation.
- Advise clients to swallow sustained-release tablets and to avoid chewing or crushing the tablets.
- Inform clients about the possible development of dependency during and after treatment and to notify the provider if indications of withdrawal occur.
- Advise clients to keep benzodiazepines in a secure place due to their potential for dependency.

Atypical anxiolytic/ nonbarbiturate anxiolytic

SELECT PROTOTYPE MEDICATION: Buspirone

PURPOSE

EXPECTED PHARMACOLOGICAL ACTION
- The exact antianxiety mechanism of this medication is unknown. This medication binds to serotonin and dopamine receptors. Dependency is much less likely than with other anxiolytics. Buspirone does not result in sedation or potentiate the effects of other CNS depressants.
- The major disadvantage is that antianxiety effects develop slowly. Initial responses take 1 week, and 2 to 6 weeks for it to reach its full effects. As a result of this pharmacological action, buspirone is taken on a scheduled basis. It is not suitable for PRN use.

THERAPEUTIC USES
- Panic disorder
- Social anxiety disorder
- Obsessive-compulsive and related disorders
- Trauma- and stressor-related disorders, PTSD

COMPLICATIONS

Dizziness, nausea, headache, lightheadedness, agitation
CLIENT EDUCATION
- Take with food to decrease nausea.
- Avoid activities that require alertness until effects are known.
- Most adverse effects are self-limiting.

Constipation
CLIENT EDUCATION: Increase fiber and fluid.

CONTRAINDICATIONS/PRECAUTIONS

- Buspirone is Pregnancy Risk Category B.
- Buspirone is not recommended for use by clients who are breastfeeding.
- Use buspirone cautiously in older adult clients and clients who have liver or kidney dysfunction.
- Buspirone is contraindicated for concurrent use with MAOI antidepressants or for 14 days after MAOIs are discontinued. Hypertensive crisis can result. Qs

INTERACTIONS

Erythromycin, ketoconazole, St. John's wort, and grapefruit can increase the effects of buspirone.
CLIENT EDUCATION
- Avoid the use of these antimicrobial agents.
- Avoid herbal preparations containing St. John's wort.
- Avoid drinking grapefruit juice.

Increased risk for serotonin syndrome with SSRIs
NURSING ACTIONS: Monitor for serotonin syndrome, fever, tremor, diarrhea, and delirium. Avoid concurrent use.

NURSING ADMINISTRATION

- Advise clients to take the medication with meals to prevent gastric irritation.
- Advise clients that effects do not occur immediately. It can take 1 week to notice the first therapeutic effects and 2 to 6 weeks for the full benefit. Take on a regular basis and not PRN. Q EBP
- Instruct clients that tolerance, dependence, or withdrawal effects are not an issue with this medication.
- Labeled for short-term treatment of anxiety, but has shown therapeutic benefit for as long as 1 year.

Selective serotonin reuptake inhibitors (SSRI antidepressants)

SELECT PROTOTYPE MEDICATION: Paroxetine

OTHER MEDICATIONS
- Sertraline
- Citalopram
- Escitalopram
- Fluoxetine
- Fluvoxamine

PURPOSE

EXPECTED PHARMACOLOGICAL ACTION

- Paroxetine selectively inhibits serotonin reuptake, allowing more serotonin to stay at the junction of the neurons.
- It does not block uptake of dopamine or norepinephrine.
- Paroxetine produces CNS stimulation, which can cause insomnia.
- The medication has a long effective half-life. Up to 4 weeks is necessary to produce therapeutic medication levels.

THERAPEUTIC USES

Paroxetine
- Generalized anxiety disorder
- Panic disorder: Decreases both the frequency and intensity of panic attacks and also prevents anticipatory anxiety about attacks
- Obsessive-compulsive disorder (OCD): Reduces manifestations by increasing serotonin
- Social anxiety disorder
- Trauma- and stressor-related disorders
- Dissociative disorders
- Depressive disorders
- Adjustment disorders

Sertraline: Panic disorder, OCD, social anxiety disorder, PTSD

Escitalopram: GAD, panic disorder, OCD

Fluoxetine: Panic disorder, OCD, PTSD

Fluvoxamine: OCD, social anxiety disorder

COMPLICATIONS

Early adverse effects

First few days/weeks: nausea, diaphoresis, tremor, fatigue, drowsiness

CLIENT EDUCATION
- Report adverse effects to the provider.
- Take the medication as prescribed.
- These effects should soon subside.

Later adverse effects

After 5 to 6 weeks of therapy: sexual dysfunction (impotence, delayed or absent orgasm, delayed or absent ejaculation, decreased sexual interest)

CLIENT EDUCATION: Report problems with sexual function (managed with dose reduction, medication holiday, changing medications).

Weight gain

CLIENT EDUCATION: Follow a well-balanced diet and exercise regularly.

GI bleeding

NURSING ACTIONS
- Use caution in clients who have a history of GI bleed or ulcers and in clients taking other medications that affect blood coagulation.
- Advise clients to report indications of bleeding (dark stool, coffee-ground emesis).

Hyponatremia

More likely in older adult clients taking diuretics ⑤

NURSING ACTIONS: Obtain baseline serum sodium, and monitor level periodically throughout treatment.

Serotonin syndrome

Agitation, confusion, disorientation, difficulty concentrating, anxiety, hallucinations, myoclonus (spastic, jerky muscle contractions), hyperreflexia, incoordination, tremors, fever, diaphoresis

NURSING ACTIONS
- Usually begins 2 to 72 hr after initiation of treatment.
- Resolves when the medication is discontinued.
- Watch for and advise clients to report any of these manifestations, which could indicate a lethal problem.

Bruxism

Grinding and clenching of teeth, usually during sleep

NURSING ACTIONS
- Report bruxism to the provider, who might switch the client to another class of medication.
- Treat bruxism with low-dose buspirone.
- Advise the client to use a mouth guard during sleep.

Withdrawal syndrome

Nausea, sensory disturbances, anxiety, tremor, malaise, unease

NURSING ACTIONS
- Minimize effects by tapering the medication slowly.
- Advise clients that, after a long period of use, the medication is tapered slowly to avoid withdrawal syndrome.
- Advise clients not to discontinue use abruptly.

Orthostatic hypotension

NURSING ACTIONS: Monitor for hypotension and advise client to change positions slowly.

Suicidal ideation

NURSING ACTIONS: Monitor and report manifestations of depression and thoughts of suicide.

CONTRAINDICATIONS/PRECAUTIONS

- Paroxetine is a Pregnancy Risk Category D medication.
- Paroxetine is contraindicated in clients taking MAOIs or a TCA.
- Clients taking paroxetine should avoid alcohol.
- Use paroxetine cautiously in clients who have liver and kidney dysfunction, seizure disorders, or a history of GI bleeding. Qs

INTERACTIONS

Use of MAOI antidepressants or TCAs can cause serotonin syndrome.
NURSING ACTIONS: Reinforce client education about this combination. Avoid concurrent use.

Antiplatelet medications and anticoagulants can increase risk for bleeding
NURSING ACTIONS: Monitor for bleeding. Avoid concurrent use.

NURSING ADMINISTRATION

- Advise clients that medications can be taken with food. Sleep disturbances are minimized by taking medication in the morning.
- Instruct clients to take the medication on a daily basis to establish therapeutic plasma levels. Q EBP
- Assist with medication regimen adherence by informing clients that it can take up to 4 weeks to achieve therapeutic effects from an SSRI.

NURSING EVALUATION OF MEDICATION EFFECTIVENESS

Depending on therapeutic intent, effectiveness is evidenced by the following.
- Verbalizing feeling less anxious and more relaxed
- Description of improved mood
- Improved memory retrieval
- Maintaining regular sleep pattern
- Greater ability to participate in social and occupational interactions
- Improved ability to cope with manifestations and identified stressors

Application Exercises

1. A nurse is collecting data from a client who is suspected of having benzodiazepine toxicity. Which of the following findings should the nurse identify as the priority to report to the provider?

    A. Drowsiness

    B. Confusion

    C. Ataxia

    D. Hypotension

2. A nurse is reinforcing teaching with a client who has a new prescription for escitalopram for treatment of generalized anxiety disorder. Which of the following statements indicates that the client understands the teaching?

    A. "I should take the medication on an empty stomach."

    B. "I will follow a low-sodium diet while taking this medication."

    C. "I need to discontinue this medication slowly."

    D. "I should stop taking the medication if it causes me to have nausea."

3. A nurse is reinforcing teaching with a client who has a new prescription for buspirone to treat anxiety. Which of the following information should the nurse include?

    A. "Take this medication on an empty stomach."

    B. "Expect optimal therapeutic effects within 24 hours."

    C. "Take this medication when needed for anxiety."

    D. "This medication has a low risk for dependency."

4. A nurse is reinforcing teaching with a client who has obsessive-compulsive disorder and a new prescription for paroxetine. Which of the following instructions should the nurse include?

    A. "It can take several weeks before you feel like the medication is helping."

    B. "Take the medication just before bedtime to promote sleep."

    C. "You should take the medication when needed for obsessive urges."

    D. "Monitor for weight gain while taking this medication."

5. A nurse is caring for a client who takes paroxetine to treat posttraumatic stress disorder and reports that he grinds his teeth during the night. The nurse should identify which of the following interventions to manage bruxism? (Select all that apply.)

    A. Concurrent administration of buspirone

    B. Administration of a different SSRI

    C. Use of a mouth guard

    D. Changing to a different class of antidepressant medication

    E. Increasing the dose of paroxetine

Application Exercises Key

1. A. Drowsiness is an indication of benzodiazepine toxicity that the nurse should monitor and report to the RN and provider. However, another finding is the priority.

    B. Confusion is an indication of benzodiazepine toxicity that the nurse should monitor and report to the RN and provider. However, another finding is the priority.

    C. Ataxia is an adverse effect of benzodiazepines that the nurse should monitor and report to the RN and provider. However, another finding is the priority.

    D. **CORRECT:** When using the airway, breathing, circulation approach to client care, the priority finding is hypotension. The nurse should report this finding to the RN and provider and prepare to assist with treatment for benzodiazepine toxicity.

    Ⓝ *NCLEX® Connection: Pharmacological Therapies, Adverse Effects/ Contraindications/Side Effects/Interactions*

2. A. The client can take this medication with food for GI distress or without food.

    B. The client is at risk for hyponatremia while taking escitalopram.

    C. **CORRECT:** When discontinuing escitalopram, the client should taper the medication slowly according to a prescribed tapered dosing schedule to reduce the risk of withdrawal syndrome.

    D. The client can expect to have nausea and drowsiness during the first days/weeks of treatment. However, these adverse effects should soon subside.

    Ⓝ *NCLEX® Connection: Pharmacological Therapies, Expected Actions/Outcomes*

3. A. The client can take this medication with food to reduce GI distress.

    B. Buspirone can take up to 3 to 6 weeks to obtain optimal therapeutic effects.

    C. The client should take buspirone on a regular, not PRN, basis because therapeutic effects occur slowly.

    D. **CORRECT:** Buspirone has a low risk for physical or psychological dependence or tolerance.

    Ⓝ *NCLEX® Connection: Pharmacological Therapies, Expected Actions/Outcomes*

4. A. **CORRECT:** Paroxetine can take 1 to 4 weeks before the client reaches full therapeutic benefit.

    B. Take paroxetine in the morning to prevent insomnia.

    C. Take paroxetine on a regular basis, rather than as-needed.

    D. Paroxetine can cause decreased appetite and weight loss.

    Ⓝ *NCLEX® Connection: Pharmacological Therapies, Expected Actions/Outcomes*

5. A. **CORRECT:** Concurrent administration of a low dose of buspirone is effective to manage the adverse effects of paroxetine.

    B. Other SSRIs also will have bruxism as an adverse effect.

    C. **CORRECT:** Using a mouth guard during sleep can decrease the risk for oral damage resulting from bruxism.

    D. **CORRECT:** Changing to different class of antidepressant medication that does not have the adverse effect of bruxism is an effective measure.

    E. Increasing the dose of paroxetine can cause bruxism to worsen.

    Ⓝ *NCLEX® Connection: Pharmacological Therapies, Adverse Effects/ Contraindications/Side Effects/Interactions*

PRACTICE Answer

Using the ATI Active Learning Template: System Disorder

ALTERATION IN HEALTH (DIAGNOSIS): Serotonin syndrome is a potentially lethal complication that usually begins 2 to 72 hr after initiation of treatment with an SSRI. The syndrome resolves when the medication is discontinued.

EXPECTED FINDINGS

*   Agitation
*   Confusion
*   Disorientation
*   Difficulty concentrating
*   Anxiety
*   Hallucinations
*   Hyperreflexia
*   Incoordination
*   Tremors
*   Fever
*   Diaphoresis

RISK FACTORS

*   Onset of treatment with an SSRI within the last 2 to 72 hr
*   Concurrent use of an SSRI with an MAOI
*   Concurrent use of an SSRI with a TCA

Ⓝ *NCLEX® Connection: Pharmacological and Parenteral Therapies, Adverse Effects/ Contraindications/Side Effects/Interactions*

CHAPTER 7 *Depressive Disorders*

Depressive disorders are a widespread problem and one of the leading causes of disability. Clients who have major depressive disorder can require hospitalization with close observation and suicide precautions until antidepressant medications reach their peak effect.

Antidepressant medications are classified into five main groups: selective serotonin reuptake inhibitors (SSRIs), serotonin-norepinephrine reuptake inhibitors (SNRIs), atypical antidepressants, tricyclic antidepressants (TCAs), and monoamine oxidase inhibitors (MAOIs).

Selective serotonin reuptake inhibitors

SELECT PROTOTYPE MEDICATION: Fluoxetine

OTHER MEDICATIONS
- Citalopram
- Escitalopram
- Paroxetine
- Sertraline
- Fluvoxamine
- Vortioxetine

PURPOSE

EXPECTED PHARMACOLOGICAL ACTION
- SSRIs selectively block reuptake of the monoamine neurotransmitter serotonin in the synaptic space, thereby intensifying the effects of serotonin.
- SSRIs are considered one of the first-line treatments for depression.
- It can take approximately 1 to 4 weeks or longer before pharmacological benefits take effect. Q EBP

THERAPEUTIC USES
- Major depression
- Obsessive-compulsive disorders
- Bulimia nervosa
- Premenstrual dysphoric disorders
- Panic disorders
- Posttraumatic stress disorder
- Social anxiety disorder
- Generalized anxiety disorder

COMPLICATIONS

Sexual dysfunction

Anorgasmia, impotence, decreased libido

CLIENT EDUCATION
- Possible adverse effects and to notify the provider if intolerable.
- Ways to manage sexual dysfunction can include lowering dosage, discontinuing medication temporarily (medication holiday), and using adjunct medications to improve sexual function (sildenafil, buspirone)
- Atypical antidepressant such as bupropion has fewer sexual dysfunction adverse effects.

CNS stimulation

Inability to sleep, agitation, anxiety

CLIENT EDUCATION
- Notify the provider. Dose can need to be lowered.
- Take dose in the morning.
- Avoid caffeinated beverages.
- Relaxation techniques to promote sleep.

Weight changes

Weight loss can occur early in therapy but can be followed by weight gain with long-term treatment.

NURSING ACTIONS
- Monitor the client's weight.
- Encourage clients to participate in regular exercise and to follow a healthy, well-balanced diet.

Serotonin syndrome

Can begin 2 to 72 hr after starting treatment and can be lethal Qs

MANIFESTATIONS
- Confusion, agitation, poor concentration, hostility
- Disorientation, hallucinations, delirium
- Seizures leading to status epilepticus
- Tachycardia leading to cardiovascular shock
- Labile blood pressure
- Diaphoresis
- Fever leading to hyperpyrexia
- Incoordination, hyperreflexia
- Nausea, vomiting, diarrhea, abdominal pain
- Coma leading to apnea (and death in severe cases)

NURSING ACTIONS

- Advise clients to observe for manifestations. If any occur, instruct the client to notify the provider and withhold the medication.
- Start symptomatic treatment (medications to create serotonin-receptor blockade and muscle rigidity, cooling blankets, anticonvulsants, artificial ventilation)
- Monitor vital signs and I&O.
- Provide safety measures to prevent injury when muscle rigidity and changes in mental status are present.
- Provide cooling blankets and tepid baths to assist with temperature regulation.

Withdrawal syndrome

Resulting in headache, nausea, visual disturbances, anxiety, dizziness, and tremors

CLIENT EDUCATION: Taper dose gradually.

Hyponatremia

More likely in older adult clients taking diuretics ⓒ

NURSING ACTIONS: Obtain baseline serum sodium, and monitor level periodically throughout treatment.

Rash

CLIENT EDUCATION: A rash is treatable with an antihistamine or withdrawal of medication.

Sleepiness, faintness, lightheadedness

CLIENT EDUCATION

- These adverse effects are not common but can occur.
- Avoid driving if these adverse effects occur. Qs

Gastrointestinal

Can cause constipation.

NURSING ACTIONS: Use caution in clients who have a history of GI bleed and ulcers, and those taking other medications that affect blood coagulation.

CLIENT EDUCATION

- Watch for manifestations of bleeding (hematemesis, bloody stools).
- Increase fiber and fluid intake.

Bruxism (teeth grinding)

NURSING ACTIONS

- Advise clients to report manifestations to the provider.
- Advise clients to use a mouth guard.
- Changing to a different classification of antidepressants or adding a low dose of buspirone can decrease this adverse effect.

CONTRAINDICATIONS/PRECAUTIONS

- These medications are Pregnancy Risk Category C, except for paroxetine, which is Category D. Qs

  Paroxetine increases the risk of birth defects. Therefore, other SSRIs are recommended. Late in pregnancy, use of SSRIs increases the risk of withdrawal manifestations or pulmonary hypertension in the newborn.

- SSRIs are contraindicated in clients taking MAOIs or TCAs. SSRIs need to be discontinued at least 2 weeks before initiating an MAOI.
- Use cautiously in clients who have liver and kidney dysfunction, cardiac disease, seizure disorders, diabetes, ulcers, and a history of GI bleeding.

INTERACTIONS

MAOIs, TCAs, and St. John's wort increase the risk of serotonin syndrome.
CLIENT EDUCATION

- MAOIs should be discontinued for 14 days prior to starting an SSRI. If already taking fluoxetine, wait 5 weeks before starting a MAOI.
- Avoid concurrent use of TCAs and St. John's wort.

Fluoxetine can displace warfarin from bound protein and result in increased warfarin levels.
NURSING ACTIONS

- Monitor PT and INR levels.
- Check for indications of bleeding and the need for dosage adjustment.

Fluoxetine can increase the levels of tricyclic antidepressants and lithium.
NURSING ACTIONS: Avoid concurrent use.

Lithium levels can be increased or decreased by concomitant use of SSRIs.
NURSING ACTIONS

- Avoid concurrent use.
- Monitor lithium levels closely.

Fluoxetine suppresses platelet aggregation and thus increases the risk of bleeding when used concurrently with NSAIDs and anticoagulants.
CLIENT EDUCATION: Monitor for indications of bleeding (bruising, hematuria) and notify the provider if they occur.

Serotonin-norepinephrine reuptake inhibitors

SELECT PROTOTYPE MEDICATION: Venlafaxine

OTHER MEDICATIONS
- Desvenlafaxine
- Duloxetine

PURPOSE

EXPECTED PHARMACOLOGICAL ACTION: SNRIs block reuptake of norepinephrine and serotonin with effects similar to the SSRIs.

THERAPEUTIC USES
- Major depression
- Generalized anxiety disorder
- Social anxiety disorder
- Panic disorder
- Pain due to fibromyalgia, osteoarthritis, low-back pain, diabetic neuropathy (duloxetine; unlabeled use for venlafaxine)

COMPLICATIONS

Nausea, anorexia, weight loss

NURSING ACTIONS: Monitor weight and food intake.

Headache, insomnia, anxiety

NURSING ACTIONS: Monitor for these findings.

Hypertension, tachycardia

NURSING ACTIONS: Monitor vital signs and report changes to the provider.

Dizziness, blurred vision

CLIENT EDUCATION: Avoid driving and use of machinery until effects are known. Qs

Withdrawal syndrome

Results in headache, nausea, visual disturbances, anxiety, dizziness, and tremors

CLIENT EDUCATION: Discontinue the medication gradually.

Risk for suicide in children and adolescents

NURSING ACTIONS: Monitor children/adolescents carefully for suicidal ideation and thought disorders. Qs

Sexual dysfunction

Anorgasmia, decreased libido, impotence, menstrual changes

CLIENT EDUCATION
- Report sexual dysfunction to the provider.
- Ways to manage sexual dysfunction can include lowering dosage, temporarily discontinuing medication (medication holiday), and using adjunct medications to improve function (sildenafil, buspirone).
- An atypical antidepressant such as bupropion has fewer effects on sexual function.

Serotonin syndrome

See complications of SSRIs

Bronchitis, dyspnea

CLIENT EDUCATION: Report respiratory findings to the provider.

CONTRAINDICATIONS/PRECAUTIONS

- These medications are Pregnancy Risk Category C. Avoid during the third trimester and avoid breastfeeding while taking an SNRI.
- SNRIs are contraindicated in clients taking SSRIs, MAOIs, or TCAs. SNRIs need to be discontinued at least 2 weeks before initiating an MAOI. Qs
- Precautions are needed for older adults, and clients who have bipolar disorder, mania, seizure disorder, recent MI, or interstitial lung disease.

INTERACTIONS

Neuroleptic malignant syndrome–like reactions if given concurrently with MAOIs
NURSING ACTIONS: Stop MAOI at least 14 days before beginning a SNRI.

NSAIDs, anticoagulants increase risk for bleeding with venlafaxine
NURSING ACTIONS: Review client's medications with provider, including over-the-counter medications.

Alcohol and other medications affecting the CNS increase risk for CNS effects
CLIENT EDUCATION: Avoid alcohol and other CNS depressants. Use caution when driving or using machinery. Qs

Kava, Valerian increase risk for CNS depression; St. John's wort can cause serotonin syndrome.
CLIENT EDUCATION: Avoid these supplements.

Atypical antidepressants

SELECT PROTOTYPE MEDICATION: Bupropion

OTHER MEDICATIONS
- Vilazodone
- Mirtazapine
- Reboxetine
- Trazodone

PURPOSE

EXPECTED PHARMACOLOGICAL ACTION: Bupropion acts by inhibiting norepinephrine and dopamine uptake. It is referred to as a norepinephrine-dopamine reuptake inhibitor.

THERAPEUTIC USES
- Treatment of depression
- Alternative to SSRIs and SNRIs for clients unable to tolerate sexual dysfunction adverse effects of these antidepressants
- Aid for smoking cessation
- Prevention of seasonal affective disorder (SAD)
- Alternative treatment choice for attention-deficit disorder (ADD)

COMPLICATIONS

Headache, dry mouth, GI distress, constipation, increased heart rate, hypertension, restlessness, insomnia

NURSING ACTIONS
- Advise clients to observe for possible adverse effects and to notify the provider if intolerable.
- Treat headache with mild analgesic.
- Advise clients to sip on fluids or chew sugarless gum to treat dry mouth and to increase dietary fiber to prevent constipation.

Nausea, vomiting, anorexia, weight loss

NURSING ACTIONS: Monitor weight and food intake.

Seizures

NURSING ACTIONS
- Avoid administering to clients at risk for seizures, such as clients who have head injuries.
- Monitor for seizures, and treat accordingly.

CONTRAINDICATIONS/PRECAUTIONS

- Bupropion is a Pregnancy Risk Category B. Qs
- Contraindicated in clients taking MAOIs
- Contraindicated for clients who have seizure disorders or eating disorders

INTERACTIONS

MAOIs such as phenelzine increase the risk of toxicity. MAOIs should be discontinued 2 weeks prior to beginning treatment with bupropion.

Other atypical antidepressants

Vilazodone

PHARMACOLOGICAL ACTION: Both blocks serotonin and works as a serotonin agonist at receptor sites (first medication to work in this way)

NURSING ACTIONS
- Contraindicated with SSRIs and SNRIs (serotonin syndrome), and other serotonin receptor agonists (buspirone, phenothiazines).
- Stop MAOI at least 14 days before starting vilazodone.
- Reinforce teaching of manifestations of serotonin syndrome to client and instruct when to notify provider.
- Monitor for suicidal ideation.
- Instruct clients to avoid grapefruit juice while taking vilazodone.
- Many adverse effects are similar to those of SSRIs and SNRIs.
- Take with food to help increase absorption.

Mirtazapine

PHARMACOLOGICAL ACTION: It increases the release of serotonin and norepinephrine by blocking presynaptic receptors, and thereby increases the amount of neurotransmitters available for impulse transmission.

NURSING ACTIONS
- Therapeutic effects can occur sooner with less sexual dysfunction than with SSRIs.
- Mirtazapine is generally well tolerated. Clients can experience sleepiness that can be exacerbated by other CNS depressants (alcohol, benzodiazepines), weight gain, and elevated cholesterol.
- Advise clients to take at bedtime; can be used as a sleep aid.

Reboxetine

- Similar results as with SSRIs.
- Generally well tolerated, but clients can experience dry mouth, decreased blood pressure, constipation, sexual dysfunction, and urinary hesitancy or retention.
- Weight gain and sleepiness do not occur.
- This medication should not be combined with an MAOI.

PHARMACOLOGICAL ACTION: Selectively inhibits the reuptake of norepinephrine, thereby increasing the amount of neurotransmitters available for impulse transmission.

Trazodone

PHARMACOLOGICAL ACTION: Moderate selective blockade of serotonin receptors, which allows more serotonin to be available for impulse transmission.

NURSING ACTIONS
- Usually used with another antidepressant agent.
- Sedation is a potential problem; can be indicated for a client who has insomnia.
- Priapism is a potential adverse effect. Instruct clients to seek medical attention immediately if this occurs.

Tricyclic antidepressants

SELECT PROTOTYPE MEDICATION: Amitriptyline

OTHER MEDICATIONS
- Imipramine
- Doxepin
- Nortriptyline
- Amoxapine
- Trimipramine
- Desipramine
- Clomipramine

PURPOSE

EXPECTED PHARMACOLOGICAL ACTION
- These medications block reuptake of norepinephrine and serotonin in the synaptic space, thereby intensifying the effects of these neurotransmitters.
- It can take approximately 10 to 14 days before TCAs begin to work, and maximum effects might not be seen for 4 to 8 weeks.

THERAPEUTIC USES
- Depression
- Depressive episodes of bipolar disorders

OTHER USES
- Neuropathic pain
- Fibromyalgia
- Anxiety disorders
- Obsessive-compulsive disorder
- Insomnia
- Attention-deficit/hyperactivity disorder (ADHD)
- Enuresis

COMPLICATIONS

Orthostatic hypotension

NURSING ACTIONS
- Instruct clients about the effects of orthostatic hypotension (lightheadedness, dizziness). If these occur, advise the client to sit or lie down. Orthostatic hypotension is minimized by changing positions slowly.
- Monitor blood pressure and heart rate for clients in the hospital for orthostatic changes before administration and 1 hr after. If a significant decrease in blood pressure or increase in heart rate is noted, do not administer the medication, and notify the provider.

Anticholinergic effects

- Dry mouth
- Blurred vision
- Photophobia
- Urinary hesitancy or retention
- Constipation
- Tachycardia

CLIENT EDUCATION
- Ways to minimize anticholinergic effects
  - Chewing sugarless gum
  - Sipping on water
  - Wearing sunglasses when outdoors
  - Eating foods high in fiber
  - Participating in regular exercise
  - Increasing fluid intake to at least 2 to 3 L a day from beverages and food sources
  - Voiding just before taking medication
- Notify the provider if effects persist.

Sedation

This effect usually diminishes over time.

CLIENT EDUCATION
- Avoid hazardous activities such as driving if sedation is excessive. Qs
- Take medication at bedtime to minimize daytime sleepiness and promote sleep.

Toxicity

Resulting in cholinergic blockade and cardiac toxicity evidenced by dysrhythmias, confusion, and agitation, followed by seizures, coma, and possible death

NURSING ACTIONS
- Obtain baseline ECG.
- Monitor vital signs frequently.
- Monitor for manifestations of toxicity.
- Notify the provider if manifestations of toxicity occur.

Decreased seizure threshold

NURSING ACTIONS: Monitor clients who have seizure disorders.

Excessive sweating

NURSING ACTIONS: Inform clients of adverse effects. Assist clients with frequent linen changes.

CONTRAINDICATIONS/PRECAUTIONS

- TCAs are Pregnancy Risk Category C.
- Contraindicated in clients who have seizure disorders or who have recently experienced a myocardial infarction.
- Use cautiously in older adult clients and clients who have coronary artery disease; diabetes, liver, kidney, or respiratory disorders; urinary retention or obstruction; angle-closure glaucoma; benign prostatic hyperplasia; or hyperthyroidism. Ⓒ
- Clients who have an increased risk for suicide should receive a 1-week supply of medication at a time due to the lethality of an overdose. Qs
- Amoxapine has been associated with tardive dyskinesia and neuroleptic malignant syndrome. Monitor for manifestations such as muscle rigidity, altered mental status, and autonomic nervous system problems (tachycardia, sweating).

INTERACTIONS

Concurrent use with MAOIs or St. John's wort can lead to serotonin syndrome.
NURSING ACTIONS: Avoid concurrent use.

Antihistamines and other anticholinergic agents have additive anticholinergic effects.
NURSING ACTIONS: Avoid concurrent use.

Increased effects of epinephrine, dopamine (direct-acting sympathomimetics) occur because uptake into the nerve terminals is blocked by TCAs, and they remain for a longer amount of time in the synaptic space.
NURSING ACTIONS: Avoid concurrent use.

TCAs decrease the effects of ephedrine, amphetamine (indirect-acting sympathomimetics) because uptake into the nerve terminals is blocked, and they are unable to reach their site of action.
NURSING ACTIONS: Avoid concurrent use.

Alcohol, benzodiazepines, opioids, and antihistamines cause additive CNS depression when used concurrently.
CLIENT EDUCATION: Avoid other CNS depressants.

Monoamine oxidase inhibitors

SELECT PROTOTYPE MEDICATION: Phenelzine

OTHER MEDICATIONS
- Isocarboxazid
- Tranylcypromine
- Selegiline (transdermal MAOI)

PURPOSE

EXPECTED PHARMACOLOGICAL ACTION

These medications block MAO in the brain, thereby increasing the amount of norepinephrine, dopamine, serotonin, and tyramine available for transmission of impulses. An increased amount of these neurotransmitters at nerve endings intensifies responses and relieves depression. However, the increase in tyramine can cause heightened blood pressure or hypertensive crisis if dietary and medication restrictions are not implemented.
- Onset of therapeutic action is not immediate, and usually takes 2 to 4 weeks.
- Less frequently used in comparison to other antidepressants due to food/drug interactions and adverse effects.

THERAPEUTIC USES

- Depression
- Bulimia nervosa
- Panic disorder
- Social anxiety disorder
- Generalized anxiety disorder
- Obsessive-compulsive disorder
- Posttraumatic stress disorder

COMPLICATIONS

CNS stimulation

Anxiety, agitation, mania, or hypomania

CLIENT EDUCATION: Observe for effects and notify the provider if they occur.

Orthostatic hypotension

NURSING ACTIONS
- Monitor blood pressure and heart rate for orthostatic changes.
- Hold medication and notify the provider of significant changes.
- Instruct the client to change positions slowly. Qs

Hypertensive crisis, severe hypertension, headache, nausea, increased heart rate, increased blood pressure

- Hypertensive crisis resulting from intake of dietary tyramine, which could lead to a cerebral vascular accident
- Severe hypertension as a result of intensive vasoconstriction and stimulation of the heart
- Headache, nausea, and increased heart rate and blood pressure

NURSING ACTIONS
- Request for the RN to administer phentolamine IV (a rapid-acting alpha-adrenergic blocker) or administer nifedipine SL.
- Provide continuous cardiac monitoring and respiratory support as indicated.

Local rash with transdermal preparation

NURSING ACTIONS
- Choose a clean, dry area for each application.
- Apply a topical glucocorticoid on the affected area.

CONTRAINDICATIONS/PRECAUTIONS

- MAOIs are Pregnancy Risk Category C. Qs
- Contraindicated in clients taking SSRIs and those who have pheochromocytoma, heart failure, cardiovascular or cerebral vascular disease, or severe kidney insufficiency.
- Use cautiously in clients who have diabetes and seizure disorders or are taking TCAs.
- Transdermal selegiline is contraindicated for clients taking carbamazepine or oxcarbazepine, which can increase blood levels of the MAOI.

INTERACTIONS

Indirect-acting sympathomimetic medications (ephedrine, amphetamine) promote the release of norepinephrine and can lead to hypertensive crisis.
CLIENT EDUCATION: Avoid over-the-counter decongestants and cold remedies, which frequently contain medications with sympathomimetic action.

Use of TCAs can lead to hypertensive crisis.
NURSING ACTIONS: Use MAOIs and TCAs cautiously.

Use of SSRIs can lead to serotonin syndrome.
NURSING ACTIONS: Avoid concurrent use.

Antihypertensives have an additive hypotensive effect.
NURSING ACTIONS
- Monitor blood pressure.
- Notify the provider if there is a significant drop in blood pressure. A reduced dosage of antihypertensive can be indicated.

Use of meperidine can lead to hyperpyrexia.
NURSING ACTIONS: Use an alternative analgesic.

Tyramine-rich foods can lead to hypertensive crisis.
- Clients will most likely experience headache, nausea, increased heart rate, and increased blood pressure.
- Tyramine-rich foods include aged cheese, pepperoni, salami, avocados, figs, bananas, smoked fish, protein dietary supplements, soups, soy sauce, some types of beer, and red wine.
- The MAOI transdermal patch does not seem to affect tyramine sensitivity due to its low dose, but tyramine restriction is recommended at higher doses.
- NURSING ACTIONS
  - Determine the client's ability to follow strict adherence to dietary restrictions.
  - Inform clients of manifestations of hypertensive crisis and to notify the provider if they occur.
  - Provide clients with written instructions regarding foods and beverages to avoid.
  - Advise clients to avoid taking any medications without approval of the provider.
  - Advise clients that dietary and medication restrictions should be continued for 2 weeks after the MAOI has been discontinued.

Concurrent use of vasopressors (phenylethylamine, caffeine) can result in hypertension.
CLIENT EDUCATION: Avoid foods (caffeinated beverages, chocolate, fava beans, ginseng) that contain these agents.

General anesthetics can enhance hypotensive effects.
CLIENT EDUCATION: MAOIs should not be used within 10 to 14 days before or after surgery.

NURSING ADMINISTRATION

- Instruct clients to take these medications as prescribed on a daily basis to establish therapeutic plasma levels.
- Assist with medication regimen adherence by informing clients that it can take 1 to 3 weeks to begin experiencing therapeutic effects. Full therapeutic effects can take 2 to 3 months. Qᴘᴄᴄ
- Instruct clients to continue therapy after achieving therapeutic effects. Sudden discontinuation of medication can result in relapse.
- Advise clients that therapy usually continues for 6 months after resolution of manifestations and can continue for 1 year or longer.
- Monitor for suicide risk. Antidepressant medications can increase a client's risk for suicide, particularly during initial treatment. Antidepressant-induced suicide is mainly associated with clients younger than 25. Qs

SSRIs and SNRIs

- Advise clients to take medication in the morning to minimize sleep disturbances.
- Advise clients to take medications with food to minimize GI disturbances.
- Advise clients about potential sexual adverse effects.
- Avoid use of MAOIs.
- Obtain baseline sodium levels for older adult clients taking diuretics, and monitor periodically. Ⓖ

Atypical antidepressants

- For all atypical antidepressant medications, avoid use with MAOIs.
- Advise clients taking bupropion for prevention of seasonal pattern depression to take medication beginning in the autumn each year and gradually taper dose and discontinue by spring.

TCAs

- Monitor for toxicity manifested by cardiac dysrhythmias.
- Administer at bedtime due to sedation and risk for orthostatic hypotension.
- Monitor for clients "cheeking" or hoarding TCAs due to potential lethality in overdose.

MAOIs

- Due to the risk for hypertensive crisis, advise clients to avoid foods with tyramine (ripe avocados or figs, fermented or smoked meats, liver, dried or cured fish, most cheeses, some types of beer and wine, and protein dietary supplements). Caffeine-containing products can also increase this risk.
- Advise clients to avoid taking any other prescription or nonprescription medications unless approved by the provider.

NURSING EVALUATION OF MEDICATION EFFECTIVENESS

Depending on therapeutic intent, effectiveness is evidenced by the following.

- Verbalized improvement in mood
- Increased hopefulness and will to live
- Ability to perform ADLs
- Improved sleeping and eating habits
- Increased interaction with peers

Application Exercises

1. A nurse is caring for a client who has major depressive disorder and a new prescription for phenelzine. Which of the following findings should the nurse identify as an adverse effect of this medication?

   A. Orthostatic hypotension

   B. Hearing loss

   C. Gastrointestinal bleeding

   D. Weight loss

2. A nurse is reinforcing teaching with a client who has major depressive disorder and a new prescription for amitriptyline. Which of the following information should the nurse include? (Select all that apply.)

   A. Expect therapeutic effects in 24 to 48 hr.

   B. Discontinue the medication after a week of improved mood.

   C. Change positions slowly to minimize dizziness.

   D. Decrease dietary fiber intake to control diarrhea.

   E. Chew sugarless gum to prevent dry mouth.

3. A nurse is reinforcing discharge teaching with a client who has posttraumatic stress disorder and a new prescription for fluoxetine. Which of the following statements should the nurse make to the client?

   A. "You may have a decreased desire for intimacy while taking this medication."

   B. "You should take this medication at bedtime to help promote sleep."

   C. "You will have fewer urinary adverse effects if you urinate just before taking this medication."

   D. "You'll need to wear sunglasses when outdoors due to the light sensitivity caused by this medication."

4. A nurse is caring for a client who has major depressive disorder and a new prescription for venlafaxine. Which of the following findings should the nurse identify as an adverse effect of the medication? (Select all that apply)

   A. Cough

   B. Dizziness

   C. Decreased libido

   D. Alopecia

   E. Hypotension

5. A nurse is caring for a client who has been taking sertraline for the past 2 days. Which of the following findings should alert the nurse to the possibility that the client is developing serotonin syndrome?

   A. Bruising

   B. Fever

   C. Tinnitus

   D. Rash

PRACTICE Active Learning Scenario

A nurse in an acute mental health clinic is caring for a client who is experiencing hypertensive crisis. The client reports taking tranylcypromine for the treatment of depression and that he ate pepperoni pizza shortly before the manifestations began. Use the ATI Active Learning Template: System Disorder and the ATI Mental Health Review Module to complete this item.

ALTERATION IN HEALTH (DIAGNOSIS)

EXPECTED FINDINGS: Identify at least three.

MEDICATIONS: Identify at least one medication that could be used for treatment.

CLIENT EDUCATION: Identify four dietary sources of tyramine the client should avoid.

Application Exercises Key

1. A. **CORRECT:** Orthostatic hypotension is an adverse of effect of MAOIs, including phenelzine.

    B. Phenelzine is more likely to cause blurred vision than hearing loss.

    C. Clients taking phenelzine are at risk for multiple adverse effects. However, these do not include GI bleeding.

    D. Clients taking phenelzine are at risk for weight gain rather than weight loss.

    Ⓝ *NCLEX® Connection: Pharmacological Therapies, Adverse Effects/ Contraindications/Side Effects/Interactions*

2. A. Therapeutic effects are expected after several weeks of taking amitriptyline.

    B. Stopping amitriptyline abruptly can result in relapse.

    C. **CORRECT:** Changing positions slowly helps prevent orthostatic hypotension, which is an adverse effect of amitriptyline.

    D. Clients should increase dietary fiber to prevent constipation, which is an adverse effect of amitriptyline.

    E. **CORRECT:** Chewing sugarless gum can minimize dry mouth, which is an adverse effect of amitriptyline.

    Ⓝ *NCLEX® Connection: Pharmacological Therapies, Expected Actions/Outcomes*

3. A. **CORRECT:** Decreased libido is a potential adverse effect of fluoxetine and other SSRIs.

    B. Clients should take fluoxetine in the morning due to CNS stimulation.

    C. Clients taking a TCA, rather than fluoxetine, should void prior to taking the medication due to the potential for urinary hesitancy or retention.

    D. Clients taking a TCA, rather than fluoxetine, should wear sunglasses when outdoors due to the potential for photophobia.

    Ⓝ *NCLEX® Connection: Pharmacological Therapies, Adverse Effects/ Contraindications/Side Effects/Interactions*

4. A. **CORRECT:** Cough and dyspnea can indicate that the client has developed bronchitis, which is an adverse effect of venlafaxine.

    B. **CORRECT:** Dizziness is a common adverse effect of venlafaxine.

    C. **CORRECT:** Sexual dysfunction (decreased libido, decreased orgasm, impotence, menstrual changes) are adverse effects of venlafaxine.

    D. Alopecia is not an adverse effect of venlafaxine.

    E. Hypertension and tachycardia are adverse effects of venlafaxine.

    Ⓝ *NCLEX® Connection: Pharmacological Therapies, Expected Actions/Outcomes*

5. A. Bleeding can result if an SSRI is administered with warfarin. However, this is not an indication of serotonin syndrome.

    B. **CORRECT:** Fever is a manifestation of serotonin syndrome, which can result from taking an SSRI such as sertraline.

    C. Tinnitus is not an indication of serotonin syndrome.

    D. A localized rash is associated with transdermal preparation. However, it is not an indication of serotonin syndrome.

    Ⓝ *NCLEX® Connection: Pharmacological Therapies, Adverse Effects/ Contraindications/Side Effects/Interactions*

PRACTICE Answer

Using the ATI Active Learning Template: System Disorder

ALTERATION IN HEALTH (DIAGNOSIS):
Hypertensive crisis results from intensive vasoconstriction due to the intake of dietary tyramine while taking an MAOI.

EXPECTED FINDINGS
- Severe hypertension
- Headache
- Nausea
- Increased heart rate

MEDICATIONS
- Phentolamine IV, a rapid-acting alpha-adrenergic blocker
- Nifedipine, a calcium channel blocker

CLIENT EDUCATION
- Aged cheeses
- Smoked or preserved fish or meats (pepperoni, salami)
- Avocados
- Figs
- Bananas
- Protein dietary supplements
- Soups containing meat extracts
- Soy sauce
- Some beers
- Red wine

Ⓝ *NCLEX® Connection: Pharmacological and Parenteral Therapies, Medication Administration*

UNIT 2   MEDICATIONS AFFECTING THE NERVOUS SYSTEM

CHAPTER 8   *Bipolar Disorders*

Bipolar disorders are primarily managed with mood-stabilizing medications such as lithium carbonate. Other medications used to treat bipolar disorders include antiepileptic drugs (AEDs), such as valproic acid, carbamazepine, lamotrigine, oxcarbazepine, and topiramate.

Atypical antipsychotics, such as olanzapine, can be useful in early treatment to promote sleep and to decrease anxiety and agitation. These medications also demonstrate mood-stabilizing properties.

Anxiolytics (clonazepam, lorazepam) can be useful in treating acute mania and managing the psychomotor agitation often seen in mania.

Antidepressant medications (bupropion, sertraline) can be useful during the depressive phase, but need to be used with caution to avoid triggering a manic cycle. These are typically prescribed in combination with a mood stabilizer to prevent rebound mania.

Mood stabilizer

SELECT PROTOTYPE MEDICATION: Lithium carbonate

PURPOSE

EXPECTED PHARMACOLOGICAL ACTION
- Lithium produces neurochemical changes in the brain, including serotonin receptor blockade.
- There is evidence that lithium can decrease neuronal atrophy or increase neuronal growth.

THERAPEUTIC USES: Lithium is used in the treatment of bipolar disorders. Lithium controls episodes of acute mania, and helps prevent the return of mania or depression.

COMPLICATIONS

Effects with therapeutic lithium levels (some resolve within a few weeks)

Gastrointestinal (GI) distress

Nausea, diarrhea, abdominal pain

NURSING ACTIONS
- Advise clients that effects are usually transient.
- Administer medication with meals or milk.

Fine hand tremors

Can interfere with purposeful motor skills and can be exacerbated by factors such as stress and caffeine

NURSING ACTIONS
- Administer beta adrenergic blocking agents such as propranolol.
- Adjust to the lowest possible dosage, give in divided doses, or use long-acting formulations.
- Advise clients to report an increase in tremors.

Polyuria, mild thirst

NURSING ACTIONS
- Use a potassium-sparing diuretic, such as spironolactone.
- Instruct clients to maintain adequate fluid intake by consuming 2,000 to 3,000 mL fluid from beverages and food sources.

Weight gain

NURSING ACTIONS: Assist clients to follow a healthy diet and regular exercise regimen.

Kidney toxicity

NURSING ACTIONS
- Monitor I&O.
- Adjust dosage, and keep dose low.
- Check baseline kidney function, and monitor kidney function periodically.

Goiter and hypothyroidism

With long-term treatment

NURSING ACTIONS
- Obtain baseline T_3, T_4, and TSH levels prior to starting treatment, and then annually.
- Advise clients to monitor for manifestations of hypothyroidism (cold, dry skin; decreased heart rate; weight gain).
- Administer levothyroxine to manage hypothyroid effects.

Bradydysrhythmia, hypotension, electrolyte imbalances

NURSING ACTIONS: Encourage clients to maintain adequate fluid and sodium intake.

Lithium toxicity

Early indications

LITHIUM LEVEL: Less than 1.5 mEq/L

- MANIFESTATIONS: Diarrhea, nausea, vomiting, thirst, polyuria, muscle weakness, fine hand tremor, slurred speech, lethargy
- NURSING ACTIONS
  - Advise clients to withhold medication and notify the provider.
  - Administer new dosage based on serum lithium levels.

Advanced indications

LITHIUM LEVEL: 1.5 to 2.0 mEq/L

- MANIFESTATIONS: Ongoing GI distress (nausea, vomiting, diarrhea); mental confusion; poor coordination; coarse tremors; sedation
- NURSING ACTIONS
  - Advise clients to withhold medication and notify the provider.
  - Administer new dosage based on serum lithium levels.
  - If manifestations are severe, it can be necessary to promote excretion.

Severe toxicity

- LITHIUM LEVEL: 2.0 to 2.5 mEq/L
  - MANIFESTATIONS: Extreme polyuria of dilute urine, tinnitus, involuntary extremity movements, blurred vision, ataxia, seizures, severe hypotension leading to coma and possibly death from respiratory complications
  - NURSING ACTIONS
    - Administer an emetic to clients who are alert.
    - Perform gastric lavage.
- LITHIUM LEVEL: Greater than 2.5 mEq/L
  - MANIFESTATIONS: Oliguria, seizures, rapid progression of manifestations leading to coma and death
  - NURSING ACTIONS: Assist in preparing client for possible hemodialysis.

CONTRAINDICATIONS/PRECAUTIONS

- Lithium is Pregnancy Risk Category D. This medication is teratogenic, especially during the first trimester.
- Discourage clients from breastfeeding if lithium therapy is necessary. Qs
- Use cautiously in clients who have impaired kidney function, heart disease, sodium depletion, or dehydration.

INTERACTIONS

Diuretics

Sodium is excreted with the use of diuretics. Reduced serum sodium decreases lithium excretion, which can lead to toxicity.

NURSING ACTIONS

- Monitor for indications of toxicity.
- Advise clients to observe for indications of toxicity and to notify the provider.
- Encourage clients to maintain a diet adequate in sodium, and to consume 2,000 mL to 3,000 mL of water each day from food and beverage sources.

NSAIDs (ibuprofen, celecoxib)

Concurrent use increases renal reabsorption of lithium, leading to toxicity.

CLIENT EDUCATION

- Avoid use of NSAIDs.
- Use aspirin as a mild analgesic.

Anticholinergics

Antihistamines and tricyclic antidepressants can induce urinary retention and polyuria, leading to abdominal discomfort.

CLIENT EDUCATION: Avoid medications that have anticholinergic effects.

NURSING ADMINISTRATION

- Monitor plasma lithium levels during treatment.
  - At initiation of treatment, monitor levels at least 5 days after starting lithium therapy and after any dosage change, until therapeutic level has been achieved; then every 1 to 3 months, depending on length of treatment and stability. QEBP
  - Older adult clients often require more frequent monitoring. ⒢
  - Lithium blood levels should be obtained in the morning, usually 12 hr after the last dose.
  - During initial treatment of a manic episode, levels should be 0.8 to 1.4 mEq/L.
  - Maintenance level range is 0.4 to 1.0 mEq/L.
  - Plasma levels 1.5 mEq/L or greater can result in toxicity.
- Monitor CBC, serum electrolytes, kidney function tests, and thyroid function tests during lithium therapy.
- Advise clients that effects begin within 7 to 14 days.
- Advise clients to take lithium as prescribed. Lithium must be administered in two to three doses daily due to a short half-life. Taking lithium with food will help decrease GI distress.
- Encourage clients to adhere to laboratory appointments needed to monitor lithium effectiveness and adverse effects. Emphasize the high risk of toxicity due to the narrow therapeutic range.

- Provide nutritional counseling. Stress the importance of adequate fluid and sodium intake. Qᴘᴄᴄ
- Instruct clients to monitor for manifestations of toxicity and when to contact the provider. Clients should withhold medication and seek medical attention for diarrhea, vomiting, or excessive sweating.
- Conditions that cause dehydration (exercising in hot weather, diarrhea) put clients at risk for lithium toxicity.

Mood-stabilizing antiepileptic drugs

SELECT PROTOTYPE MEDICATIONS
- Carbamazepine
- Valproic acid
- Lamotrigine

Oxcarbazepine and topiramate are less frequently used and recommended for maintenance treatment of bipolar disorder.

PURPOSE

EXPECTED PHARMACOLOGICAL ACTION: AEDs help treat and manage bipolar disorders by various mechanisms.
- Slowing the entrance of sodium and calcium back into the neuron, thus extending the time it takes for the nerve to return to its active state
- Potentiating the inhibitory effects of gamma butyric acid (GABA)
- Inhibiting glutamic acid (glutamate), which in turn suppresses CNS excitation

THERAPEUTIC USES: Treatment and prevention of relapse of mania and depressive episodes. Especially useful for clients who have mixed mania and rapid-cycling bipolar disorders.

COMPLICATIONS

CARBAMAZEPINE

Central nervous system (CNS) effects

Cognitive function is minimally affected, but CNS effects can include nystagmus, double vision, vertigo, staggering gait, and headache.

NURSING ACTIONS
- Administer low doses initially, then gradually increase dosage.
- Instruct clients to avoid driving and other activities that require alertness at the beginning of treatment. Qₛ
- Advise clients that CNS effects should subside within a few weeks.
- Administer dose at bedtime.

Hematologic effects

Leukopenia, anemia, thrombocytopenia, pancytopenia

NURSING ACTIONS
- Obtain baseline CBC and platelets, and perform ongoing monitoring.
- Observe for indications of bruising and bleeding of gums.
- Monitor for sore throat, fatigue, and other indications of infection.

Teratogenesis

CLIENT EDUCATION: Avoid use during pregnancy.

Hypo-osmolality

Promotes secretion of ADH, which inhibits water excretion by the kidneys and places older adult clients who have heart failure at risk for fluid overload Ⓖ

NURSING ACTIONS
- Monitor serum sodium.
- Monitor for edema, decrease in urine output, and hypertension.

Skin disorders

Dermatitis, rash, and Stevens-Johnson syndrome, which is potentially life-threatening

NURSING ACTIONS
- Treat mild reactions with anti-inflammatory or antihistamine medications.
- Advise clients to wear sunscreen.
- Instruct clients to notify the provider if Stevens-Johnson syndrome rash occurs and to withhold medication.

Hepatotoxicity

Evidenced by anorexia, nausea, vomiting, fatigue, abdominal pain, and jaundice

NURSING ACTIONS
- Check baseline liver function.
- Monitor liver function regularly.
- Advise clients to observe for indications and to notify the provider if they occur.
- Avoid using in children younger than 2 years old.
- Administer lowest effective dose.

LAMOTRIGINE

Double or blurred vision, dizziness, headache, nausea, vomiting

NURSING ACTIONS: Caution clients about performing activities requiring concentration.

Serious skin rashes

Include Stevens-Johnson syndrome

CLIENT EDUCATION: Withhold medication and notify the provider if rash occurs.

VALPROIC ACID

GI effects

Nausea, vomiting, indigestion

CLIENT EDUCATION
- Manifestations are usually self-limiting.
- Take medication with food or switch to enteric-coated pills.

Hepatotoxicity

Evidenced by anorexia, nausea, vomiting, fatigue abdominal pain, jaundice

NURSING ACTIONS
- Check baseline liver function.
- Monitor liver function regularly.
- Advise clients to observe for indications and to notify the provider if they occur.
- Avoid using in children younger than 2 years old.
- Administer lowest effective dose.

Pancreatitis

Evidenced by nausea, vomiting, and abdominal pain

NURSING ACTIONS
- Advise clients to observe for indications and to notify the provider immediately if they occur.
- Monitor amylase levels.
- Discontinue medication if pancreatitis develops.

Thrombocytopenia

NURSING ACTIONS
- Advise clients to observe for manifestations, such as bruising, and to notify the provider if these occur.
- Monitor platelet counts.

Teratogenesis

CLIENT EDUCATION: Avoid use during pregnancy.

Weight gain

CLIENT EDUCATION: Follow a healthy low-calorie diet, engage in regular exercise, and monitor weight.

CONTRAINDICATIONS/PRECAUTIONS

- These medications are Pregnancy Risk Category D and can result in birth defects. Lamotrigine is Pregnancy Risk Category C, but can cause cleft lip and palate if taken during the first trimester.
- Carbamazepine is contraindicated in clients who have bone marrow suppression or bleeding disorders. Qs
- Valproic acid is contraindicated in clients who have liver disorders.
- Monitor plasma valproic acid and carbamazepine levels while undergoing treatment.

INTERACTIONS

CARBAMAZEPINE

Oral contraceptives, warfarin

Concurrent use causes a decrease in the effects of these medications due to stimulation of hepatic drug-metabolizing enzymes.

NURSING ACTIONS
- Advise clients to use an alternate form of birth control.
- Monitor for therapeutic effects of warfarin.
- Dosages might need to be adjusted.

Grapefruit

Inhibits metabolism, thus increasing carbamazepine levels.

CLIENT EDUCATION: Avoid consuming grapefruit or products that contain grapefruit.

Phenytoin and phenobarbital

Decrease the effects of carbamazepine by stimulating metabolism

NURSING ACTIONS
- Monitor phenytoin and phenobarbital levels.
- Adjust dosage of medications as prescribed.

LAMOTRIGINE

Carbamazepine, phenytoin, and phenobarbital

These promote liver drug-metabolizing enzymes, thereby decreasing the effect of lamotrigine.

NURSING ACTIONS
- Monitor for therapeutic effects.
- Adjust dosage of medications as prescribed.

Valproic acid

Inhibits medication-metabolizing enzymes and thus increases the half-life of lamotrigine

NURSING ACTIONS
- Monitor for adverse effects
- Adjust dosage of medications as prescribed.

VALPROIC ACID

Phenytoin and phenobarbital

Serum levels of these medications are increased when used concurrently with valproic acid.

NURSING ACTIONS
- Monitor phenytoin and phenobarbital levels.
- Adjust dosage of medications as prescribed.

NURSING EVALUATION OF MEDICATION EFFECTIVENESS

Depending on therapeutic intent, effectiveness is evidenced by the following.

- Relief of acute manic manifestations (flight of ideas, excessive talking, agitation) or depressive manifestations (fatigue, poor appetite, psychomotor retardation)
- Mood stability
- Ability to perform ADLs
- Improved sleeping and eating habits
- Appropriate interaction with peers

PRACTICE Active Learning Scenario

A nurse is reinforcing discharge teaching with a client who has a new diagnosis of bipolar disorder. The client has a new prescription for lithium carbonate 600 mg PO three times a day. Use the ATI Active Learning Template: Medication to complete this item.

CLIENT EDUCATION: Include three adverse effects the nurse should include.

Application Exercises

1. A nurse is reviewing a client's laboratory results and notes a lithium level of 2.1 mEq/L. Which of the following actions should the nurse plan to take?
   - A. Perform immediate gastric lavage.
   - B. Assist in preparing the client for hemodialysis.
   - C. Administer half a dose at the next scheduled time.
   - D. Request a stat repeat of the laboratory test.

2. A nurse is reinforcing medication teaching with a client who has bipolar disorder and a new prescription for lithium carbonate. Which of the following information should the nurse include?
   - A. Avoid the use of acetaminophen for headaches.
   - B. Restrict intake of foods rich in sodium.
   - C. Decrease fluid intake to less than 1,500 mL daily
   - D. Limit aerobic activity in hot weather.

3. A nurse is collecting data from a client who has bipolar disorder and is taking lithium carbonate. The nurse should identify which of the following findings as a possible indication of toxicity?
   - A. Severe hypertension
   - B. Coarse tremors
   - C. Constipation
   - D. Muscle spasms

4. A nurse is reinforcing medication teaching with a client who has bipolar disorder and a new prescription for valproic acid. The nurse should instruct the client to have which of the following laboratory tests completed periodically? (Select all that apply.)
   - A. Thrombocyte count
   - B. Hematocrit
   - C. Amylase
   - D. Liver function tests
   - E. Potassium

5. A nurse is planning to reinforce ing with a female client who has bipolar disorder and a new prescription for carbamazepine. Which of the following statements should the nurse include? (Select all that apply.)
   - A. "This medication can safely be taken during pregnancy."
   - B. "Eliminate grapefruit juice from your diet."
   - C. "You will need to have your blood count monitored periodically."
   - D. "Notify your provider if you develop a rash."
   - E. "Avoid driving for the first few days after starting this medication."

Application Exercises Key

1. A. **CORRECT:** Gastric lavage is indicated for a client who has severe toxicity, as evidenced by a plasma lithium level of 2.1 mEq/L. This action will lower the client's lithium level.

   B. Hemodialysis is indicated for a client who has a plasma lithium level greater than 2.5 mEq/L.

   C. Administering half dose of lithium will worsen the level of toxicity.

   D. There is no indication that the client needs another laboratory test, and this action can delay needed treatment.

   Ⓝ *NCLEX® Connection: Pharmacological Therapies, Adverse Effects/ Contraindications/Side Effects/Interactions*

2. A. The client should use acetaminophen, rather than NSAIDs such as ibuprofen, for headaches because NSAIDs can cause increased blood levels of lithium.

   B. The client should increase, rather than decrease, sodium intake to reduce the risk for toxicity.

   C. The client should increase, rather than decrease, fluid intake to reduce the risk for toxicity.

   D. **CORRECT:** The client should avoid activities that have the potential to cause sodium/water depletion, which can increase the risk for toxicity.

   Ⓝ *NCLEX® Connection: Pharmacological Therapies, Expected Actions/Outcomes*

3. A. Severe hypotension, rather than hypertension, is an indication of toxicity.

   B. **CORRECT:** Coarse tremors are an indication of toxicity.

   C. Diarrhea, rather than constipation, is an indication of toxicity.

   D. Muscle weakness, rather than muscle spasm, is an indication of lithium toxicity.

   Ⓝ *NCLEX® Connection: Pharmacological Therapies, Expected Actions/Outcomes*

4. A. **CORRECT:** Treatment with valproic acid can result in thrombocytopenia. The client's thrombocyte count should be monitored periodically.

   B. Treatment with valproic acid is not known to have an effect on a client's hematocrit.

   C. **CORRECT:** Treatment with valproic acid can result in pancreatitis. The client's amylase should be monitored periodically.

   D. **CORRECT:** Treatment with valproic acid can result in hepatotoxicity. The client's liver function should be monitored periodically.

   E. Treatment with valproic acid is not known to have an effect on a client's potassium.

   Ⓝ *NCLEX® Connection: Pharmacological Therapies, Expected Actions/Outcomes*

5. A. Carbamazepine is a Pregnancy Category Risk D medication. The client should be instructed to avoid pregnancy while taking carbamazepine.

   B. **CORRECT:** Grapefruit juice affects carbamazepine metabolism and should be avoided.

   C. **CORRECT:** Carbamazepine blood levels and the CBC should be monitored during therapy. The client is at risk for bone marrow depression while taking carbamazepine and should notify the provider of a sore throat or other manifestations of an infection.

   D. **CORRECT:** Carbamazepine can cause Stevens-Johnson syndrome, which can be fatal. The client should notify the provider promptly if a rash occurs.

   E. **CORRECT:** CNS effects (drowsiness, dizziness) can occur early in treatment with carbamazepine. The client should avoid activities requiring alertness until these effects subside.

   Ⓝ *NCLEX® Connection: Pharmacological Therapies, Expected Actions/Outcomes*

PRACTICE Answer

Using the ATI Active Learning Template: Medication

CLIENT EDUCATION

- Gastrointestinal distress: nausea, diarrhea, abdominal pain
- Fine hand tremors
- Polyuria
- Mild thirst
- Weight gain
- Kidney toxicity
- Goiter and hypothyroidism
- Bradydysrhythmias
- Hypotension
- Electrolyte imbalances

Ⓝ *NCLEX® Connection: Pharmacological and Parenteral Therapies, Medication Administration*

UNIT 2   MEDICATIONS AFFECTING THE NERVOUS SYSTEM

CHAPTER 9   *Psychotic Disorders*

Schizophrenia spectrum disorders are the primary reason for the administration of antipsychotic medications. The clinical course of schizophrenia usually involves acute exacerbations with intervals of semi-remission.

Medications are used to treat positive symptoms related to behavior, thought, perception, and speech (agitation, bizarre behavior, delusions, hallucinations, flight of ideas, illogical thinking patterns, tangential speech patterns), negative symptoms (social withdrawal, lack of emotion, lack of energy [anergia], flattened affect, decreased motivation, decreased pleasure in activities), and cognitive manifestations (disordered thinking, reduced ability to focus, and memory difficulties).

The goals of psychopharmacological treatment for schizophrenia spectrum and other psychotic disorders include suppressing acute episodes, preventing acute exacerbations, and maintaining the highest possible level of functioning. Q**EBP**

Antipsychotics: First-generation (conventional)

- These medications control mainly positive symptoms of psychotic disorders.
- Potency refers to the size of the dose needed to elicit a given response. A medication with high potency requires a smaller dose to relieve manifestations, while a medication with low potency requires a larger dose.

SELECT PROTOTYPE MEDICATIONS
- Chlorpromazine: low potency
- Haloperidol: high potency

OTHER MEDICATIONS
- Thioridazine: low potency
- Chlorpromazine: low potency
- Perphenazine: medium potency
- Loxapine: medium potency
- Haloperidol: high potency
- Fluphenazine: high potency
- Thiothixene: high potency

PURPOSE

EXPECTED PHARMACOLOGICAL ACTION
- Block dopamine (D_2), acetylcholine, histamine, and norepinephrine receptors in the brain and periphery.
- Inhibit psychotic manifestations, believed to be a result of D_2 blockade in the brain.

THERAPEUTIC USES
- Acute and chronic psychotic disorders
- Schizophrenia spectrum disorders
- Bipolar disorders (primarily the manic phase)
- Tourette syndrome
- Agitation
- Prevention of nausea/vomiting through blocking of dopamine in the chemoreceptor trigger zone of the medulla

INDICATIONS
- Clients who can tolerate the adverse effects
- Clients who are violent or particularly aggressive

FORMULATIONS
- Tablets
- Oral solution
- Depot preparations (used for clients who have difficulty adhering to medication regimen)
  - Therapeutic effect occurs up to several weeks following the first depot injection.
    - Haloperidol decanoate IM every 4 weeks
    - Fluphenazine decanoate IM, subcutaneous every 2 weeks

COMPLICATIONS

EXTRAPYRAMIDAL SIDE EFFECTS (EPSs)

Acute dystonia

- The client experiences severe spasms of the tongue, neck, face, eyes, or back. This is a crisis situation, which requires rapid treatment. Q**s**
- Can develop within the first few hours or days after administration of the first dose.

NURSING ACTIONS: Treat with anticholinergic agents, such as benztropine or diphenhydramine.

Parkinsonism

Findings include mask-like face, bradykinesia, rigidity, shuffling gait, drooling, and tremors.

NURSING ACTIONS
- Observe for parkinsonism within 1 month of initiation of therapy.
- Treat with benztropine, diphenhydramine, or amantadine. Discontinue these medications to determine if they are still needed. If manifestations return, administer atypical antipsychotic.

Akathisia

The client is unable to stand still or sit, and is continually pacing and agitated.

NURSING ACTIONS
- Observe for akathisia within 2 months of the initiation of treatment.
- Manage effects with beta blocker, benzodiazepine, or anticholinergic medication.

Tardive dyskinesia (TD)

- Manifestations include involuntary movements of the tongue and face, such as lip-smacking, which cause speech and eating disturbances.
- Can also include involuntary movements of arms, legs, or trunk.
- The Abnormal Involuntary Movement Scale (AIMS) is used to monitor for manifestations.
- TD is a late EPS that can occur months to years after the start of therapy, and can improve following medication change but is often permanent.

NURSING ACTIONS
- Administer the lowest dosage possible to control manifestations.
- Evaluate the client after 12 months of therapy and then every 3 months. If indications of TD appear, dosage should be lowered or the client should be switched to an atypical agent.

OTHER ADVERSE EFFECTS

Neuroleptic malignant syndrome

! Life-threatening medical emergency

Manifestations include sudden high-grade fever, blood pressure fluctuations, dysrhythmias, muscle rigidity, diaphoresis, drooling, and change in level of consciousness developing into coma. Qs

NURSING ACTIONS
- Stop antipsychotic medication.
- Monitor vital signs.
- Apply cooling blankets.
- Administer antipyretics (aspirin, acetaminophen).
- Increase fluid intake.
- Diazepam is administered to control anxiety as well as reduce blood pressure and heart rate.
- Dantrolene and bromocriptine are administered to induce muscle relaxation.
- Wait 2 weeks before resuming therapy. Consider lowering the dosage or switching to an atypical agent.

Anticholinergic effects

More likely to occur with low-potency first-generation antipsychotics
- Dry mouth
- Blurred vision
- Photophobia
- Urinary hesitancy/retention
- Constipation
- Tachycardia

NURSING ACTIONS
Suggest strategies to decrease anticholinergic effects.
- Chewing sugarless gum
- Sipping water
- Avoiding hazardous activities
- Wearing sunglasses when outdoors
- Eating foods high in fiber
- Participating in regular exercise
- Maintaining fluid intake of 2 to 3 L water daily from food and beverage sources
- Voiding just before taking medication

Neuroendocrine effects

Effects include gynecomastia (breast enlargement), galactorrhea, and menstrual irregularities.

CLIENT EDUCATION: Observe for manifestations and notify the provider if these occur.

Seizures

- The greatest risk for developing seizures is existing seizure disorders.
- An increase in antiseizure medication can be necessary.

CLIENT EDUCATION: Report seizure activity to the provider.

Skin effects

Effects include photosensitivity resulting in severe sunburn, and contact dermatitis from handling medications.

CLIENT EDUCATION
- Avoid excessive exposure to sunlight, use sunscreen, and wear protective clothing.
- Avoid direct contact with medication.

Orthostatic hypotension

- More likely to occur with low-potency first-generation antipsychotics
- Clients should develop tolerance in 2 to 3 months.

NURSING ACTIONS
- In the hospital setting, monitor blood pressure and heart rate for orthostatic changes. If a significant decrease in blood pressure or increase in heart rate is noted, do not administer the medication, and notify the provider.
- Instruct clients about the indications of postural hypotension (lightheadedness, dizziness). If these occur, advise the client to sit or lie down. Orthostatic hypotension can be minimized by getting up or changing positions slowly.

Sedation

CLIENT EDUCATION
- Effects should diminish within a few weeks.
- This medication can be taken at bedtime to avoid daytime sleepiness.
- Do not drive until sedation has subsided. Qs

Sexual dysfunction

- Common in men and women
- Client might need a lower dosage or to be switched to a high-potency agent.

NURSING ACTIONS
- Advise clients of possible adverse effects.
- Encourage clients to report adverse effects to the provider.

Agranulocytosis

NURSING ACTIONS
- Advise clients to observe for indications of infection (fever, sore throat) and to notify the provider if these occur.
- If indications of infection appear, monitor the WBC count. Medication should be discontinued if laboratory tests indicate the presence of infection.

Severe dysrhythmias

NURSING ACTIONS
- Obtain baseline ECG and potassium level prior to treatment and periodically throughout the treatment period.
- Avoid concurrent use with other medications that prolong QT interval.

Liver impairment

NURSING ACTIONS
- Check baseline liver function.
- Monitor liver function regularly.
- Advise clients to observe for indications (anorexia, nausea, vomiting, fatigue, abdominal pain, jaundice) and to notify the provider.

CONTRAINDICATIONS/PRECAUTIONS

- Contraindicated in clients in a coma, and clients who have severe depression, Parkinson's disease, prolactin-dependent cancer of the breast, and severe hypotension.
- Contraindicated in older clients who have dementia. Antipsychotics for dementia-related psychosis are associated with increased mortality. ⓖ
- Use cautiously in clients who have glaucoma, paralytic ileus, prostate enlargement, heart disorders, liver or kidney disease, and seizure disorders.
- Newborns exposed to antipsychotics in the third trimester of pregnancy can develop extrapyramidal symptoms or manifestations of withdrawal.

INTERACTIONS

Anticholinergic agents

Concurrent use with other anticholinergic medications will increase anticholinergic effects.

CLIENT EDUCATION: Avoid over-the-counter medications that contain anticholinergic agents, such as sleep aids.

CNS depressants

Alcohol, opioids, and antihistamines have additive CNS depressant effects.

CLIENT EDUCATION
- Avoid alcohol and other medications that cause CNS depression.
- Avoid hazardous activities, such as driving.

Levodopa

By activating dopamine receptors, levodopa counteracts the effects of antipsychotic agents.

NURSING ACTIONS: Avoid concurrent use of levodopa and other direct dopamine receptor agonists.

NURSING ADMINISTRATION

- Use the Abnormal Involuntary Movement Scale (AIMS) to screen for the presence of EPS. QEBP
- Monitor clients to differentiate between EPSs and worsening of psychotic disorder.
- Administer anticholinergics, beta blockers, and benzodiazepines to control early EPSs. If adverse effects are intolerable, the client can be switched to a low-potency or an atypical antipsychotic agent.
- Advise clients that antipsychotic medications do not cause addiction.
- Advise clients to take medication as prescribed and on a regular schedule.
- Advise clients that some therapeutic effects can be noticeable within a few days, but significant improvement can take 2 to 4 weeks, and possibly several months for full effects.
- Consider depot preparations administered IM once every 2 to 4 weeks for clients who have difficulty maintaining medication regimen. Inform the client that lower doses can be used with depot preparations, which will decrease the risk of adverse effects and the development of tardive dyskinesia. QPCC
- Start oral administration with twice-a-day dosing, then switch to daily dosing at bedtime to decrease daytime drowsiness and promote sleep.

Antipsychotics: Second- and third-generation (atypical)

- These agents are often chosen as first-line treatment for schizophrenia.
- Although first- and second-generation have the same efficacy, second-generation medications are more expensive.

SELECT PROTOTYPE MEDICATION:
Risperidone (second-generation antipsychotic)

OTHER MEDICATIONS (9.1)
- Olanzapine
- Quetiapine
- Ziprasidone
- Clozapine
- Asenapine
- Lurasidone
- Paliperidone
- Iloperidone
- Aripiprazole (third-generation)

PURPOSE

EXPECTED PHARMACOLOGICAL ACTION
- Second-generation antipsychotic agents work mainly by blocking serotonin, and to a lesser degree, dopamine receptors. These medications also block receptors for norepinephrine, histamine, and acetylcholine.
- The third-generation medication (aripiprazole) works by stabilizing the dopamine system as both an agonist and antagonist.

THERAPEUTIC USES
- Schizophrenia spectrum disorders (negative and positive symptoms)
- Psychotic episodes induced by levodopa therapy
- Bipolar disorders
- Impulse control disorders

9.1 Other atypical antipsychotic agents

Olanzapine
FORMULATIONS: Tablets, orally disintegrating tablets, short-acting injectable, extended-release injection

COMPLICATIONS
- Low risk of EPS
- High risk for diabetes mellitus, weight gain, and dyslipidemia
- Other adverse effects: leukopenia, sedation, orthostatic hypotension, anticholinergic effects

Quetiapine
FORMULATIONS: Tablets, extended-release tablets

COMPLICATIONS
- Low risk of EPS
- Moderate risk for diabetes mellitus, weight gain, and dyslipidemia
- Other effects: cataracts, sedation, orthostatic hypotension, anticholinergic effects
- Clients should have baseline eye exam and then every 6 months.
- ECG changes and QT prolongation can lead to torsades de pointes

Ziprasidone
Affects both dopamine and serotonin; can be used for clients who have concurrent depression

FORMULATIONS: Capsules, short-acting injectable

COMPLICATIONS
- Low risk of EPS, diabetes mellitus, weight gain, dyslipidemia
- Other effects: sedation, orthostatic hypotension, anticholinergic effects, rash
- ECG changes and QT prolongation can lead to torsades de pointes.

Clozapine
The first atypical antipsychotic developed. Despite its effectiveness for schizophrenia spectrum disorders, it is no longer considered a first-line medication because of its serious adverse effects.

FORMULATIONS: Tablets, orally disintegrating tablets

COMPLICATIONS
- Low risk of EPS
- High risk of weight gain, diabetes mellitus, dyslipidemia
- Agranulocytosis can occur. Obtain baseline ANC (absolute neutrophil count) and WBC and monitor throughout treatment per protocol.
- Monitor for indications of infection (fever, sore throat, lesions in mouth), and notify the provider if manifestations occur. Qs
- Other adverse effects: sedation, hypersalivation, orthostatic hypotension, and anticholinergic effects
- Pregnancy Risk Category B

Asenapine
FORMULATION: Sublingual tablets

COMPLICATIONS
- Drowsiness, prolonged QT interval, EPS (higher doses)
- Causes temporary numbing of the mouth
- Low risk of diabetes mellitus, weight gain, dyslipidemia, anticholinergic effects

Lurasidone
FORMULATION: Tablets

COMPLICATIONS
- Common adverse effects: sedation, akathisia, parkinsonism, nausea, agitation, anxiety
- Low risk for diabetes mellitus, weight gain, dyslipidemia
- Does not cause anticholinergic effects or prolong the QT interval
- Pregnancy Risk Category B

Paliperidone
FORMULATIONS: Extended-release tablets, extended-release injections

COMPLICATIONS
- High risk for diabetes mellitus, weight gain, dyslipidemia
- Other adverse effects: sedation, prolonged QT interval, orthostatic hypotension, anticholinergic effects, mild EPS

Iloperidone
FORMULATION: Tablets

COMPLICATIONS
- Common adverse effects: dry mouth, sedation, fatigue, nasal congestion
- Significant risk for weight gain, prolonged QT interval, orthostatic hypotension
- Advise clients to follow titration schedule during initial therapy to minimize hypotension.
- Low risk for diabetes mellitus, dyslipidemia, EPS

Aripiprazole (third-generation antipsychotic)
FORMULATIONS: Tablets, orally disintegrating tablets, oral solution, sustained-release injectable

COMPLICATIONS
- Common adverse effects: headache, agitation, nervousness, anxiety, insomnia, nausea, vomiting, dizziness
- Low risk of EPS
- Low risk of weight gain, diabetes, dyslipidemia and orthostatic hypotension
- Does not prolong QT interval

ADVANTAGES

- Relief of both the positive and negative symptoms of the disease
- Decrease in affective manifestations (depression, anxiety) and suicidal behaviors
- Improvement of neurocognitive deficits, such as poor memory
- Fewer or no EPSs, including TD, because of less dopamine blockade
- Fewer anticholinergic adverse effects because most atypical antipsychotics, with the exception of clozapine, cause little or no blockade of cholinergic receptors
- Less relapse compared to first-generation antipsychotics.

FORMULATIONS

- IM depot preparations: Use for clients who have difficulty with medication regimen.
- Therapeutic effect occurs up to several weeks following the first depot injection.

COMPLICATIONS

Diabetes mellitus

New onset of diabetes mellitus or loss of glucose control in clients who have diabetes (referred to as metabolic syndrome and also includes weight gain and dyslipidemia)

NURSING ACTIONS
- Obtain baseline fasting blood glucose and monitor throughout treatment.
- Instruct client to report indications (increased thirst, urination, and appetite).

Weight gain

CLIENT EDUCATION: Follow a healthy low-calorie diet, engage in regular exercise, and monitor weight gain.

Dyslipidemia

Increases risk for hypertension and other cardiovascular disease

NURSING ACTIONS: Obtain baseline fasting lipid panel and monitor at least every 6 months.

Seizures

The greatest risk for developing seizures is existing seizure disorders.

CLIENT EDUCATION
- Report seizure activity to the provider.
- Avoid driving or hazardous activities if a seizure has occurred.

Orthostatic hypotension

NURSING ACTIONS
- Monitor blood pressure and heart rate for orthostatic changes.
- Instruct clients to change positions slowly.

Anticholinergic effects

Include urinary hesitancy or retention, nasal congestion, constipation, and dry mouth

NURSING ACTIONS
- Monitor for effects and report occurrence to the provider.
- Educate clients about measures to relieve dry mouth, such as sipping fluids.

Agitation, dizziness, sedation, sleep disruption

NURSING ACTIONS
- Monitor for effects and report to the provider if they occur.
- Administer alternative medication if prescribed.

EPSs (parkinsonism, acute dystonia, akathisia, tardive dyskinesia)

The risk for EPS is low but not absent.

NURSING ACTIONS
- Monitor for and reinforce with clients how to recognize EPSs.
- Use AIMS tool to screen for EPSs.

Neuroendocrine

NURSING ACTIONS
- Advise clients to observe for galactorrhea, gynecomastia, and amenorrhea, and to notify the provider if these occur.
- Obtain prolactin level if indicated.

Sexual dysfunction (anorgasmia, impotence, low libido)

CLIENT EDUCATION
- Observe for possible sexual adverse effects and notify the provider if they are intolerable.
- Ways to manage sexual dysfunction can include using adjunct medications to improve sexual function (sildenafil).

CONTRAINDICATIONS/PRECAUTIONS

- Risperidone and most other atypical antipsychotics are Pregnancy Risk Category C.
- Lurasidone and clozapine are Category B.
- Contraindicated for clients who have dementia. All atypical antipsychotic medications can cause death related to stroke or infection. Ⓖ
- Clients should avoid use of alcohol.
- Use cautiously in clients who have cardiovascular or cerebrovascular disease, seizures, or diabetes mellitus. Obtain a fasting blood glucose for clients who have diabetes mellitus, and monitor blood glucose carefully.

INTERACTIONS

Immunosuppressive medications

Immunosuppressants, such as anticancer medications, can further suppress immune function in clients taking clozapine.

NURSING ACTIONS: Avoid use in clients taking clozapine.

Alcohol, opioids, antihistamines

Have additive CNS depressant effects.

CLIENT EDUCATION
- Avoid alcohol and medications that cause CNS depression.
- Avoid hazardous activities, such as driving.

Antipsychotic agents

By activating dopamine receptors, levodopa counteracts the effects of antipsychotic agents.

NURSING ACTIONS: Avoid concurrent use of levodopa and other direct dopamine receptor agonists.

Tricyclic antidepressants, amiodarone, clarithromycin

Prolong QT interval and thus increase the risk of cardiac dysrhythmias in clients taking ziprasidone

NURSING ACTIONS: Atypical antipsychotics that prolong the QT interval should not be used concurrently with other medications that have the same effect.

Barbiturates, phenytoin

Stimulate hepatic medication-metabolizing enzymes and thereby decrease medication levels of aripiprazole, quetiapine, and ziprasidone

NURSING ACTIONS: Monitor medication effectiveness.

Fluconazole

Inhibits hepatic medication-metabolizing enzymes and thereby increases levels of aripiprazole, quetiapine, and ziprasidone

NURSING ACTIONS: Monitor for adverse effects or toxicity.

NURSING ADMINISTRATION

- Clients often require oral preparations until effectiveness is achieved. Advise clients that low doses of medication are given initially and are then gradually increased. Qᴘᴄᴄ
- Use oral disintegrating tablets for clients who might attempt to "cheek" (or pocket) tablets or have difficulty swallowing them.
- Advise clients taking asenapine to avoid eating or drinking for 10 min after each dose.
- Administer lurasidone and ziprasidone with food (at least 350 calories) to increase absorption.
- The cost of antipsychotic medications can be a factor for some clients. Determine the need for case management intervention. Qᴛᴄ

NURSING EVALUATION OF MEDICATION EFFECTIVENESS

Depending on therapeutic intent, effectiveness can be evidenced by improvement in the following.
- Positive and negative manifestations (prevention of acute psychotic symptoms, absence of hallucinations, delusions, anxiety, and hostility)
- Ability to perform ADLs
- Ability to interact socially with peers
- Sleeping and eating habits

Application Exercises

1. A nurse is reinforcing teaching with a client who has schizophrenia about strategies to cope with anticholinergic effects of fluphenazine. Which of the following strategies should the nurse include?

   A. Take the medication in the morning to prevent insomnia.

   B. Chew sugarless gum to moisten the mouth.

   C. Use cooling measures to decrease fever.

   D. Take an antacid to relieve nausea.

2. A nurse is collecting data from a client who recently began taking haloperidol. Which of the following findings should the nurse identify as the highest priority to report to the provider?

   A. Shuffling gait

   B. Neck spasms

   C. Drowsiness

   D. Sexual dysfunction

3. A nurse is reinforcing discharge teaching with a client who has a new prescription for clozapine. Which of the following statements should the nurse include?

   A. "You should have a high-carbohydrate snack between meals and at bedtime."

   B. "You are likely to develop hand tremors if you take this medication for a long period of time."

   C. "You may experience temporary numbness of your mouth after each dose."

   D. "You should have your white blood cell count monitored every week."

4. A nurse is reinforcing teaching with a male client who has schizophrenia and is taking risperidone. Which of the following statements should the nurse include?

   A. "Add extra snacks to your diet to prevent weight loss."

   B. "Notify the provider if you develop breast enlargement."

   C. "You may begin to have mild seizures while taking this medication."

   D. "This medication is likely to increase your libido."

5. A nurse is collecting data from a client who has schizophrenia and is taking chlorpromazine. In which of the following manifestations should the nurse expect the most improvement? (Select all that apply.)

   A. Disorganized speech

   B. Bizarre behavior

   C. Impaired social interactions

   D. Hallucinations

   E. Decreased motivation

PRACTICE Active Learning Scenario

A nurse is caring for a client who has neuroleptic malignant syndrome.

Use the ATI Active Learning Template: System Disorder to complete this item to include the following sections.

DESCRIPTION OF DISORDER/DISEASE PROCESS

DATA COLLECTION: Identify at least four expected objective findings.

MEDICATIONS: Identify two medications indicated for treatment and their purpose.

NURSING CARE: Identify at least three interventions.

Application Exercises Key

1. A. Insomnia is not an anticholinergic effect.

    B. **CORRECT:** Chewing sugarless gum can help the client cope with dry mouth, which is a potential anticholinergic effect of fluphenazine.

    C. Fever is not an anticholinergic effect.

    D. Nausea is not an anticholinergic effect.

    Ⓝ *NCLEX® Connection: Pharmacological Therapies, Expected Actions/Outcomes*

2. A. Shuffling gait is an indication of parkinsonism and should be reported to the provider. However, this is not the greatest risk to the client and is therefore not the priority finding.

    B. **CORRECT:** Neck spasms are an indication of acute dystonia, which is a crisis situation requiring rapid treatment. This is the greatest risk to the client and is therefore the priority finding.

    C. Drowsiness is an adverse effect of haloperidol and should be reported to the provider. However, this is not the greatest risk to the client.

    D. Sexual dysfunction is an adverse effect of haloperidol and should be reported to the provider. However, this is not the greatest risk to the client.

    Ⓝ *NCLEX® Connection: Pharmacological Therapies, Adverse Effects/ Contraindications/Side Effects/Interactions*

3. A. Clozapine increases the client's risk of developing diabetes mellitus and weight gain. It is not recommended to increase carbohydrate intake.

    B. Clozapine has a low risk of EPS such as hand tremors.

    C. Asenapine, rather than clozapine, causes temporary numbing of the mouth.

    D. **CORRECT:** Due to the risk for agranulocytosis, weekly monitoring of the client's WBC count is recommended while taking clozapine.

    Ⓝ *NCLEX® Connection: Pharmacological Therapies, Expected Actions/Outcomes*

4. A. Risperidone and other atypical antidepressants cause weight gain. The client should be taught to maintain a lower-calorie balanced diet.

    B. **CORRECT:** Gynecomastia (breast enlargement) and galactorrhea can occur due to an increase in prolactin levels while taking risperidone. The client should inform the provider if these manifestations occur.

    C. Seizures are not an adverse effect of risperidone.

    D. Sexual dysfunction, causing decreased libido and impotence are adverse effects of risperidone.

    Ⓝ *NCLEX® Connection: Pharmacological Therapies, Expected Actions/Outcomes*

5. A. **CORRECT:** A client who takes a conventional antipsychotic medication, such as chlorpromazine, should have the greatest improvement in positive symptoms such as disorganized speech.

    B. **CORRECT:** A client who takes a conventional antipsychotic medication, such as chlorpromazine, should have the greatest improvement in positive symptoms such as bizarre behavior.

    C. Conventional antipsychotic medications, such as chlorpromazine, have less effect on negative symptoms such as impaired social interactions.

    D. **CORRECT:** A client who takes a conventional antipsychotic medication, such as chlorpromazine, should have the greatest improvement in positive symptoms such as hallucinations.

    E. Conventional antipsychotic medications, such as chlorpromazine, have less effect on negative symptoms such as decreased motivation.

    Ⓝ *NCLEX® Connection: Pharmacological Therapies, Expected Actions/Outcomes*

PRACTICE Answer

Using the ATI Active Learning Template: System Disorders

DESCRIPTION OF DISORDER/DISEASE PROCESS: Neuroleptic malignant syndrome is a potential adverse effect of first-generation (conventional) antipsychotic medications that most commonly occurs within the first 2 weeks of treatment.

DATA COLLECTION
- Sudden high fever
- Blood pressure fluctuations
- Drooling
- Diaphoresis
- Dysrhythmias
- Muscle rigidity
- Changes in level of consciousness
- Coma

MEDICATIONS
- Aspirin: antipyretic
- Acetaminophen: antipyretic
- Dantrolene: induces muscle relaxation
- Bromocriptine: induces muscle relaxation

NURSING CARE
- Notify the provider immediately.
- Withhold the conventional antipsychotic medication.
- Monitor vital signs.
- Apply cooling blankets.
- Increase fluid intake.
- Discuss with the provider the need to wait 2 weeks before resuming therapy.
- Discuss with the provider the possible need to switch to an atypical agent.

Ⓝ *NCLEX® Connection: Pharmacological and Parenteral Therapies, Expected Actions/Outcomes*

UNIT 2   MEDICATIONS AFFECTING THE NERVOUS SYSTEM

CHAPTER 10 *Medications for Children and Adolescents Who Have Mental Health Issues*

Various medications are used to manage behavioral disorders in children and adolescents (attention deficit-hyperactivity disorder, conduct disorder, intermittent explosive disorder, autism spectrum disorders). Pharmacological management is most effective when accompanied by techniques to modify behavior.

Central nervous system stimulants

10.1 Select prototypes and other medications

	SHORT-ACTING	INTERMEDIATE-ACTING	LONG-ACTING
Methylphenidate	3 to 5 hr	6 to 8 hr	8 to 12 hr
Dexmethylphenidate	4 to 5 hr	n/a	12 hr
Dextroamphetamine	4 to 6 hr	n/a	6 to 10 hr
Amphetamine mixture	4 to 6 hr	n/a	10 to 12 hr
Lisdexamfetamine dimesylate	n/a	n/a	10 to 12 hr

PURPOSE

EXPECTED PHARMACOLOGICAL ACTION: Raise the levels of norepinephrine and dopamine in the central nervous system (CNS).

THERAPEUTIC USES
- ADHD
- Conduct disorder
- Narcolepsy
- Obesity

COMPLICATIONS

CNS stimulation

Insomnia, restlessness

NURSING ACTIONS: Administer the last dose before 4 p.m. Q̇EBP

CLIENT EDUCATION: Observe for effects and notify the provider if they occur.

Decreased appetite, weight loss, growth suppression

NURSING ACTIONS
- Monitor the client's weight and compare to baseline height and weight.
- Administer medication during or immediately after meals.
- Promote good nutrition in children.
- Consult with prescriber about possible "medication holidays."

CLIENT EDUCATION: Encourage children to eat at regular meal times and avoid unhealthy foods for snacks.

Cardiovascular effects

- Dysrhythmias, chest pain, high blood pressure
- These medications can increase the risk of sudden death in clients who have heart abnormalities.

NURSING ACTIONS: Monitor vital signs and ECG.

CLIENT EDUCATION: Observe for effects (shortness of breath, chest pain, dizziness) and notify the provider if they occur.

Development of psychotic manifestations

Such as hallucinations and paranoia

CLIENT EDUCATION: Report manifestations immediately and discontinue the medication if they occur.

Physical tolerance and withdrawal reaction

Headache, nausea, vomiting, muscle weakness, depression

CLIENT EDUCATION: Do not stop taking medication suddenly; doing so can lead to depression and severe fatigue. Withdraw medication gradually.

Hypersensitivity skin reaction to transdermal methylphenidate

Hives, papules

NURSING ACTIONS: Remove the patch and notify the provider.

Toxicity

Dizziness, palpitations, hypertension, hallucinations, seizures

NURSING ACTIONS
- Treat hallucinations with chlorpromazine.
- Treat seizures with diazepam.
- Administer fluids.

CONTRAINDICATIONS/PRECAUTIONS

- Use with caution in clients who are pregnant (Pregnancy Risk Category C), breastfeeding, or have hypertension or depression.
- These medications are contraindicated in clients who have a history of substance use disorder, hypertension, hyperthyroidism, cardiovascular disorders, glaucoma, severe anxiety, and psychosis.

INTERACTIONS

Concurrent use of MAOIs can cause hypertensive crisis.
NURSING ACTIONS: Avoid concurrent use. Do not use within 14 days of MAOIs.

Concurrent use of caffeine can increase CNS stimulant effects.
CLIENT EDUCATION: Avoid foods and beverages that contain caffeine.

Methylphenidate inhibits metabolism of phenytoin, warfarin, and phenobarbital, leading to increased serum levels.
- Concurrent use of these medications is done with caution.
- NURSING ACTIONS: Monitor clients for adverse effects (CNS depression, toxicity, indications of bleeding).

OTC cold and decongestant medications with sympathomimetic action can increase CNS stimulant effects.
CLIENT EDUCATION: Avoid use of OTC medications.

CLIENT EDUCATION

- Swallow sustained-release tablets whole. Do not chew or crush the tablets.
- It is important to administering the medication on a regular schedule.
- For transdermal medication, place the patch on one hip daily in the morning and leave it in place no longer than 9 hr. Alternate hips daily.
- ADHD is not cured by medication. Management with an overall treatment plan that includes family therapy and cognitive-behavioral therapy will improve outcomes. Q EBP
- These medications have specific handling procedures controlled by federal law. Handwritten prescriptions are required for medication refills.
- Learn safety and storage of medications.
- These medications have a high potential for development of a substance use disorder, especially in adolescents. Use strictly as prescribed.
- Avoid activities that require alertness until medication effects are known.

NURSING EVALUATION OF MEDICATION EFFECTIVENESS

Depending on therapeutic intent, effectiveness is evidenced by the following.
- Improvement of manifestations of ADHD, such as increased ability to focus and complete tasks, interact with peers, and manage impulsivity
- Improved ability to stay awake

Norepinephrine selective reuptake inhibitors

SELECT PROTOTYPE MEDICATION: Atomoxetine

OTHER MEDICATION: Bupropion

PURPOSE

EXPECTED PHARMACOLOGICAL ACTION
- Block reuptake of norepinephrine at synapses in the CNS. Atomoxetine is not a stimulant medication.
- Bupropion blocks the synaptic reuptake of norepinephrine and dopamine. It is considered a second-line medication for ADHD.

THERAPEUTIC USES
- ADHD
- Depression

COMPLICATIONS

Atomoxetine is usually tolerated well with minimal adverse effects.

Appetite suppression, weight loss, growth suppression

NURSING ACTIONS
- Obtain baseline height and weight prior to treatment. Monitor weight at regular intervals.
- Administer medication with or without meals.
- Encourage children to eat at regular meal times and avoid unhealthy foods for snacks.

Gastrointestinal effects

Nausea, vomiting

CLIENT EDUCATION: Take with food if these occur.

Suicidal ideation

In children and adolescents

NURSING ACTIONS: Monitor for indications of depression.

CLIENT EDUCATION: Report change in mood, excessive sleeping, agitation, and irritability. Q s

Hepatotoxicity

CLIENT EDUCATION: Report indications of liver damage (flu-like manifestations, yellowing skin, abdominal pain).

Seizure activity

NURSING ACTIONS
- Use low doses, and monitor for seizure activity.
- Do not use in clients who have a seizure disorder.

CONTRAINDICATIONS/PRECAUTIONS

- Use cautiously in clients who have cardiovascular and hepatic disorders, and hypo/hypertension.
- Atomoxetine is contraindicated in clients who have angle-closure glaucoma, heart failure, and jaundice.
- Bupropion increases seizure risk at high dosages. It is contraindicated in clients who have seizure risk factors and eating disorders.

INTERACTIONS

Concurrent use of MAOIs can cause hypertensive crisis.

NURSING ACTIONS: Avoid concurrent use. Do not use within 14 days of MAOIs.

Paroxetine, fluoxetine, and quinidine gluconate inhibit hepatic metabolizing enzymes, thereby increasing levels of atomoxetine.
- NURSING ACTIONS: Reduce dosage of atomoxetine if used concurrently with these medications.
- CLIENT EDUCATION: Remind clients to watch for and report increased adverse reactions of atomoxetine.

NURSING ADMINISTRATION

- Note any changes in the child's behavior related to dosing and timing of medications.
- Administer the medication as a daily dose in the morning, or in two divided doses (morning and afternoon), with or without food.
- Instruct clients that therapeutic effects can take 1 to 3 weeks to fully develop.

NURSING EVALUATION OF MEDICATION EFFECTIVENESS

Depending on therapeutic intent, effectiveness is evidenced by improvement of manifestations of ADHD (increase in ability to focus and complete tasks, interact with peers, and manage impulsivity).

Tricyclic antidepressants

SELECT PROTOTYPE MEDICATION: Desipramine

OTHER MEDICATIONS
- Imipramine
- Clomipramine

PURPOSE

EXPECTED PHARMACOLOGICAL ACTION: These medications block reuptake of the monoamine neurotransmitters norepinephrine and serotonin in the synaptic space, thereby intensifying the effects that these neurotransmitters produce.

THERAPEUTIC USES IN CHILDREN
- Depression
- Autism spectrum disorder
- ADHD (considered less effective than CNS stimulants and used as second-line treatment for ADHD)
- Panic, social phobia, separation anxiety disorder
- Obsessive compulsive disorder (OCD)

COMPLICATIONS

Orthostatic hypotension

NURSING ACTIONS: Monitor blood pressure with first dose.

CLIENT EDUCATION: Change positions slowly. **Qs**

Anticholinergic effects

Dry mouth, blurred vision, photophobia, urinary hesitancy or retention, constipation, tachycardia

CLIENT EDUCATION
- Ways to minimize anticholinergic effects include the following.
  - Chewing sugarless gum
  - Sipping on water
  - Avoiding activities that require alertness
  - Wearing sunglasses when outdoors
  - Eating foods high in fiber
  - Participating in regular exercise
  - Increasing fluid intake to 2 to 3 L/day from beverages or food sources
  - Voiding just before taking medication
- Notify the provider if anticholinergic effects are intolerable.

Weight gain

NURSING ACTIONS: Monitor client weight.

CLIENT EDUCATION: Participate in regular exercise and follow a healthy, low-calorie diet.

Sedation

CLIENT EDUCATION
- Adverse effects usually diminish over time.
- Avoid activities that require alertness, such as driving, if sedation is excessive.
- Take medication at bedtime to minimize daytime sleepiness and to promote sleep.

Toxicity

Resulting in cholinergic blockade and cardiac toxicity evidenced by dysrhythmias, confusion, and agitation, followed by seizures and coma

NURSING ACTIONS
- Give clients who are acutely ill a 1-week supply of medication.
- Obtain baseline ECG.
- Monitor vital signs frequently.
- Monitor for toxicity and notify the provider if indications of toxicity occur.

Decreased seizure threshold

NURSING ACTIONS: Monitor clients who have seizure disorders.

Excessive sweating

NURSING ACTIONS
- Inform clients of this adverse effect.
- Assist with frequent linen changes.

CONTRAINDICATIONS/PRECAUTIONS

- Use cautiously in clients who have seizure disorders; diabetes mellitus; liver, kidney and respiratory disorders; or hyperthyroidism.
- Contraindicated in clients who have closed-angle glaucoma, and acute MI.

INTERACTIONS

Concurrent use of monoamine oxidase inhibitors (MAOIs) causes hypertension.
NURSING ACTIONS
- Avoid concurrent use.
- Do not use within 14 days of MAOIs.

Antihistamines and other anticholinergic agents have additive anticholinergic effects.
NURSING ACTIONS: Avoid concurrent use.

Tricyclic antidepressants (TCAs) block uptake of epinephrine and norepinephrine (direct-acting sympathomimetics) in the synaptic space, leading to decreased intensity of their effects.
NURSING ACTIONS: Avoid concurrent use.

TCAs inhibit uptake of ephedrine and amphetamine (indirect-acting sympathomimetics) and reduce their ability to get to the site of action in the nerve terminal, leading to decreased responses to these medications.
NURSING ACTIONS: Avoid concurrent use.

Alcohol, benzodiazepines, opioids, and antihistamines cause additive CNS depression when used concurrently.
CLIENT ACTIONS: Avoid concurrent use with CNS depressants.

NURSING ADMINISTRATION

- Instruct the client's parents to administer this medication as prescribed on a daily basis to establish therapeutic plasma levels.
- Assist with medication regimen compliance by informing clients and parents that it can take 2 to 3 weeks to experience therapeutic effects. Full therapeutic effects can take 2 to 3 months.
- Instruct clients and parents the importance of continuing therapy after improvement in manifestations. Sudden discontinuation of the medication can result in relapse.
- Take medication at bedtime to prevent daytime drowsiness.
- Give only 1 week worth of medication at a time for an acutely ill client. Tricyclics have high lethality in overdosage. Qs

NURSING EVALUATION OF MEDICATION EFFECTIVENESS

Depending on therapeutic intent, effectiveness is evidenced by the following.

For depression
- Verbalized improvement in mood
- Improved sleeping and eating habits
- Increased interaction with peers

For autism spectrum disorder: Decreased anger, agitation, and compulsive behavior

For ADHD
- Less hyperactivity
- Greater ability to pay attention

Alpha₂ adrenergic agonists

SELECT PROTOTYPE MEDICATION: Guanfacine

OTHER MEDICATION: Clonidine

PURPOSE

EXPECTED PHARMACOLOGICAL ACTION: The action of alpha$_2$ adrenergic agonists is not completely understood. However, they are known to activate presynaptic alpha$_2$ adrenergic receptors within the brain.

THERAPEUTIC USES: ADHD

COMPLICATIONS

CNS effects

Sedation, drowsiness, fatigue

NURSING ACTIONS: Monitor for these adverse effects and report their occurrence to the provider.

CLIENT EDUCATION: Avoid activities that require alertness.

Cardiovascular effects

Hypotension, bradycardia

NURSING ACTIONS: Monitor blood pressure and pulse especially during initial treatment.

CLIENT EDUCATION: Do not abruptly discontinue medication, which can cause rebound hypertension.

Weight gain

NURSING ACTIONS: Monitor client weight.

CLIENT EDUCATION: Participate in regular exercise and follow a healthy, well-balanced diet.

CONTRAINDICATIONS/PRECAUTIONS

- Extended-release clonidine is contraindicated for children younger than 6 years old.
- Use cautiously in clients who have cardiac disease, cerebrovascular disease, or kidney or liver impairment, and older adults.

INTERACTIONS

CNS depressants, including alcohol, can increase CNS effects.
NURSING ACTIONS: Avoid concurrent use.

Antihypertensives can worsen hypotension.
NURSING ACTIONS: Avoid concurrent use.

Foods with high-fat content increase guanfacine absorption.
CLIENT EDUCATION: Avoid taking medication with a high-fat meal. QEBP

NURSING ADMINISTRATION

- Monitor use of alcohol and CNS depressants, especially for adolescent clients.
- Instruct clients to not chew, crush, or split extended-release preparations.
- Monitor blood pressure and pulse at baseline, with initial treatment, and with each dosage change.
- Advise clients to avoid abrupt discontinuation of medication, which can result in rebound hypertension. Medication should be tapered according to a prescribed dosage schedule when discontinuing treatment.

NURSING EVALUATION OF MEDICATION EFFECTIVENESS

Depending on therapeutic intent, effectiveness is evidenced by improvement of manifestations of ADHD, such as increase in ability to focus and complete tasks, interact with peers, and manage impulsivity.

Antipsychotics: Atypical

SELECT PROTOTYPE MEDICATION: Risperidone

OTHER MEDICATIONS
- Olanzapine
- Quetiapine
- Aripiprazole

PURPOSE

EXPECTED PHARMACOLOGICAL ACTION

- Second-generation antipsychotic agents (risperidone, olanzapine, quetiapine) work mainly by blocking serotonin, and to a lesser degree, dopamine receptors. These medications also block receptors for norepinephrine, histamine, and acetylcholine.
- Aripiprazole is a third-generation antipsychotic and acts as a dopamine system stabilizer. It blocks dopamine and serotonin receptors, and also is a partial agonist at these receptors. Thus, net effects on receptor activity depend on how much dopamine and serotonin is present.

THERAPEUTIC USES

- Autism spectrum disorder
- Conduct disorder
- Posttraumatic stress disorder (PTSD)
- Relief of psychotic manifestations
- Intermittent explosive disorder

COMPLICATIONS

Diabetes mellitus

New onset of diabetes mellitus or loss of glucose control in clients who have diabetes

NURSING ACTIONS: Obtain baseline fasting blood glucose and monitor periodically throughout treatment.

CLIENT EDUCATION: Report indications such as increased thirst, urination, and appetite.

Weight gain

CLIENT EDUCATION: Follow a healthy, low-calorie diet; engage in regular exercise; and monitor weight gain.

Hypercholesterolemia

With increased risk for hypertension and other cardiovascular disease

NURSING ACTIONS: Obtain a baseline fasting lipid profile and then monitor every 6 months while treatment continues.

Orthostatic hypotension

NURSING ACTIONS: Monitor blood pressure with first dose.

CLIENT EDUCATION: Change positions slowly.

Anticholinergic effects

Urinary hesitancy or retention, dry mouth

NURSING ACTIONS: Monitor for these adverse effects and report their occurrence to the provider.

CLIENT EDUCATION: Use measures to relieve dry mouth, such as sipping fluids throughout the day.

Agitation, dizziness, sedation, sleep disruption

NURSING ACTIONS: Administer an alternative medication if prescribed.

CLIENT EDUCATION: Monitor for these adverse effects and report their occurrence to the provider. Avoid activities that require alertness until effects are known.

Mild extrapyramidal adverse effects, such as tremor

NURSING ACTIONS: Monitor for and instruct clients to recognize extrapyramidal adverse effects. These are usually dose-related.

Agranulocytosis, neutropenia

NURSING ACTIONS: Monitor WBC periodically.

CLIENT EDUCATION: Monitor and report manifestations of an infection, such as a sore throat. Qs

Hyperprolactinemia

NURSING ACTIONS: Monitor and report gynecomastia and amenorrhea.

CONTRAINDICATIONS/PRECAUTIONS

- Be aware of possible alcohol use in the adolescent client. Instruct clients to avoid the use of alcohol.
- Use cautiously in clients who have cardiovascular disease, seizures, dehydration, kidney/hepatic disease, or diabetes mellitus. Obtain a baseline fasting glucose for clients who have diabetes mellitus and monitor carefully.

INTERACTIONS

Alcohol, opioids, and antihistamines cause additive CNS depressant effects.
CLIENT EDUCATION
- Avoid alcohol and other medications that cause CNS depression.
- Avoid hazardous activities, such as driving.

By activating dopamine receptors, levodopa counteracts effects of antipsychotic agents.
NURSING ACTIONS: Avoid concurrent use of levodopa and other direct dopamine receptor agonists.

Tricyclic antidepressants, amiodarone, and clarithromycin prolong QT interval and thus increase the risk of cardiac dysrhythmias.
NURSING ACTIONS: Avoid concurrent use.

Barbiturates promote hepatic medication-metabolizing enzymes, thereby decreasing medication levels of quetiapine.
NURSING ACTIONS: Monitor medication effectiveness.

Medications that inhibit CYP3A4, such as fluconazole, inhibit hepatic medication-metabolizing enzymes, thereby increasing medication levels of aripiprazole, quetiapine, and ziprasidone.
NURSING ACTIONS: Monitor for adverse effects.

NURSING ADMINISTRATION

- Administer by oral or IM route.
  - Risperidone is available in an oral solution and quick-dissolving tablets for ease in administration.
  - Olanzapine is available in an orally disintegrating tablet for ease in administration.
- Advise clients that doses of medication are low initially and then gradually increased.

NURSING EVALUATION OF MEDICATION EFFECTIVENESS

Depending on therapeutic intent, effectiveness is evidenced by the following.

For autism spectrum disorder
- Reduction of hyperactivity and agitation
- Improvement in mood

For conduct disorder: decrease in aggressiveness

For ADHD: reduction in hyperactivity and impulsivity

Selective serotonin reuptake inhibitors

SELECT PROTOTYPE MEDICATION: Fluoxetine

OTHER MEDICATION: Sertraline

PURPOSE

EXPECTED PHARMACOLOGICAL ACTION: Selectively blocks the reuptake of serotonin, intensifying monoamine effects in the CNS.

THERAPEUTIC USES
- Autism spectrum disorder
- Obsessive compulsive disorder
- Major depressive disorder
- Intermittent explosive disorder
- Bulimia nervosa

COMPLICATIONS

Serotonin syndrome

Agitation, confusion, hallucinations

NURSING ACTIONS: Do not use within 14 days of MAOIs. Monitor for effects and discontinue.

Weight gain

CLIENT EDUCATION: Follow a healthy, low-calorie diet; engage in regular exercise; and monitor weight gain.

Withdrawal syndrome (dizziness, nausea, tremors)

NURSING ACTIONS: Do not discontinue abruptly.

Suicidal ideation

NURSING ACTIONS: Monitor and report any thoughts of suicide.

Extrapyramidal effects (ataxia, tremors)

NURSING ACTIONS: Monitor and report manifestations.

Dizziness, fatigue, insomnia, agitation

NURSING ACTIONS: Reduce dosage if needed.

CLIENT EDUCATION: Avoid activities that require alertness until effects are known.

Sexual dysfunction (impotence, decreased libido)

CLIENT EDUCATION: This is a possible adverse effect.

Dysrhythmias

NURSING ACTIONS: Monitor for dysrhythmias. Reduce dosage as needed.

CONTRAINDICATIONS/PRECAUTIONS

- Pregnancy Risk Category C: Can cause abstinence syndrome and pulmonary hypertension in the newborn.
- Use cautiously in clients who are breastfeeding or who have narrow-angle glaucoma.

INTERACTIONS

Concurrent use of MAOIs and other medications that can cause serotonin syndrome (SNRIs, buspirone, phenothiazines) increases the risk for serotonin syndrome.
NURSING ACTIONS
- Avoid concurrent use.
- Do not use within 14 days of MAOIs.

Elevation of plasma levels of TCAs and lithium
NURSING ACTIONS
- Avoid concurrent use.
- Monitor for toxicity.

Antiplatelet medications and anticoagulants increase risk for bleeding.
NURSING ACTIONS
- Avoid concurrent use.
- Monitor for bleeding.

NURSING ADMINISTRATION

- Administer orally with or without meals.
- Therapeutic effects can take 1 to 4 weeks.
- Notify provider if pregnancy is suspected.

NURSING EVALUATION OF MEDICATION EFFECTIVENESS

Depending on therapeutic intent, effectiveness is evidenced by the following.
- Improvement in mood, decreased manifestations of obsessive compulsive disorder, decrease in aggressiveness
- **For depression**
  - Verbalized improvement in mood
  - Improved sleeping and eating habits
  - Increased interaction with peers
- **For autism spectrum disorder, intermittent explosive disorder:** Decreased anger, agitation, and compulsive behavior

Application Exercises

1. A nurse is reinforcing teaching with the parents of a child who has autism spectrum disorder and a new prescription for desipramine. The nurse should instruct the parents that which of the following adverse effects is the priority to report to the provider?

    A. Constipation

    B. Suicidal thoughts

    C. Photophobia

    D. Dry mouth

2. A nurse is reinforcing teaching with an adolescent client who has obsessive-compulsive disorder and a new prescription for clomipramine. Which of the following instructions should the nurse include to minimize an adverse effect of his medication?

    A. Wear sunglasses when outdoors.

    B. Check your temperature daily.

    C. Take this medication in the morning.

    D. Add extra calories to your diet.

3. A nurse is caring for a school-age child who has a new prescription for atomoxetine. For which of the following adverse effects should the nurse monitor?

    A. Kidney toxicity

    B. Liver damage

    C. Seizure activity

    D. Adrenal insufficiency

4. A nurse is reinforcing teaching with the parents of a school-age child who has ADHD about methylphenidate. Which of the following instructions should the nurse include?

    A. Crush the tablets and mix with fruit juice.

    B. Administer the last dose before 4 p.m.

    C. Expect the child to gain weight while taking the medication.

    D. Administer the medication at least 2 hr before meals.

5. A nurse is reinforcing teaching with a school-age child who has ADHD and his parents about lisdexamfetamine. Which of the following information should the nurse include? (Select all that apply.)

    A. An adverse effect of this medication is CNS stimulation.

    B. Administer the medication 1 hr before bedtime.

    C. Monitor blood pressure while taking this medication.

    D. Therapeutic effects of this medication will take 1 to 3 weeks to fully develop.

    E. This medication raises the levels of dopamine in the brain.

PRACTICE Active Learning Scenario

A nurse in a pediatric mental health clinic is caring for a client who has a new prescription for risperidone for the treatment of conduct disorder. Use the ATI Active Learning Template: Medication to complete this item.

COMPLICATIONS: Identify at least four adverse effects of this medication.

NURSING INTERVENTIONS: Identify at least four nursing interventions to prevent or minimize the adverse effects of this medication.

Application Exercises Key

1. A. The client is at risk for constipation due to the anticholinergic effects of desipramine. The client should increase fluid intake to reduce the risk of constipation. However, another adverse effect is the priority.

   B. **CORRECT:** The greatest risk to this client is injury from a suicide attempt. Desipramine can cause suicidal thoughts and behaviors, which puts the client at risk. The parents should monitor and report any indication of increased depression or thoughts of suicidal behavior.

   C. The client is at risk for photophobia due to the anticholinergic effects of desipramine. The client should wear sunglasses when exposed to sunlight. However, another adverse effect is the priority.

   D. The client is at risk for dry mouth because of the anticholinergic effects of desipramine. The client should increase fluids and use hard candy to reduce dry mouth. However, another adverse effect is the priority.

   Ⓝ *NCLEX® Connection: Pharmacological Therapies, Adverse Effects/ Contraindications/Side Effects/Interactions*

2. A. **CORRECT:** Wearing sunglasses when outdoors will decrease photophobia, an anticholinergic effect associated with TCA use.

   B. Checking the client's temperature daily is not necessary while taking a TCA.

   C. The client should take this medication at bedtime to prevent daytime sleepiness.

   D. Following a low-calorie diet plan will help prevent weight gain, an adverse effect of TCAs.

   Ⓝ *NCLEX® Connection: Pharmacological Therapies, Expected Actions/Outcomes*

3. A. Atomoxetine can cause urinary retention but does not cause kidney toxicity.

   B. **CORRECT:** Liver damage is an adverse effect of atomoxetine. Monitor for manifestations such as jaundice, upper abdominal tenderness, darkening of urine, and elevated liver enzymes.

   C. Bupropion increases seizure risk at high dosages. Seizure activity is not an adverse effect of atomoxetine.

   D. Atomoxetine can cause suicidal ideation and mood swings. Adrenal insufficiency is not an adverse effect of atomoxetine.

   Ⓝ *NCLEX® Connection: Pharmacological Therapies, Adverse Effects/ Contraindications/Side Effects/Interactions*

4. A. The nurse should instruct the parents to administer the tablets whole and not crush the tablets or allow the child to chew them.

   B. **CORRECT:** The nurse should instruct the parents to administer the last dose of methylphenidate before 4 p.m. to minimize insomnia.

   C. The nurse should instruct the parents that the child can have a decreased appetite and weight loss while taking methylphenidate.

   D. The nurse should instruct the parents to administer methylphenidate with or immediately following meals to decrease GI upset.

   Ⓝ *NCLEX® Connection: Pharmacological Therapies, Expected Actions/Outcomes*

5. A. **CORRECT:** An adverse effect of lisdexamfetamine is CNS stimulation, such as insomnia and restlessness.

   B. Administer lisdexamfetamine daily in the morning to reduce insomnia.

   C. **CORRECT:** The nurse should instruct the client to monitor blood pressure due to potential cardiovascular effects of lisdexamfetamine.

   D. Therapeutic effects of lisdexamfetamine begin immediately and last 10 to 12 hr.

   E. **CORRECT:** Lisdexamfetamine, a CNS stimulant, works by raising the levels of norepinephrine and dopamine in the CNS.

   Ⓝ *NCLEX® Connection: Pharmacological Therapies, Expected Actions/Outcomes*

PRACTICE Answer

Using the ATI Active Learning Template: Medication

COMPLICATIONS

- New onset of diabetes mellitus or loss of glucose control in clients who have diabetes
- Weight gain
- Hypercholesterolemia
- Orthostatic hypotension
- Anticholinergic effects (urinary hesitancy or retention, dry mouth)
- Agitation
- Dizziness
- Sedation
- Sleep disruption
- Tremors
- Agranulocytosis, neutropenia
- Hyperprolactinemia

NURSING INTERVENTIONS

- Obtain fasting blood glucose prior to and periodically throughout treatment.
- Instruct the client to report indications of diabetes mellitus, including increased thirst, urination, and appetite.
- Advise clients to follow a healthy, low-calorie diet.
- Recommend regular exercise.
- Monitor weight throughout treatment.
- Monitor fasting lipid profile every 6 months throughout treatment.
- Monitor blood pressure with first dose and instruct client to change positions slowly.
- Encourage the client to sip fluids throughout the day.
- Monitor and report manifestations of an infection, such as a sore throat.
- Monitor and report gynecomastia and amenorrhea.

Ⓝ *NCLEX® Connection: Pharmacological and Parenteral Therapies, Adverse Effects/ Contraindications/Side Effects/Interactions*

CHAPTER 11 *Substance Use Disorders*

Abstinence syndrome occurs when clients abruptly withdraw from a substance to which they are physically dependent.

Clients who have a substance use disorder can experience tolerance and withdrawal. Tolerance requires increased amounts of the substance to achieve the desired effect. Withdrawal is physiological manifestations that occur when the concentration of the substance in the client's bloodstream declines.

Withdrawing from a substance that has the potential to cause physical dependence can cause abstinence syndrome. The client can experience distressing manifestations that can lead to coma and death.

Major substances associated with substance use disorder include alcohol, caffeine, cannabis, hallucinogens, inhalants, opioids, sedatives/hypnotics/anxiolytics, stimulants, tobacco, and other or unknown substances (anabolic steroids, betel nut, unidentified black market substances).

Substance withdrawal depends on the substance and can produce a variety of manifestations (gastrointestinal distress, neurological and behavioral changes, cardiovascular changes, seizures).

Medications to support withdrawal/abstinence from alcohol

- Effects of withdrawal can start anywhere from 4 to 72 hr after the last intake of alcohol depending on the client's frequency and amount of alcohol intake. These withdrawal effects can continue 5 to 7 days.
- Manifestations
  - Nausea
  - Vomiting
  - Tremors
  - Restlessness and inability to sleep
  - Depressed mood or irritability
  - Increased heart rate, blood pressure, respiratory rate, and temperature
  - Diaphoresis
  - Tonic-clonic seizures
  - Illusions
- Alcohol withdrawal delirium can occur 2 to 3 days after cessation of alcohol, and is considered a medical emergency. Findings include severe disorientation, psychotic manifestations (auditory or visual hallucinations), severe hypertension, and cardiac dysrhythmias that can progress to death. Qs

WITHDRAWAL

Benzodiazepines

First-line treatment for treatment of alcohol withdrawal

EXAMPLES: Chlordiazepoxide, diazepam, lorazepam, clorazepate, oxazepam

INTENDED EFFECTS
- Maintenance of vital signs within expected limits
- Decrease in the risk of seizures
- Decrease in the intensity of withdrawal manifestations
- Substitution therapy during alcohol withdrawal

NURSING ACTIONS
- Administer around the clock or PRN.
- Obtain baseline vital signs.
- Monitor vital signs and neurological status on an ongoing basis.
- Maintain seizure precautions.

Adjunct medications to treatment with benzodiazepines

Effectiveness is minimal if used as monotherapy for the management of alcohol withdrawal. To achieve intended effects, they should be used as an adjunct to benzodiazepines.

EXAMPLES: Carbamazepine, clonidine, propranolol, atenolol

INTENDED EFFECTS
- Decrease in seizures and withdrawal manifestations: carbamazepine
- Depression of autonomic response (decrease in blood pressure, heart rate): clonidine, propranolol, atenolol
- Decrease in craving: propranolol, atenolol

NURSING ACTIONS
- Maintain seizure precautions.
- Obtain baseline vital signs, and continue to monitor on an ongoing basis.
- Check heart rate prior to administration of propranolol and withhold if less than 60/min.

ABSTINENCE MAINTENANCE (FOLLOWING WITHDRAWAL)

Disulfiram

INTENDED EFFECTS
- Disulfiram is a daily oral medication that is a type of aversion (behavioral) therapy.
- Disulfiram used concurrently with alcohol causes acetaldehyde syndrome.
  - Manifestations include nausea, vomiting, weakness, flushing, headaches, sweating, chest pain, palpitations, and hypotension.
  - Acetaldehyde syndrome can progress to respiratory depression, cardiovascular suppression, seizures, and death.

NURSING ACTIONS
- Inform clients of the dangers and potentially fatal reaction of drinking any alcohol.
- Advise clients to avoid any products that contain alcohol (cough syrups, sauces, mouthwash, aftershave lotion, colognes, hand sanitizer).
- Monitor liver function tests to detect hepatotoxicity.
- Encourage clients to wear a medical alert bracelet.
- Encourage clients to participate in a 12-step self-help program.
- Advise clients that the potential for acetaldehyde syndrome with alcohol ingestion persists for 2 weeks following discontinuation of disulfiram.
- Inform the client of the need to wait at least 12 hr after the last drink of alcohol before taking the initial dose of disulfiram.

Naltrexone

- Clients must abstain from alcohol before starting naltrexone.
- Adverse effects include nausea, sedation, headache, and anxiety.

INTENDED EFFECTS: Naltrexone is a pure opioid antagonist that suppresses the craving and pleasurable effects of alcohol (also used for opioid withdrawal).

NURSING ACTIONS
- Assist in obtaining an accurate history to determine whether clients are also dependent on opioids. Concurrent use of naltrexone and opiates results in withdrawal reactions. Qs
- Advise clients to take the medication with meals to decrease gastrointestinal distress.
- Suggest monthly IM injections of depot naltrexone for clients who have difficulty adhering to an oral treatment regimen.

Acamprosate

INTENDED EFFECTS: Acamprosate decreases unpleasant effects resulting from abstinence (dysphoria, anxiety, restlessness).

CLIENT EDUCATION
- Diarrhea can result.
- Maintain adequate fluid intake, and receive adequate rest.
- Take medication three times per day with meals.
- Avoid use in pregnancy.

Medications to support withdrawal/abstinence from opioids

Characteristic withdrawal syndrome occurs within 1 hr to several days after cessation of substance use.
- Findings include agitation, insomnia, flu-like manifestations, rhinorrhea, yawning, sweating, piloerection, abdominal cramping, and diarrhea.
- Manifestations are non–life-threatening, although suicidal ideation can occur.

Methadone

INTENDED EFFECTS
- Methadone is an oral opioid agonist used for substitution therapy (methadone substitution) to replace the opioid to which the client has a physical dependence.
  - Methadone substitution prevents abstinence syndrome from occurring and removes the need for the client to obtain illegal substances.
  - Dependence is transferred from the illegal opioid to methadone.
  - Once the client is effectively substituting methadone for the opioid, the dose of methadone is tapered gradually.

- Methadone is also used for withdrawal, long-term maintenance, and suppressive therapy.
  - In suppressive therapy, the client is given gradually increasing doses of methadone to promote tolerance. Tolerance to high doses of methadone results in a lack of pleasurable effects from opioids resulting in the client's decreased desire to use opioids.

NURSING ACTIONS
- Observe the client to make sure the dosage is adequate to suppress withdrawal. (Client's report of prior opiate usage can be unreliable.)
- Inform clients that the methadone dose must be slowly tapered to produce a withdrawal with minimal adverse effects.
- Encourage clients to participate in a 12-step self-help program. Qpcc
- Inform clients that medication must be administered from an approved treatment center.

Clonidine

INTENDED EFFECTS
- Clonidine assists with withdrawal effects related to autonomic hyperactivity (diarrhea, nausea, vomiting).
- Clonidine therapy does not reduce the craving for opioids.

NURSING ACTIONS
- Obtain baseline vital signs.
- Advise clients to avoid activities that require mental alertness until drowsiness subsides.
- Encourage clients to chew sugarless gum or suck on hard candy, as well as sip small amounts of water or suck on ice chips to treat dry mouth.
- Assist in identifying clients who are at risk for overuse of clonidine. If taken in high doses, clonidine can cause euphoria and hallucinations. Some clients combine clonidine with benzodiazepines, opioids, or cocaine to achieve increased effects of these substances.

Buprenorphine

INTENDED EFFECTS
- Buprenorphine is an agonist-antagonist opioid used for withdrawal and maintenance.
- It is substituted for the opioid to which the client has a physical dependence and prevents withdrawal manifestations.
- It decreases feelings of craving and can be effective in maintaining adherence.
- It is considered safer than methadone due to a decreased risk for respiratory depression and potential for dependence.
- Unlike methadone, a primary care provider can prescribe and dispense buprenorphine.
- Buprenorphine is available alone or combined with naloxone.

NURSING ACTIONS: Administer sublingually (tablets or films).

Medications to support withdrawal/abstinence from nicotine

Abstinence syndrome is evidenced by irritability, nervousness, restlessness, insomnia, and difficulty concentrating.

Bupropion

INTENDED EFFECTS: Decreases nicotine craving and manifestations of withdrawal

NURSING ACTIONS
- To treat dry mouth, encourage clients to chew sugarless gum or suck on hard candy as well as sip small amounts of water or suck on ice chips.
- Advise clients to avoid caffeine and other CNS stimulants to control insomnia and agitation
- Avoid use in clients who have an increased risk for seizures.
- Advise clients that bupropion can cause weight loss, thus limiting weight gain related to smoking cessation.

Nicotine replacement therapy

INTENDED EFFECTS
- These nicotine replacements are pharmaceutical product substitutes for the nicotine in cigarettes or chewing tobacco.
- The use of nicotine replacement therapy approximately doubles the success rate of smoking cessation.

CLIENT EDUCATION
- Avoid using any nicotine products while pregnant or breastfeeding.
- **Nicotine lozenge**
  - Allow the lozenge to slowly dissolve in the mouth (20 to 30 min).
  - Do not chew or swallow the lozenge.
  - Avoid oral intake 15 min prior to or during lozenge use.
  - Follow product directions for dosage strength and recommended titration.
  - Limit lozenge use to five in a 6 hr period or a maximum of 20/day.
  - Monitor for adverse effects which include dyspepsia, irritation of the mouth, nausea, and hiccups.
  - Ask the client when the first cigarette is smoked each day. Higher dosages are indicated for clients who smoke within 30 min of waking.
- **Nicotine gum**
  - Use of nicotine gum is not recommended for longer than 6 months.
  - Chew gum slowly and intermittently over 30 min.
  - Avoid eating or drinking 15 min prior to and while chewing the gum.
  - Monitor for adverse effects (soreness of the throat and mouth, jaw discomfort, hiccups, belching).
  - Ask the client how many cigarettes are smoked each day. Dosing is based on total cigarettes smoked per day.

- **Nicotine patch**
  - Clients should apply a nicotine patch to an area of clean, dry, and hair-free skin each day.
  - Instruct the client to apply patch to upper body or upper arm.
  - Instruct the client to change the site each day and to avoid reusing the site for at least 1 week.
  - Advise clients to avoid using any nicotine products while the patch is on.
  - Follow product directions for dosage times.
  - Advise clients that nicotine patches can be purchased without a prescription.
  - Reinforce recommended dosages with the client. Dosing typically begins with a larger patch (higher amounts of nicotine) and gradually decreases to a smaller patch (lower amounts of nicotine).
  - Remove the patch prior to an MRI scan, and replace when the scan is completed.
  - Adverse effects can include mild erythema, itching, and burning sensation underneath the patch
  - Advise clients to stop using patches and notify the provider if severe local skin reactions occur.
- **Nicotine nasal spray**
  - Provides pleasurable effects of smoking due to rapid rise of nicotine in the client's blood level.
  - One spray in each nostril delivers the amount of nicotine in one cigarette.
  - Advise client to follow product instructions for dosage frequency.
  - Monitor for adverse effects (sneezing, rhinitis, irritation of the nasal passages and throat, coughing, watery eyes).
  - Not recommended for clients who have disorders affecting the upper respiratory system (chronic sinus problems, allergies, asthma).
- **Nicotine inhaler**
  - Simulates smoking by puffing on the inhaler, which delivers nicotine.
  - Contains menthol, which creates sensation in the back of the throat similar to smoking.
  - Advise clients to gradually taper use over 2 to 3 months and then discontinue. Qᴱᴮᴾ
  - Avoid in clients who have asthma.
  - Monitor for adverse effects (throat irritation and burning sensation of the mouth, dyspepsia, coughing).

Varenicline

INTENDED EFFECTS

- Varenicline is a nicotinic receptor agonist that promotes the release of dopamine to simulate the pleasurable effects of nicotine.
- Reduces cravings for nicotine as well as the severity of withdrawal manifestations.
- Reduces the incidence of relapse by blocking the desired effects of nicotine.

NURSING ACTIONS

- Instruct clients to take medication after a meal.
- Monitor blood pressure during treatment.
- Monitor clients who have diabetes mellitus for loss of glycemic control.
- Follow instructions for titration to minimize adverse effects.
- Advise clients to notify the provider of nausea, vomiting, insomnia, new-onset depression, or suicidal thoughts.
- Can cause neuropsychiatric effects (unpredictable behavior, mood changes, and thoughts of suicide).
- Due to potential adverse effects, varenicline is banned for use in clients who are commercial truck or bus drivers, air traffic controllers, or airplane pilots. Qs

---

For all medication classifications in this chapter.

NURSING EVALUATION OF MEDICATION EFFECTIVENESS

Depending on therapeutic intent, effectiveness is evidenced by the following.
- Absence of injury
- Decreased cravings for substance
- Abstinence from substance
- Regular attendance at self-help group
- Improved coping skills to replace substance usage

Application Exercises

1. A nurse is reinforcing teaching for a client who is withdrawing from alcohol and has a new prescription for propranolol. Which of the following information should the nurse include?

   A. Increases the risk for seizure activity

   B. Provides a form of aversion therapy

   C. Decreases cravings

   D. Results in mild hypertension

2. A nurse is assisting with a staff education session to discuss medications used during the care of a client experiencing alcohol withdrawal. Which of the following medications should the nurse include in the discussion? (Select all that apply.)

   A. Lorazepam

   B. Diazepam

   C. Disulfiram

   D. Naltrexone

   E. Acamprosate

3. A nurse is reinforcing teaching for a client who has a new prescription for clonidine to assist with maintenance of abstinence from opioids. The nurse should instruct the client to monitor for which of the following adverse effects?

   A. Diarrhea

   B. Dry mouth

   C. Insomnia

   D. Hypertension

4. A nurse is reinforcing teaching with a female client who has tobacco use disorder about nicotine replacement therapy. Which of the following statements indicates that the client understands the teaching?

   A. "I should avoid eating right before I chew a piece of nicotine gum."

   B. "I will need to stop using the nicotine gum after 1 year."

   C. "I know that nicotine gum is a safe alternative to smoking if I become pregnant."

   D. "I must chew the nicotine gum quickly for about 15 minutes."

5. A nurse in an acute mental health facility is assisting with the care of a client who is experiencing withdrawal from opioid use and has a new prescription for clonidine. Which of the following actions should the nurse identify as the priority?

   A. Administer clonidine on the prescribed schedule.

   B. Provide ice chips at the client's bedside.

   C. Educate the client on the effects of clonidine.

   D. Obtain baseline vital signs.

PRACTICE Active Learning Scenario

A nurse is reinforcing teaching with a client who has tobacco use disorder about a new prescription for varenicline to promote smoking cessation. Use the ATI Active Learning Template: Medication to complete this item.

EXPECTED PHARMACOLOGICAL ACTION

THERAPEUTIC USES

COMPLICATIONS: Identify at least three adverse effects.

CLIENT EDUCATION: Identify at least two teaching points.

EVALUATION OF MEDICATION EFFECTIVENESS: Identify a client outcome to indicate medication effectiveness.

Application Exercises Key

1. A. Seizure activity is a potential effect of alcohol withdrawal. However, propranolol does not increase this risk.

   B. Disulfiram, rather than propranolol, provides a form of aversion therapy.

   C. **CORRECT:** Propranolol is an adjunct medication used during withdrawal to decrease the client's craving for alcohol.

   D. Propranolol is an antihypertensive medication that can result in hypotension rather than hypertension.

   Ⓝ *NCLEX® Connection: Pharmacological Therapies, Expected Actions/Outcomes*

2. A. **CORRECT:** Lorazepam is a benzodiazepine used during alcohol withdrawal to decrease anxiety and reduce the risk for seizures.

   B. **CORRECT:** Diazepam is a benzodiazepine used during alcohol withdrawal to decrease anxiety and reduce the risk for seizures.

   C. Disulfiram is administered to assist the client in maintaining abstinence from alcohol following withdrawal.

   D. Naltrexone is administered to assist the client in maintaining abstinence from alcohol following withdrawal.

   E. Acamprosate decreases unpleasant effects, such as anxiety or restlessness, resulting from abstinence.

   Ⓝ *NCLEX® Connection: Pharmacological Therapies, Expected Actions/Outcomes*

3. A. Constipation, rather than diarrhea, is a common adverse effect associated with clonidine use.

   B. **CORRECT:** Dry mouth is a common adverse effect associated with clonidine use.

   C. Sedation, rather than insomnia, is a common adverse effect associated with clonidine use.

   D. Clonidine is more likely to cause hypotension than hypertension.

   Ⓝ *NCLEX® Connection: Pharmacological Therapies, Expected Actions/Outcomes*

4. A. **CORRECT:** The client should avoid eating or drinking 15 min prior to and while chewing the nicotine gum.

   B. The client should not use nicotine gum for longer than 6 months.

   C. The client should avoid all nicotine products, including nicotine gum, while pregnant or breastfeeding.

   D. The client should chew the nicotine gum slowly and intermittently over 30 min.

   Ⓝ *NCLEX® Connection: Pharmacological Therapies, Expected Actions/Outcomes*

5. A. The nurse should administer clonidine according to the schedule prescribed to maintain therapeutic medication levels. However, there is another action the nurse should take first.

   B. The nurse should provide the client with ice chips because clonidine can cause the client to have a dry mouth. However, there is another action the nurse should take first.

   C. The nurse should reinforce teaching with the client as needed to ensure understanding about clonidine's therapeutic effects, adverse effects, and administration. However, there is another action the nurse should take first.

   D. **CORRECT:** The first action the nurse should take using the nursing process is to collect data from the client. Therefore, the nurse should first obtain baseline vital signs prior to administering the medication.

   Ⓝ *NCLEX® Connection: Pharmacological Therapies, Expected Actions/Outcomes*

PRACTICE Answer

Using the ATI Active Learning Template: Medication

EXPECTED PHARMACOLOGICAL ACTION: Varenicline is a nicotinic receptor agonist that promotes the release of dopamine to simulate the pleasurable effects of nicotine.

THERAPEUTIC USES: Varenicline is indicated to reduce nicotine cravings and block the desired effects of nicotine in clients who have tobacco use disorder.

COMPLICATIONS
- New-onset hypertension
- Loss of glycemic control in clients who have diabetes mellitus
- Nausea
- Vomiting
- Insomnia
- New-onset depression
- Suicidal thoughts

CLIENT EDUCATION
- Clients who are commercial truck or bus drivers, airplane pilots, or air traffic controllers should not take varenicline.
- Take medication after a meal.
- Titrate as prescribed to minimize adverse effects.
- Notify the provider if adverse effects occur.

EVALUATION OF MEDICATION EFFECTIVENESS
- The client will maintain smoking cessation.
- The client will report reduced cravings for nicotine.

Ⓝ *NCLEX® Connection: Pharmacological and Parenteral Therapies, Medication Administration*

UNIT 2   MEDICATIONS AFFECTING THE NERVOUS SYSTEM

CHAPTER 12 *Chronic Neurologic Disorders*

Chronic neurologic disorders include Parkinson's disease (PD) and seizure disorders. Medications for treating chronic neurologic disorders help manage manifestations and improve quality of life.

Cholinesterase inhibitors

Cholinesterase inhibitors are anticholinesterase agents and have two categories.

Irreversible inhibitors (echothiophate): Therapeutic effects have a long duration and primarily treat glaucoma. Pralidoxime reverses the effects of echothiophate.

Reversible inhibitors: Therapeutic effects have a moderate duration (2 to 4 hr). They treat Alzheimer's disease and PD, and reverse the effects of nondepolarizing neuromuscular blocking agents.

SELECT PROTOTYPE MEDICATION: Neostigmine (reversible inhibitor)

OTHER MEDICATIONS
- Physostigmine
- Edrophonium
- Donepezil

PURPOSE

EXPECTED PHARMACOLOGICAL ACTION

Cholinesterase inhibitors prevent the enzyme cholinesterase from inactivating acetylcholine (ACh), thereby increasing the amount of ACh available at receptor sites. Transmission of nerve impulses increases at all sites responding to ACh as a transmitter.

THERAPEUTIC USES

12.1 Therapeutic uses for cholinesterase inhibitors	NEOSTIGMINE	ECHOTHIOPHATE	PHYSOSTIGMINE	EDROPHONIUM	DONEPEZIL
Reversal of muscarinic antagonists			✓		
Treatment of myasthenia gravis	✓				
Treatment of glaucoma			✓		
Reversal of nondepolarizing neuromuscular blocking agents	✓			✓	
Treatment of Alzheimer's disease					✓
Treatment of Parkinson's disease					✓

COMPLICATIONS

Excessive muscarinic stimulation

Increased gastrointestinal (GI) motility, increased GI secretions, diaphoresis, increased salivation, bradycardia, urinary urgency, miosis, spasm of accommodation (focusing of the lens for near vision)

NURSING ACTIONS
- Inform clients of potential adverse effects. If effects become intolerable, instruct them to notify the provider.
- Treat severe adverse effects with atropine.

Cholinergic crisis

Excessive muscarinic stimulation and respiratory depression from neuromuscular blockade

NURSING ACTIONS
- Provide respiratory support through mechanical ventilation and oxygen, and administer atropine to reverse muscarinic stimulation.
- Have resuscitation equipment available. Qs

CONTRAINDICATIONS/PRECAUTIONS

- Pregnancy Risk Category C
- Obstruction of the GI and renal systems
- Use cautiously with clients who have seizure disorders, hyperthyroidism, peptic ulcer disease, asthma, bradycardia, or hypotension.

INTERACTIONS

Atropine counteracts the effects of cholinesterase inhibitors.
- Atropine treats toxicity from cholinesterase inhibitors (increased muscarinic stimulation and respiratory depression).
- NURSING ACTIONS: Monitor clients closely and assist with mechanical ventilation until they have regained full muscle function.

Neostigmine and edrophonium reverse the neuromuscular blockade that nondepolarizing neuromuscular blocking agents cause after surgical procedures and overdose.
NURSING ACTIONS: Monitor for the return of respiratory function. Support respiratory function as necessary. When treating an overdose, assist with mechanical ventilation until the return of full muscle function.

Succinylcholine is a depolarizing short-acting neuromuscular blocker for use during surgical procedures.
- Cholinesterase inhibitors increase the neuromuscular blockage of depolarizing neuromuscular blockers.
- NURSING ACTIONS: Avoid concurrent use.

NURSING ADMINISTRATION

- Neostigmine dosing is PO, IM, IV, or subcutaneous.
- Neostigmine bromide is a PO tablet; neostigmine methylsulfate is an injectable preparation.
- Inform clients that dosage is very individual, starts at very low doses, and requires titration until they achieve desirable muscle function.
- Advise clients to wear a medical alert bracelet.

NURSING EVALUATION OF MEDICATION EFFECTIVENESS

Indications of effectiveness include the following.
- Recovery of muscle strength
- Improved cognition
- Slow disease progression

Anti-Parkinson's medications

SELECT PROTOTYPE MEDICATIONS

Dopaminergic medications promote dopamine synthesis, activate dopamine receptors, prevent dopamine breakdown, promote dopamine release, or block the degradation of levodopa.
- **A dopamine synthesis medication** (levodopa) is available in combination with a dopamine agonist (carbidopa) as levodopa/carbidopa.
  - Levodopa crosses the blood-brain barrier, whereas dopamine alone cannot cross this barrier and has a very short half-life. Dopaminergic nerve terminals take up levodopa, convert it to dopamine (DA), and, once in the synaptic space, cause stimulation of DA receptors.
  - Carbidopa augments levodopa by decreasing the amount of levodopa that undergoes conversion to DA in the intestine and periphery. This results in larger amounts of levodopa reaching the CNS.

Dopamine agonists activate dopamine receptors: pramipexole, bromocriptine, and ropinirole, a first-line supplement to levodopa. Apomorphine is a rescue medication for "off" times.
- Catecholamine-O-methyltransferase (COMT) inhibitors enhance the effect of levodopa by blocking its breakdown: entacapone, tolcapone
- Monoamine oxidase-B (MAO-B) prevents dopamine breakdown: selegiline, rasagiline
- Dopamine releaser prevents dopamine reuptake: amantadine
- Anticholinergic medications block the muscarinic receptors, which assist in maintaining balance between dopamine and acetylcholine receptors in the brain.
- Dopamine agonists, COMT inhibitors, MAO-B inhibitors, dopamine releasers, and centrally acting anticholinergic antagonists concurrently increase the beneficial effects of levodopa/carbidopa.

PURPOSE

EXPECTED PHARMACOLOGICAL ACTION

These medications do not halt the progression of PD. However, they do offer relief from dyskinesias (bradykinesia, resting tremors, muscle rigidity) and an increase in the ability to perform ADLs by maintaining the balance between dopamine and acetylcholine in the extrapyramidal system.

THERAPEUTIC USES

Levodopa/carbidopa

- Most effective for PD treatment, but the beneficial effects diminish by the end of year 5.
- "Wearing off" times occur at the end of the dose cycle or can occur at any time, even at high dose levels, lasting minutes to several hours.
- Full therapeutic effects can take several months to develop.

Dopamine agonists

Pramipexole, ropinirole, apomorphine
- Monotherapy in early-stage PD and in conjunction with levodopa/carbidopa in late-stage PD to allow for lower dosages of levodopa/carbidopa
- More often for younger clients who are better able to tolerate daytime drowsiness and postural hypotension

Bromocriptine, an ergot derivative, has poor tolerance and a high incidence of valvular heart injury.

Dopamine releaser

Amantadine releases dopamine stores from the neurons, prevents dopamine reuptake, and can block cholinergic and glutamate receptors.

COMT inhibitors

Beneficial in combination with levodopa/carbidopa to inhibit the metabolism of levodopa in the intestines and peripheral tissues: entacapone, tolcapone

MAO-B inhibitors

First-line medications in combination with levodopa/carbidopa for decreasing the "wear-off" effect

Selegiline can preserve the dopamine levodopa produces and prolong the effects of levodopa but only up to 1 or 2 years.

Rasagiline preserves dopamine in the brain and does not undergo the conversion into amphetamine or methamphetamine that selegiline does.

Centrally acting anticholinergics

Centrally acting anticholinergic antagonists diminish cholinergic effects (neuron excitability) due to decreased dopamine: benztropine, trihexyphenidyl

ADVERSE EFFECTS

Levodopa/carbidopa

Usually dose-dependent

Nausea, vomiting, drowsiness
NURSING ACTIONS
- Administer with food, in small doses, at the start of treatment and if GI effects occur.
- Avoid administering with foods high in protein because they delay absorption and reduce the therapeutic effect, thus causing an "off" episode.
- Advise clients to eat protein in several small portions during the day.
- Advise clients to avoid vitamin preparations and foods containing pyridoxine (wheat germ, green vegetables, bananas, whole-grain cereals, liver, legumes), which reduce the therapeutic effects of levodopa/carbidopa.
- Additional carbidopa can help alleviate nausea and vomiting.

Dyskinesias (head bobbing, tics, grimacing, tremors)
- The provider might have to decrease the dosage, but the decrease can result in resumption of PD manifestations.
- Surgical or electrical stimulation can help.

NURSING ACTIONS: Administer amantadine (releases and uptakes DA) to decrease dyskinesias.

Orthostatic (postural) hypotension
NURSING ACTIONS
- Monitor blood pressure.
- Instruct clients about indications of orthostatic hypotension (lightheadedness, dizziness) and to avoid sudden changes of position.

Cardiovascular effects from beta$_1$ stimulation
- Tachycardia, palpitations, dysrhythmias
- NURSING ACTIONS
  - Monitor vital signs.
  - Monitor ECG.
  - Notify the provider if manifestations occur.
  - Use cautiously with clients who have cardiovascular disorders.

Psychosis
- Visual hallucinations, nightmares, paranoid ideation
- NURSING ACTIONS
  - Administer second-generation antipsychotic medications, such as clozapine, to decrease psychotic effects without increasing the manifestations of PD.
  - Second-generation antipsychotic medications do not block dopamine receptors in the striatum.
  - Avoid concurrent use of conventional antipsychotic agents, such as haloperidol, which block dopamine receptors.
  - Check for the concurrent use of antidepressant MAOI medications, which can result in hypertensive crisis. Do not use levodopa/carbidopa within 2 weeks of MAOI use.

Discoloration of sweat and urine
CLIENT EDUCATION: This finding is harmless.

Activation of malignant melanoma
Do not administer this medication to clients who have skin lesions the provider has not diagnosed.

Dopamine agonists

Sudden inability to stay awake
CLIENT EDUCATION: Notify the provider immediately if this occurs.

Daytime sleepiness
CLIENT EDUCATION
- There is a potential for drowsiness. Avoid activities that require alertness.
- Avoid other CNS depressants such as alcohol.

Orthostatic hypotension
NURSING ACTIONS: Inform clients about manifestations (lightheadedness, dizziness) and advise them to avoid sudden changes of position.

Psychosis
- Visual hallucinations, nightmares, especially in older adults
- NURSING ACTIONS: Administer second-generation antipsychotic medications, such as clozapine, if manifestations occur.

Impulse control disorder
- Gambling, shopping, binge eating, hypersexuality
- NURSING ACTIONS
  - Manifestations appear 9 months after the initial dose. Manifestations subside after discontinuing the medication.
  - Screen for compulsive behavior before initiating therapy.

Dyskinesias (head bobbing, tics, grimacing, tremors)
A decrease in the dosage of the medication is necessary.

Nausea
CLIENT EDUCATION: Take the medication with food (slows absorption of the medication).

Dopamine releaser

CNS effects (confusion, dizziness, restlessness)
CLIENT EDUCATION: Avoid activities that require alertness while taking the medication.

Atropine-like effects
- Dry mouth, blurred vision, mydriasis (dilated pupils), urinary hesitancy or retention, constipation
- NURSING ACTIONS
  - Advise clients to observe for manifestations and notify the provider.
  - Monitor I&O, and ask clients about hesitancy or urinary retention.
  - Advise clients to chew gum, eat high-fiber foods, and increase fluid intake to 2 to 3 L/day from beverages and food.

Discoloration of skin (livedo reticularis)
CLIENT EDUCATION: Discoloration of the skin will subside after discontinuing the medication.

COMT inhibitors

Same as for pramipexole in combination with levodopa/carbidopa
Interventions are the same as for pramipexole in combination with levodopa/carbidopa.

GI: vomiting, diarrhea, constipation
NURSING ACTIONS: Treat adverse effects according to manifestations.

Discoloration of urine to a yellow-orange
CLIENT EDUCATION: The urine color change is harmless.

Rhabdomyolysis (muscle pain, tendon weakness)
CLIENT EDUCATION: Monitor and report manifestations to the provider immediately.

Liver failure
NURSING ACTIONS
- Monitor liver function periodically.
- Monitor for manifestations of liver failure (nausea, fatigue, jaundice, abdominal pain).
- Use with caution with hepatic impairment.

MAO-B inhibitors

Insomnia (selegiline)
NURSING ACTIONS: Administer selegiline no later than noon to reduce the risk of insomnia.

Hypertensive crisis resulting from consuming foods containing tyramine
CLIENT EDUCATION: Avoid eating foods that contain tyramine (avocados, soybeans, figs, smoked meats, dried or cured fish, cheese, yeast products, beer, chianti wine, chocolate, caffeinated beverages).

Hypertensive crisis and death from some medications
NURSING ACTIONS: Provide a list of medications to avoid (meperidine, fluoxetine, MAOIs, antidepressants, sympathomimetics).

Nausea, diarrhea
CLIENT EDUCATION: Take the medication with meals and limit their protein intake to increase absorption

Centrally acting anticholinergics

Nausea, vomiting
CLIENT EDUCATION: Take the medication with food but avoid high-protein snacks.

Atropine-like effects
- Dry mouth, blurred vision, mydriasis (dilated pupils), urinary retention, constipation
- NURSING ACTIONS
  - Advise clients to observe for manifestations and notify the provider if they occur.
  - Monitor I&O, and ask clients about urinary retention.
  - Advise clients to chew gum, eat foods high in fiber, and increase fluid intake to 2 to 3 L/day from beverage and food sources.
  - Advise clients to schedule periodic eye examinations to measure for increased intraocular pressure that can result in glaucoma.

Antihistamine effects (sedation, drowsiness)
NURSING ACTIONS
- Advise clients to avoid activities that require alertness while taking the medication.
- Avoid administering to older adult clients due to CNS adverse effects (sedation, confusion, delusions, hallucinations).

CLIENT EDUCATION

- Family members should assist clients with the medication at home.
- Notify the provider if sudden loss of the effects of medication occurs.
- Effects might not be noticed for several weeks to several months.
- Medication "holidays" require monitoring in a health care facility.
- Avoid high-protein meals and snacks.
- Avoid pregnancy when taking levodopa or pramipexole.
- The use of pramipexole with cimetidine can increase the amount of pramipexole in the blood.
- Do not stop taking medications abruptly.

NURSING EVALUATION OF MEDICATION EFFECTIVENESS

Indications of effectiveness include the following.
- Absence of tremors
- Less irritability
- Less stiffness
- Increase in the ability to perform ADLs

Antiepileptics (AEDs)

TRADITIONAL ANTIEPILEPTIC MEDICATIONS

- Phenobarbital
- Primidone
- Phenytoin
- Carbamazepine: also for treating bipolar disorder, trigeminal and glossopharyngeal neuralgias
- Valproic acid: also for treating bipolar disorder, migraine headaches
- Ethosuximide

NEWER ANTIEPILEPTIC MEDICATIONS

- Lamotrigine
- Levetiracetam
- Topiramate
- Oxcarbazepine
- Gabapentin
- Pregabalin
- Tiagabine
- Zonisamide
- Lacosamide
- Vigabatrin
- Ezogabine

OTHER MEDICATIONS: Benzodiazepines for treating status epilepticus (acute prolonged seizures)
- Diazepam
- Lorazepam

PURPOSE

EXPECTED PHARMACOLOGICAL ACTION

AEDs control seizure disorders by various mechanisms.
- Slowing the entrance of sodium and calcium back into the neuron, thus extending the time it takes for the nerve to return to its active state and slows the frequency of neuron firing
- Suppressing neuronal firing, which decreases seizure activity and prevents propagation of seizure activity into other areas of the brain
- Decreasing seizure activity by enhancing the inhibitory effects of gamma butyric acid (GABA)

- Phenytoin is a hydantoin medication that suppresses partial seizure and primary generalized seizure activity in the affected neurons.
- Carbamazepine treats partial seizures and tonic–clonic seizures and has no therapeutic effect on absence seizures.
- Valproic acid treats all types of seizures.

COMPLICATIONS

TRADITIONAL ANTIEPILEPTIC MEDICATIONS

Barbiturates: phenobarbital, primidone

CNS effects
- Adults: drowsiness, sedation, depression
- Older adults: confusion, anxiety
- Children: irritability, hyperactivity
- NURSING ACTIONS
  - Advise clients to observe for manifestations and to notify the provider if they occur.
  - Advise clients to avoid activities that require alertness, such as driving.
  - Never administer primidone with phenobarbital because phenobarbital is an active metabolite. The liver metabolizes primidone and converts it to phenobarbital.
  - Contraindications include porphyria, severe respiratory illness, liver disease, and kidney impairment.
  - Providers generally prescribe primidone with phenytoin or carbamazepine.
  - Avoid administering other CNS depressants (alcohol, benzodiazepines, opioids).

12.2 Antiepileptic medications

Traditional antiepileptic medications	PHENOBARBITAL	PRIMIDONE	PHENYTOIN	CARBAMAZEPINE	VALPROIC ACID	ETHOSUXIMIDE	Newer antiepileptic medications	LAMOTRIGINE	LEVETIRACETAM	TOPIRAMATE	OXCARBAZEPINE	GABAPENTIN	PREGABALIN	TIAGABINE	ZONISAMIDE	LACOSAMIDE	VIGABATRIN	EZOGABINE
Simple partial, complex partial, secondarily generalized seizures	✓	✓	✓	✓	✓			✓	✓	✓	✓	✓	✓	✓	✓	✓	✓	✓
Primary generalized seizures — Tonic-clonic	✓	✓	✓	✓	✓			✓	✓	✓								
Primary generalized seizures — Absence					✓	✓		✓										
Primary generalized seizures — Myoclonic					✓			✓	✓	✓								

Toxicity
- Nystagmus, ataxia, respiratory depression, coma, pinpoint pupils, hypotension, death
- NURSING ACTIONS
  - Withhold the medication and notify the provider. Administer oxygen and maintain respiratory function with ventilatory support.
  - Monitor vital signs.
  - Have resuscitation equipment available.

Decreased synthesis of vitamins K and D, decreased effectiveness of warfarin
NURSING ACTIONS: Monitor laboratory values (INR, calcium, vitamin D).

Hydantoins: phenytoin

CNS effects
- Nystagmus, sedation, ataxia, double vision, cognitive impairment
- NURSING ACTIONS: Monitor for CNS effects, and notify the provider if they occur.

Gingival hyperplasia
- Softening and overgrowth of gum tissue, tenderness, bleeding gums
- CLIENT EDUCATION: Use good oral hygiene (dental flossing, massaging gums). Folic acid supplements can decrease the occurrence.

Skin rash
NURSING ACTIONS: Withhold the medication and notify the provider if a rash develops.

Cardiovascular effects: dysrhythmias, hypotension
- Clients should receive phenytoin at a slow IV rate (no faster than 50 mg/min) and in a dilute solution to prevent adverse cardiovascular effects.
- Contraindications include sinus bradycardia, sinoatrial block, and Stokes-Adams syndrome.

Endocrine and other effects
- Coarsening of facial features, hirsutism, interference with vitamin D metabolism
- CLIENT EDUCATION
  - Report changes.
  - Consume adequate amounts of calcium and vitamin D.

Interference with vitamin K-dependent clotting factors causing bleeding in newborns
NURSING ACTIONS: Administer prophylactic vitamin K to clients who are pregnant for 1 month before delivery.

Purple glove syndrome
- Rare effect causing edema and discoloration of the hands and arms
- NURSING ACTIONS: Withhold the medication and notify the provider.

Carbamazepine

CNS effects
- Nystagmus, double vision, vertigo, staggering gait, and headache can occur, but the medications minimally affect cognitive function.
- Providers prescribe low doses initially and then gradually increase the dosage.

NURSING ACTIONS: Administer the medication at bedtime.

Hematologic effects
- Leukopenia, anemia, thrombocytopenia
- NURSING ACTIONS
  - Document a baseline CBC and platelet count. Perform ongoing monitoring of CBC and platelets.
  - Observe for bruising, bleeding of gums, sore throat, fever, pallor, weakness, and infection.
  - Do not administer to clients who have bone marrow suppression or bleeding disorders.

Hypo-osmolarity
- Carbamazepine promotes the secretion of ADH, which inhibits water excretion by the kidneys and places clients who have heart failure at risk for fluid overload.
- NURSING ACTIONS
  - Monitor sodium levels periodically.
  - Monitor for edema, a decrease in urine output, and hypertension.

Skin disorders
- Dermatitis, rash, Stevens-Johnson syndrome
- NURSING ACTIONS
  - Treat mild reactions with anti-inflammatory or antihistamine medications.
  - Withhold the medication and notify the provider when there is a severe reaction.

Valproic acid

GI effects (nausea, vomiting, indigestion)
CLIENT EDUCATION: Take the medication with food. The enteric-coated formulation can reduce GI effects.

Hepatotoxicity (anorexia, abdominal pain, jaundice)
NURSING ACTIONS
- Document baseline liver function and monitor liver function periodically.
- Advise clients to observe for manifestations of hepatotoxicity (anorexia, nausea, vomiting, abdominal pain, jaundice) and to notify the provider if they occur.
- Do not administer to children younger than 2 years.
- Administer the lowest effective dose.
- Do not administer to clients who have liver disease.

Pancreatitis (nausea, vomiting, abdominal pain)
NURSING ACTIONS
- Advise clients to observe for manifestations and to notify the provider immediately if these occur.
- Monitor amylase levels.
- Withhold the medication and notify the provider if pancreatitis develops.

Thrombocytopenia
NURSING ACTIONS
- Advise clients to observe for manifestations such as bruising, and to notify the provider if they occur.
- Monitor platelet counts and bleeding times.

CNS effects from hyperammonemia
- Vomiting, lethargy, impaired cognitive alertness
- NURSING ACTIONS
  - Monitor blood ammonia levels periodically.
  - Withhold the medication and notify the provider if hyperammonemia develops.

Ethosuximide

GI effects (nausea, vomiting)
NURSING ACTIONS: Administer with food.

CNS effects (sleepiness, lightheadedness, fatigue)
Providers usually prescribe a low initial dosage.

CLIENT EDUCATION: Avoid hazardous activities, such as driving.

Note: Ethosuximide only treats absence seizures.

NEWER ANTIEPILEPTIC MEDICATIONS

Lamotrigine

CNS effects
- Dizziness, somnolence, aphasia, double or blurred vision, headache, nausea, vomiting, depression
- NURSING ACTIONS
  - Lamotrigine has a therapeutic effect on absence seizures and all other forms of seizures.
  - Avoid activities that require alertness until the medication's effects have stabilized.
  - Withhold the medication and notify the provider if manifestations are severe.
  - Monitor for suicidal ideation.

Aseptic meningitis (inflammation of the meninges without bacterial infection)
- Effects include headache, fever, stiff neck, nausea, vomiting, rash, and sensitivity to light.
- NURSING ACTIONS
  - Monitor for and report manifestations to the provider.
  - Withhold the medication and notify the provider if aseptic meningitis develops.

Skin disorders
- Can include life-threatening rashes (Stevens-Johnson syndrome, toxic epidermal necrolysis)
- Concurrent use with valproic acid increases the risk of skin disorders.
- NURSING ACTIONS
  - Treat mild reactions with anti-inflammatory or antihistamine medications.
  - Withhold the medication and notify the provider if there is a severe reaction.

Levetiracetam

CNS effects
- Dizziness, asthenia (loss of strength, weakness) agitation, anxiety, depression, suicidal ideation
- NURSING ACTIONS
  - Withhold the medication and notify the provider if there is a severe reaction.
  - Monitor for suicidal ideation.

Topiramate

CNS effects
- Somnolence, dizziness, ataxia, nervousness, diplopia, confusion, impaired cognitive function
- NURSING ACTIONS: Withhold the medication and notify the provider if there is a severe reaction.

Reduced sweating and increased body temperature
CLIENT EDUCATION: Monitor amount of strenuous activity while taking the medication.

Metabolic acidosis
NURSING ACTIONS
- Monitor serum bicarbonate levels.
- Advise clients to report hyperventilation, fatigue, or anorexia.
- Withhold the medication and notify the provider if these manifestations develop.

Angle-closure glaucoma
NURSING ACTIONS
- Inform the client of the manifestations of glaucoma (ocular pain, redness, blurring of vision).
- Advise clients to have periodic eye examinations to measure intraocular pressure.

Oxcarbazepine

CNS effects
- Dizziness, drowsiness, double vision, nystagmus, headache, nausea, vomiting, ataxia
- Providers usually prescribe a low initial dosage.
- NURSING ACTIONS
  - Advise clients to avoid activities that require alertness, such as driving.
  - Monitor sodium levels for clients who have nausea and vomiting.

Skin disorders
- Can include life-threatening rashes (Stevens-Johnson syndrome, toxic epidermal necrolysis)
- NURSING ACTIONS
  - Treat mild reactions with anti-inflammatory or antihistamine medications.
  - Withhold the medication and notify the provider if there is a severe reaction.

Hyponatremia (nausea, drowsiness, headache, confusion)
NURSING ACTIONS
- Monitor sodium levels.
- Use caution with clients receiving diuretic medication because of the high risk for hyponatremia.

Multiorgan hypersensitivity reactions
- Fever and rash with some of the following: lymphadenopathy, hepatorenal syndrome, hematologic abnormalities
- NURSING ACTIONS: Withhold the medication and notify the provider if manifestations develop.

Gabapentin

CNS effects
- Somnolence, dizziness, ataxia, fatigue, nystagmus, peripheral edema (diminishing with time)
- Gabapentin has a therapeutic effect only on partial seizures.

CLIENT EDUCATION: Avoid driving if drowsy.

Pregabalin

CNS effects: Somnolence, dizziness, adverse cognitive effects, headache
NURSING ACTIONS
- Advise clients to avoid driving if drowsy.
- Withhold the medication and notify the provider if there is a severe reaction.

Weight gain, peripheral edema, dry mouth
NURSING ACTIONS
- Monitor daily weight, and report a significant increase to the provider.
- Advise clients to chew gum or suck on hard candy to increase salivation.

Hypersensitivity reactions (angioedema)
CLIENT EDUCATION: Stop taking the medication and contact the provider immediately if manifestations develop.

CONTRAINDICATIONS/PRECAUTIONS

TRADITIONAL ANTIEPILEPTIC MEDICATIONS

Barbiturates: phenobarbital, primidone

Pregnancy (due to increased risk of fetal malformations): Pregnancy Risk Category D: Administer only if the benefits outweigh the risks.

NURSING ACTIONS: Inform the client of the potential risks with pregnancy and to consult with the provider.

Hydantoins: phenytoin

Pregnancy
- Teratogenic: Cleft lip and palate, heart defects, developmental deficiencies
- Pregnancy Risk Category D: Administer only if the benefits outweigh the risks.

Carbamazepine

Pregnancy
- Birth defects: Spina bifida, neural tube defects, delays in growth
- Pregnancy Risk Category D: Administer only if the benefits outweigh the risks.

Valproic acid

Pregnancy
- Teratogenic: Cleft lip and palate, heart defects
- Pregnancy Risk Category D: Administer only if the benefits outweigh the risks.

NEWER ANTIEPILEPTIC MEDICATIONS

Lamotrigine

Pregnancy
- Teratogenic: Cleft lip and palate (low risk), heart defects
- Pregnancy Risk Category C: Administer only if the benefits outweigh the risks.

Topiramate

Pregnancy
- Teratogenic: Cleft lip and palate, heart defects
- Pregnancy Risk Category D: Administer only if the benefits outweigh the risks.

Oxcarbazepine

Pregnancy
- Teratogenic: Cleft lip and palate, heart defects
- Pregnancy Risk Category C: Administer only if the benefits outweigh the risks.

Pregabalin

Pregnancy
- Birth defects: Skeletal and visceral malformations
- Pregnancy Risk Category C: Administer only if the benefits outweigh the risks.

INTERACTIONS

TRADITIONAL ANTIEPILEPTIC MEDICATIONS

Barbiturates: phenobarbital, primidone

Decreased effectiveness of oral contraceptives
CLIENT EDUCATION: Use other forms of contraception.

Hydantoins: phenytoin

Phenytoin causes a decrease in the effects of oral contraceptives, warfarin, and glucocorticoids due to stimulation of hepatic medication-metabolizing enzymes.
NURSING ACTIONS
- Advise a dosage adjustment by the provider or an alternative form of birth control.
- Monitor for therapeutic effects of warfarin and glucocorticoids (INR, blood glucose levels). The provider might have to adjust dosages.

Alcohol (acute ingestion), diazepam, isoniazid, cimetidine, and valproic acid increase phenytoin levels.
NURSING ACTIONS
- Advise clients to avoid drinking alcohol.
- Monitor serum levels.

Carbamazepine, phenobarbital, and chronic alcohol use decrease phenytoin levels.
CLIENT EDUCATION: Avoid drinking alcohol.

Additive CNS depressant effects can occur with concurrent use of CNS depressants (barbiturates, alcohol).
CLIENT EDUCATION: Avoid concurrent use of alcohol and other CNS depressants.

Carbamazepine

Carbamazepine causes a decrease in the effects of oral contraceptives and warfarin due to stimulation of hepatic medication-metabolizing enzymes.
NURSING ACTIONS
- Advise a dosage adjustment by the provider or an alternative form of birth control.
- Monitor for therapeutic effects of warfarin with PT and INR. The provider might have to adjust the dosage.

Grapefruit juice inhibits metabolism, and thus increases carbamazepine levels.
CLIENT EDUCATION: Avoid drinking grapefruit juice.

Phenytoin and phenobarbital decrease the effects of carbamazepine.
NURSING ACTIONS: Avoid concurrent use.

Valproic acid

Concurrent use of valproic acid increases the levels of phenytoin and phenobarbital.
NURSING ACTIONS: Monitor phenytoin and phenobarbital levels. The provider might have to adjust the dosages.

NEWER ANTIEPILEPTIC MEDICATIONS

Topiramate

Phenytoin and carbamazepine can decrease topiramate levels. Topiramate can increase phenytoin levels.
NURSING ACTIONS: Consult the provider before administering phenytoin or carbamazepine with topiramate.

Oxcarbazepine

Oxcarbazepine decreases oral contraceptive levels.
CLIENT EDUCATION: Use an alternate form of contraception.

Phenytoin levels increase with oxcarbazepine.
NURSING ACTIONS: Consult the provider before administering oxcarbazepine with phenytoin.

Concurrent alcohol consumption depresses the CNS.
CLIENT EDUCATION: Avoid alcohol.

Pregabalin

Benzodiazepines, alcohol, and opioids intensify CNS effects.
CLIENT EDUCATION: Avoid medications that affect the CNS.

CLIENT EDUCATION

- Monitor therapeutic plasma levels of medications and be aware of therapeutic levels for each medication. Notify the provider of results.
- Antiepileptic medications control seizures but do not cure the disorder.
- Keep a seizure frequency diary to monitor the effectiveness of therapy.
- Take medications as prescribed and do not stop taking medications without consulting the provider. Sudden cessation of medication therapy can trigger seizures.
- Avoid activities that require alertness (driving, operating heavy machinery) until they have seizure control and they know how the medication affects them.
- Carry extra medication when traveling to avoid interruption of treatment.
- Avoid pregnancy, because these medications can cause birth defects and congenital abnormalities.
- Phenytoin doses are individual. Dosing usually starts twice a day and can be once-a-day with an extended-release form once the provider establishes the maintenance dose.
- Phenytoin has a narrow therapeutic range, and strict adherence to the medication regimen is imperative to prevent toxicity or therapeutic failure.

NURSING EVALUATION OF MEDICATION EFFECTIVENESS

Indications of effectiveness include the following.
- Absence or decreased occurrence of seizures
- Ability to perform ADLs
- Absence of injury

Application Exercises

1. A nurse in the postanesthesia recovery unit is assisting with the care of a client who received a nondepolarizing neuromuscular blocking agent and has muscle weakness. The nurse should anticipate a prescription for which of the following medications?

   A. Neostigmine

   B. Naloxone

   C. Dantrolene

   D. Vecuronium

2. A nurse is reinforcing teaching with a client who has early Parkinson's disease and a new prescription for pramipexole. The nurse should instruct the client to monitor for which of the following adverse effects of this medication?

   A. Hallucinations

   B. Increased salivation

   C. Diarrhea

   D. Discoloration of urine

3. A nurse is reinforcing teaching with a client who has a new prescription for levodopa/carbidopa for Parkinson's disease. Which of the following instructions should the nurse include?

   A. Increase intake of protein-rich foods.

   B. Expect muscle twitching to occur.

   C. Take this medication with food.

   D. Anticipate relief of manifestations in 24 hr.

4. A nurse is preparing to administer a medication to a client who has absence seizures. The nurse should anticipate administering which of the following medications? (Select all that apply.)

   A. Phenytoin

   B. Ethosuximide

   C. Gabapentin

   D. Carbamazepine

   E. Valproic acid

   F. Lamotrigine

5. A nurse is reviewing a new prescription for oxcarbazepine with a female client who has partial seizures. Which of the following instructions should the nurse include? (Select all that apply.)

   A. "Use caution if the doctor prescribes a diuretic medication."

   B. "Consider using another form of birth control if you are taking oral contraceptives."

   C. "Chew gum to increase saliva production."

   D. "Avoid driving until you see how the medication affects you."

   E. "Notify the doctor if you develop a skin rash."

PRACTICE Active Learning Scenario

A nurse is contributing to the plan of care for a client who has tonic-clonic seizures and a new prescription for phenytoin. Considering the adverse effects and nursing interventions, what should the nurse suggest for inclusion in the plan of care?

Use the ATI Active Learning Template: Medication to complete this item to include the following:

THERAPEUTIC USES: Describe.

COMPLICATIONS: Describe two adverse effects and two medication interactions.

NURSING INTERVENTIONS: Include two interventions that relate to the two adverse effects, and two interventions that relate to the two medication interactions.

Application Exercises Key

1. A. **CORRECT:** Neostigmine is a cholinesterase inhibitor that reverses the effects of nondepolarizing neuromuscular blockers.

   B. Naloxone reverses the effects of opioids.

   C. Dantrolene acts on skeletal muscles to reduce metabolic activity and treat malignant hyperthermia.

   D. Vecuronium is an intermediate-acting nondepolarizing neuromuscular blocker.

   Ⓝ *NCLEX® Connection: Pharmacological Therapies, Adverse Effects/ Contraindications/Side Effects/Interactions*

2. A. **CORRECT:** Pramipexole can cause hallucinations within 9 months of the initial dose and might require discontinuation.

   B. Increased salivation is an adverse effect of cholinesterase inhibitors. Dry mouth is an adverse effect of pramipexole.

   C. Constipation is an adverse effect of pramipexole.

   D. Discoloration of urine is an adverse effect of COMT inhibitors and not an adverse effect of pramipexole.

   Ⓝ *NCLEX® Connection: Pharmacological Therapies, Adverse Effects/ Contraindications/Side Effects/Interactions*

3. A. The client should avoid protein-rich foods, which can result in decreased therapeutic effects of levodopa.

   B. The client should monitor and report muscle twitching, which can indicate toxicity.

   C. **CORRECT:** The client should take this medication with food to reduce GI effects.

   D. The client should anticipate relief of manifestations to take several weeks to months.

   Ⓝ *NCLEX® Connection: Pharmacological Therapies, Expected Actions/Outcomes*

4. A. Phenytoin treats partial seizures and tonic-clonic seizures and has no therapeutic effect on absence seizures.

   B. **CORRECT:** Ethosuximide's only therapeutic use is to treat absence seizures.

   C. Gabapentin treats partial seizures and has no therapeutic effect on absence seizures.

   D. Carbamazepine treats partial seizures and tonic-clonic seizures and has no therapeutic effect on absence seizures.

   E. **CORRECT:** Valproic acid has a therapeutic effect on absence seizures and all other forms of seizures.

   F. **CORRECT:** Lamotrigine has a therapeutic effect on absence seizures and all other forms of seizures.

   Ⓝ *NCLEX® Connection: Pharmacological Therapies, Expected Actions/Outcomes*

5. A. **CORRECT:** Taking diuretic medications when taking oxcarbazepine requires caution because of the high risk for hyponatremia.

   B. **CORRECT:** Clients taking oxcarbazepine should use an alternate form of contraception because oxcarbazepine decreases oral contraceptive levels.

   C. Oxcarbazepine does not cause dry mouth. Pregabalin is an example of an antiepileptic medication that causes dry mouth.

   D. **CORRECT:** The client should avoid driving if CNS effects of dizziness, drowsiness, and double vision develop.

   E. **CORRECT:** The client should notify the provider if a skin rash occurs because life-threatening skin disorders can develop.

   Ⓝ *NCLEX® Connection: Pharmacological Therapies, Expected Actions/Outcomes*

PRACTICE Answer

Using the ATI Active Learning Template: Medication

THERAPEUTIC USES: Phenytoin is a hydantoin medication that suppresses partial seizure and primary generalized seizure activity in the affected neurons.

COMPLICATIONS

- CNS effects
- Gingival hyperplasia
- Teratogenic birth defects
- Decreases effectiveness of oral contraceptives, warfarin, and glucocorticoids
- Causes stimulation of hepatic medication-metabolizing enzymes
- Alcohol (acute use), diazepam, cimetidine, and valproic acid increase phenytoin levels.
- Carbamazepine, phenobarbital, and chronic alcohol use decrease phenytoin levels.
- Additive CNS depressant effects can occur with concurrent use of CNS depressants.

NURSING INTERVENTIONS

- Instruct the client to refrain from alcohol and other medications that cause CNS depression (barbiturates).
- Encourage the client to use dental floss and massage gums daily.
- Instruct the client to avoid pregnancy and use an alternate form of contraception.
- Monitor INR if on warfarin and blood glucose levels if taking a glucocorticoid.
- Monitor therapeutic effects of warfarin and glucocorticoids.
- Never abruptly discontinue antiepileptic medications.
- Advise clients to avoid use of alcohol and other CNS depressants.
- Monitor serum phenytoin levels.

Ⓝ *NCLEX® Connection: Pharmacological and Parenteral Therapies, Adverse Effects/Contraindications/Side Effects/Interactions*

UNIT 2   MEDICATIONS AFFECTING THE NERVOUS SYSTEM

CHAPTER 13   # Eye and Ear Disorders

Eye disorders

Glaucoma is a common preventable cause of blindness. Damage to the optic nerve occurs when aqueous humor does not exit from the anterior chamber of the eye. This results in buildup of aqueous humor, increased intraocular pressure (IOP), and loss of vision.

TYPES OF GLAUCOMA

Primary open-angle glaucoma (POAG)

- POAG is the most common form of glaucoma.
- Peripheral vision loss occurs gradually, with central visual field loss occurring if damage to the optic nerve continues.
- Clients typically do not have pain or other manifestations until there is widespread damage. Manifestations include halos around lights, loss of peripheral vision, and headaches.
- IOP should be less than 20 mm Hg. IOP greater than 20 mm Hg is a major risk factor for POAG. However, it can occur at therapeutic IOP levels.
- Treatment includes medication therapy to reduce IOP. Surgical intervention is necessary if medication does not reduce IOP.
- The following medications treat POAG.
  ○ Beta adrenergic blockers
  ○ Alpha$_2$ adrenergic agonists
  ○ Prostaglandin analogs
  ○ Cholinergic agonists
  ○ Carbonic anhydrase inhibitors

Angle-closure (narrow-angle) glaucoma

- This is an acute disorder with a sudden onset, resulting in irreversible blindness within 1 to 2 days without emergency treatment.
- Findings include an acute onset of ocular pain, seeing halos around lights, brow pain, nausea, blurry vision, and photophobia. Buildup of aqueous humor displaces the iris and damages the optic nerve.
- Treatment includes medication therapy to reduce IOP, with subsequent corrective surgery for restoration of the iris.
- Although several other classes of glaucoma medications treat angle-closure glaucoma, osmotic agents are first-line medications for controlling the disorder until corrective surgery can repair the damage.

Beta adrenergic blockers

NONSELECTIVE BETA BLOCKERS (have both beta$_1$ and beta$_2$ properties)
- Timolol
- Carteolol
- Metipranolol
- Levobunolol

CARDIOSELECTIVE BETA$_1$ BLOCKERS: Betaxolol

PURPOSE

EXPECTED PHARMACOLOGICAL ACTION

Beta blockers decrease IOP by decreasing the amount of aqueous humor the ciliary body produces.

THERAPEUTIC USES

- Topical beta blockers treat POAG, often in combination with other topical medications, to lower IOP.
- Occasionally, these medications treat acute closed-angle glaucoma on an emergency basis.

COMPLICATIONS

Stinging discomfort

Temporary effect immediately after instillation of the drops

CLIENT EDUCATION: This effect is transient.

Occasional conjunctivitis, blurry vision, photophobia, dry eyes

CLIENT EDUCATION: Report these effects to the provider.

Systemic effects of beta blockade on the heart and lungs

CLIENT EDUCATION
- An overdose could cause or increase the chance of systemic effects.
- When taking beta$_1$ blockers, monitor for bradycardia. Notify the provider for a heart rate less than 60/min.

CONTRAINDICATIONS/PRECAUTIONS

- Chronic respiratory disease is a contraindication because these medications can constrict the airway and cause bronchospasm.
- Sinus bradycardia and AV heart block are contraindications for using beta blockers.
- Clients who have heart failure require caution when using beta blockers.

INTERACTIONS

Oral beta blockers and calcium channel blockers can increase cardiovascular and respiratory effects.
NURSING ACTIONS: Instruct clients to inform the provider if they are taking any of these medications.

Beta blockers can interfere with some effects of insulin.
NURSING ACTIONS: Advise clients who have diabetes mellitus to monitor their blood glucose.

NURSING ADMINISTRATION

- Instill one drop in the affected eye once or twice daily.
- Review the technique for instilling eye drops. Instruct a family member in the technique if necessary. Qᴘᴄᴄ
- Use sterile technique when handling the applicator portion of the container. Avoid touching any part of the applicator, and keep the lid in place when not in use.
- Hold gentle pressure on the nasolacrimal duct for 30 to 60 seconds immediately after instilling the drop(s) to prevent or minimize systemic effects.
- Monitor heart rate and rhythm. Qs

Alpha₂ adrenergic agonists

SELECT PROTOTYPE MEDICATION: Brimonidine

OTHER MEDICATION: Apraclonidine

ALPHA₂ AGONIST/BETA BLOCKER COMBINATION: Brimonidine and timolol

PURPOSE

EXPECTED PHARMACOLOGICAL ACTION

Brimonidine decreases the production and can also increase the outflow of aqueous humor to lower IOP.

THERAPEUTIC USES

- Brimonidine is a first-line medication for long-term topical treatment of POAG.
- Apraclonidine provides short-term therapy for POAG only and is a preoperative medication for laser eye surgeries.

COMPLICATIONS

Stinging, pruritus

- Localized stinging, pruritus of the conjunctiva
- Sensation that a foreign body is in the eye

NURSING ACTIONS: Advise clients not to rub their eyes.

Dilated pupils, blurry vision, headache, dry mouth

CLIENT EDUCATION: Report these effects.

Reddened sclera

Due to blood-vessel engorgement

NURSING ACTIONS: Inform clients of the possibility of this effect.

Hypotension, drowsiness

Brimonidine crosses the blood-brain barrier, which can cause drowsiness, fatigue, and hypotension.

CLIENT EDUCATION: Use caution with driving and other tasks. Inform the provider if dizziness or weakness occurs.

CONTRAINDICATIONS/PRECAUTIONS

Advise clients who wear soft contact lenses to administer brimonidine after removing the lenses. They should not insert lenses for at least 15 min after administration to prevent absorption of the medication into the lens. Qᴘᴄᴄ

INTERACTIONS

Antihypertensive medications can intensify hypotension from brimonidine.
NURSING ACTIONS: Instruct clients to inform the provider if they are taking any antihypertensive medications.

MAO inhibitors can decrease the effects of brimonidine and cause hypertensive crisis.
NURSING ACTIONS: Instruct clients to inform the provider if they are taking MAO inhibitors.

NURSING ADMINISTRATION

- Review the technique for administering eye drops and minimizing systemic effects.
- Monitor blood pressure for hypotension or hypertension.

Prostaglandin analogs

SELECT PROTOTYPE MEDICATION: Latanoprost

OTHER MEDICATIONS
- Travoprost
- Bimatoprost

PURPOSE

EXPECTED PHARMACOLOGICAL ACTION

Latanoprost reduces IOP by increasing aqueous humor outflow through relaxation of ciliary muscles.

THERAPEUTIC USES

These agents are topical firstline medications for clients who have POAG and ocular hypertension. (13.1)

COMPLICATIONS

Bulging of ocular blood vessels

NURSING ACTIONS: Inform clients about the possibility of this effect.

Increased pigmentation

Permanently increased harmless brown pigmentation of the iris (can also cause pigmentation of lids, lashes)

NURSING ACTIONS: Inform clients about the possibility of this effect.

Stinging, burning, reddened conjunctivae

NURSING ACTIONS: Instruct clients not to rub their eyes.

Blurry vision

CLIENT EDUCATION: Report this effect to the provider.

Migraine

Rare adverse effect

CLIENT EDUCATION: Report this effect to the provider.

Carbonic anhydrase inhibitor (systemic)

SELECT PROTOTYPE MEDICATION: Acetazolamide

OTHER MEDICATION: Methazolamide

PURPOSE

EXPECTED PHARMACOLOGICAL ACTION

Reduce the production of aqueous humor by causing diuresis through kidney effects

THERAPEUTIC USES

- Quickly lower IOP in clients for whom other medications have been ineffective.
- Acetazolamide, a nonantimicrobial sulfonamide, is an emergency medication for use prior to surgery for acute angle-closure glaucoma and as a second-line medication for treating POAG.
- Acetazolamide also treats acute altitude sickness, seizures, and heart failure (as a diuretic).

> ### 13.1 Second-line topical medications for glaucoma
>
> #### Direct-acting cholinergic (muscarinic) agonist
>
> PROTOTYPE: Pilocarpine
>
> PURPOSE
> - Second-line treatment for POAG; lowers IOP indirectly through ciliary contraction
> - Also for emergency treatment of acute angle-closure glaucoma
>
> ADVERSE EFFECTS
> - Retinal detachment
> - Parasympathetic effects, such as bradycardia, increase in saliva, sweating, bronchospasm, pupil constriction
> - Decreased visual acuity, brow ache, eye pain
>
> #### Carbonic anhydrase inhibitors
>
> PROTOTYPE: Dorzolamide
>
> Also available in combination with timolol
>
> PURPOSE
> - Second-line treatment for POAG; decreases aqueous humor production
> - Timolol/dorzolamide combination increases the effect of both medications.
>
> ADVERSE EFFECTS
> - Local allergic reactions
> - Blurry vision, dry eyes, tearing, stinging, photophobia

COMPLICATIONS

Severe allergic reactions

- Possible anaphylaxis
- Possible cross-sensitivity with sulfonamides

NURSING ACTIONS
- Inform clients about manifestations of allergic reaction and to notify the provider if they occur.
- Ask about sulfonamide allergy.

Serious blood disorders

Rare serious blood disorders, such as bone marrow depression

CLIENT EDUCATION: Recognize and immediately report effects.

Gastrointestinal (GI) effects

Adverse GI effects (nausea, vomiting, diarrhea)

CLIENT EDUCATION: Report these effects and weight loss to the provider.

Electrolyte depletion (sodium, potassium), dehydration, altered liver function

NURSING ACTIONS: Prepare clients for the need to have laboratory testing regularly. Weigh daily, monitor for postural hypotension, and encourage a fluid intake of to 2 to 3 L/day, unless there are fluid restrictions.

Generalized flu-like manifestations

Headache, fever, body aches

NURSING ACTIONS: Inform clients about possible manifestations.

Central nervous system disturbances

Paresthesias of extremities, fatigue, sleepiness, seizures (rare)

NURSING ACTIONS
- Inform clients about possible manifestations.
- The provider might discontinue the medication.

Glucose disturbances

In clients who have diabetes mellitus

NURSING ACTIONS: Instruct clients who have diabetes to monitor blood glucose and watch for indications of hypo- or hyperglycemia.

CONTRAINDICATIONS/PRECAUTIONS

- Acetazolamide is pregnancy risk category C.
- Clients should only take this medication during lactation after evaluation by the provider.

INTERACTIONS

Serious effects, such as metabolic acidosis, can occur with high-dose aspirin.
NURSING ACTIONS: Question clients about aspirin use, and notify the provider.

Acetazolamide can increase the risk of toxic effects of quinidine.
CLIENT EDUCATION: Notify the provider of concurrent use and watch for indications of toxicity, such as a decrease in heart rate.

Acetazolamide can decrease lithium levels.
NURSING ACTIONS: Instruct clients taking lithium to watch for increased indications of mania. Monitor lithium levels regularly.

Acetazolamide can increase osteomalacia, an adverse effect of phenytoin.
NURSING ACTIONS: Instruct clients taking phenytoin to watch for bone pain or weakness and report these effects to the provider.

Sodium bicarbonate increases the risk of kidney stones.
NURSING ACTIONS: Question clients about the use of sodium bicarbonate and other over-the-counter antacids.

NURSING ADMINISTRATION

Acetazolamide is available orally as a tablet or a capsule. It is also available for parenteral administration.

NURSING EVALUATION OF MEDICATION EFFECTIVENESS

Indications of effectiveness include reduced IOP.

Ear disorders

Acute otitis media

- This disorder occurs most often in young children.
- A bacterial or a viral infection causes a buildup of fluid in the middle ear (middle-ear effusion) and middle-ear inflammation.
- The major indication is an acute onset of pain. Objective findings include erythema, bulging of the tympanic membrane, pulling on the ears, loss of appetite, and fever.
- Treatment for bacterial infection, especially in infants and young children, is an antibiotic. Treatment for viral infection is to manage the manifestations.

> Because of the increase in antibiotic-resistant bacteria, the current trend is to administer medications for pain relief (acetaminophen, ibuprofen), observe children over age 2 for 48 to 72 hr, and prescribe antibiotics if the infection does not resolve or worsens over several days. Q_EBP

- Yearly influenza and pneumococcal immunizations can help reduce the incidence of acute otitis media in infants and children.

MEDICATIONS FOR TREATING OTITIS MEDIA
- Oral penicillins
- Other antimicrobials, oral or parenteral
- Pain medication

Otitis externa

- A bacterial infection of the external auditory canal causes otitis externa (swimmer's ear).
- Any object that abrades or leaves moisture in the ear canal facilitates colonization of bacteria and the onset of otitis externa.
- Manifestations include an acute onset of pain, especially with movement of the pinna, itching, diminished hearing, and purulent discharge.
- Treatment usually resolves the infection within 10 days.
- Topical antimicrobial and anti-inflammatory combinations treat otitis externa.

Antimicrobials

SELECT PROTOTYPE MEDICATION: Amoxicillin

OTHER MEDICATION: Amoxicillin/clavulanate PO

Antibiotics that treat acute otitis media in clients who have a type II penicillin allergy (mild) or penicillin-resistant otitis media
- Ceftriaxone IM, IV (severe illness)
- Cefdinir PO
- Cefuroxime PO, IM, IV
- Cefpodoxime PO

Antibiotics that treat acute otitis media in clients who have a type I penicillin allergy (severe)
- Ceftriaxone IM, IV (severe illness)
- Azithromycin PO, IV
- Clindamycin PO, IM, IV (macrolide antibiotic)

PURPOSE

EXPECTED PHARMACOLOGICAL ACTION: Eradication of infection

THERAPEUTIC USES: Otitis media and various other bacterial infections

COMPLICATIONS

Possible allergic reaction

- Most common risk when taking penicillins
- Clients might require skin testing for sensitivity.

NURSING ACTIONS: Question clients about penicillin or other antibiotic allergies.

Nausea, vomiting, diarrhea

Usually less with amoxicillin than with ampicillin

CLIENT EDUCATION: Inform the provider of severe diarrhea, especially in an infant or young child.

Superinfection

With other microbes, such as *Candida albicans*, which causes oral candidiasis

CLIENT EDUCATION: Report indications of a new infection to the provider.

CONTRAINDICATIONS/PRECAUTIONS

- An allergy to penicillin is a contraindication for receiving amoxicillin.
- Clients who have an allergy to cephalosporins require caution when receiving amoxicillin.
- Infants younger than 3 months of age require caution when receiving amoxicillin due to their immature renal system and the increased risk for toxicity. Qpcc

NURSING ADMINISTRATION

- Administer amoxicillin three times daily PO, with or without food.
- As with all antibiotics, instruct clients to take the full course of medication.

NURSING EVALUATION OF MEDICATION EFFECTIVENESS

Indications of effectiveness include the following.
- Reduction of discomforts (fever, earache)
- Absence of infection
- Absence of the recurrence of infection

Fluoroquinolone antibiotic plus steroid medication

SELECT PROTOTYPE MEDICATION: Ciprofloxacin plus hydrocortisone otic drops

OTHER MEDICATIONS
- Acetic acid 2% solution otic drops
- Ciprofloxacin plus dexamethasone otic drops
- Ofloxacin otic drops

PURPOSE

EXPECTED PHARMACOLOGICAL ACTION

The bactericidal effect of ciprofloxacin and the anti-inflammatory effect of hydrocortisone should decrease pain, edema, and erythema in the ear canal.

THERAPEUTIC USES

Treat otitis externa topically

COMPLICATIONS

CNS effects

Dizziness, lightheadedness, tremors, restlessness, convulsions

CLIENT EDUCATION: Inform the provider if any of these occur.

Rash

NURSING ACTIONS: Question clients about allergies to fluoroquinolone antibiotics or steroids (dexamethasone, cortisone).

NURSING ADMINISTRATION

- Review the method for instilling otic drops.
- Inform clients that movement of the tragus or pinna might cause pain when instilling otic drops.
- Warm the medication by gently rolling the container between the hands before instilling drops. Cold drops can cause dizziness. Gently shake medication that is in suspension form.
- Place clients on the unaffected side.
- Keep clients in a side-lying position for 5 min with the affected ear up after instilling drops. Place a small piece of cotton in the ear. Avoid packing it tightly. Remove the cotton after 15 min.
- Warn clients not to instill otic medications in the eyes or swallow them. Qs
- Instruct clients to prevent otitis externa by
  - Keeping foreign bodies, such as cotton swabs, out of the ear canal, and avoiding the use of manual measures to remove cerumen.
  - Drying the ear canal after bathing or swimming, using a towel, and tilting the head to promote drainage.
  - Avoiding the use of earplugs, except while swimming.

NURSING EVALUATION OF MEDICATION EFFECTIVENESS

Indications of effectiveness include the resolution of manifestations.

Application Exercises

1. A nurse is showing a client who has a new prescription for timolol how to insert eye drops. The nurse should instruct the client to press on which of the following areas to prevent systemic absorption of the medication?

   A. Bony orbit

   B. Nasolacrimal duct

   C. Conjunctival sac

   D. Outer canthus

2. A nurse is reinforcing teaching with a client who has a new prescription for brimonidine ophthalmic drops and wears soft contact lenses. Which of the following instructions should the nurse include?

   A. "This medication can stain your contact lenses."

   B. "This medication can make your pupils constrict."

   C. "This medication can absorb into your contact lenses."

   D. "This medication can slow your heart rate."

3. A nurse in an urgent care center is reviewing the medical record of a client who is undergoing evaluation for angle-closure glaucoma. Which of the following findings is an indication of this disorder?

   A. Insidious onset of painless loss of vision

   B. Gradual reduction in peripheral vision

   C. Severe pain around the eyes

   D. Intraocular pressure 12 mm Hg

4. A nurse is reinforcing teaching with a client about preventing otitis externa. Which of the following instructions should the nurse include?

   A. Clean ears with a cotton-tipped swab daily.

   B. Place earplugs in the ears right before sleeping at night.

   C. Use a cool water irrigation solution to remove earwax.

   D. Tip head to each side to remove water from the ears after showering.

5. A nurse in a provider's office is reinforcing teaching with the parent of a toddler about how to administer ear drops. Which of the following instructions should the nurse include? (Select all that apply.)

   A. "Place your son on his unaffected side when you are ready to put in the drops."

   B. "Warm the medication by gently rolling it between your hands for a few minutes."

   C. "Gently shake the medication if it is in suspension form."

   D. "Keep your son on his side for 5 minutes after you put in the drops."

   E. "Tightly pack your son's ear with cotton after you put in the drops."

PRACTICE Active Learning Scenario

A nurse in a provider's office is reinforcing teaching with a client who has a prescription for ciprofloxacin/hydrocortisone about the medication and how to prevent otitis externa. Use the ATI Active Learning Template: Medication to complete this item.

THERAPEUTIC USES: Identify two therapeutic effects of the medication.

MEDICATION ADMINISTRATION: Identify two actions to prevent otitis externa.

Application Exercises Key

1. A. Pressing on the bony orbit will not prevent systemic absorption of the medication.

   B. **CORRECT:** Pressing on the nasolacrimal duct blocks the lacrimal punctum and prevents systemic absorption of the medication.

   C. Pressing on the conjunctival sac will not prevent systemic absorption of the medication.

   D. Pressing on the outer canthus will not prevent systemic absorption of the medication.

   (N) *NCLEX® Connection: Pharmacological Therapies, Expected Actions/Outcomes*

2. A. Rifampin can stain soft contact lenses. Brimonidine does not stain contact lenses.

   B. Brimonidine can cause mydriasis or dilated pupils.

   C. **CORRECT:** Brimonidine can absorb into soft contact lenses. The client should remove contact lenses, then instill the medication and wait at least 15 min before putting contact lenses back in.

   D. Beta adrenergic blockers, such as timolol, can slow the heart rate. Brimonidine can cause hypertension or hypotension.

   (N) *NCLEX® Connection: Pharmacological Therapies, Expected Actions/Outcomes*

3. A. Acute-angle glaucoma is painful and has a sudden onset.

   B. Gradual loss of peripheral vision is a manifestation of primary open-angle glaucoma.

   C. **CORRECT:** Severe pain around eyes that radiates over the face is a manifestation of acute angle-closure glaucoma.

   D. An IOP of 12 mm Hg is within the expected reference range. Elevated IOP is a manifestation of angle-closure glaucoma.

   (N) *NCLEX® Connection: Pharmacological Therapies, Medication Administration*

4. A. The client should not insert anything in the ear because this can push cerumen into the eardrum, damage the epithelium, or puncture the eardrum.

   B. The client should wear earplugs only when swimming to reduce the risk for otitis externa.

   C. The client should not use a cool irrigation solution to remove cerumen. Cool fluid can cause vertigo, dizziness, and nausea.

   D. **CORRECT:** The client should remove water from the ear after showering or swimming to reduce the risk for otitis externa.

   (N) *NCLEX® Connection: Pharmacological Therapies, Expected Actions/Outcomes*

5. A. **CORRECT:** The parent should have the child on his unaffected side to allow access to the affected ear and to promote drainage of the medication by gravity into the ear.

   B. **CORRECT:** The parent should warm the medication by rolling it between his hands. Administering the medication cold can cause dizziness.

   C. **CORRECT:** The parent should gently shake medication that is in suspension form to disperse the medication evenly.

   D. **CORRECT:** The parent should keep the child on his side to promote drainage of the medication by gravity into the ear.

   E. The parent should loosely pack the child's ear with cotton.

   (N) *NCLEX® Connection: Pharmacological Therapies, Expected Actions/Outcomes*

PRACTICE Answer

Using ATI Active Learning Template: Medication

THERAPEUTIC USES: The bactericidal effects of ciprofloxacin and the anti-inflammatory effects of hydrocortisone decrease pain, edema, and erythema in the ear.

MEDICATION ADMINISTRATION
- Keep foreign bodies out of the ear canal.
- Avoid manual measures to remove cerumen.
- Use a towel to dry the ear canal after bathing or swimming.
- Avoid using earplugs except while swimming.

(N) *NCLEX® Connection: Pharmacological and Parenteral Therapies, Medication Administration*

CHAPTER 14

Miscellaneous Central Nervous System Medications

Neuromuscular blocking agents have various uses, including causing muscle relaxation during general anesthesia, controlling seizures during electroconvulsive therapy, and suppressing the gag reflex during endotracheal intubation. Medications include succinylcholine and vecuronium.

Muscle relaxants and antispasmodic agents can affect both the central and peripheral nervous systems. These medications treat spasticity due to muscle injury, cerebral palsy, spinal cord injury, and multiple sclerosis. They include diazepam, baclofen, and dantrolene. Bethanechol, a **muscarinic agonist**, treats urinary retention. Oxybutynin, a **muscarinic antagonist**, treats neurogenic bladder.

Neuromuscular blocking agents

SELECT PROTOTYPE MEDICATION
- **Depolarizing** neuromuscular blockers: Succinylcholine
- **Nondepolarizing** neuromuscular blockers: Pancuronium

OTHER MEDICATIONS: Nondepolarizing neuromuscular blockers
- Atracurium
- Cisatracurium
- Rocuronium
- Vecuronium

PURPOSE

EXPECTED PHARMACOLOGICAL ACTION

Nondepolarizing neuromuscular blocking agents block acetylcholine (ACh) at the neuromuscular junction, resulting in muscle relaxation and hypotension. They do not cross the blood–brain barrier, so clients achieve complete paralysis without loss of consciousness or decreased pain sensation.

Succinylcholine

- Mimics ACh by binding with cholinergic receptors at the neuromuscular junction. This medication fills the cholinergic receptors, preventing ACh from binding with them, and causes sustained depolarization of the muscle, resulting in muscle paralysis.
- Succinylcholine has a short duration of action due to degradation by the plasma enzyme pseudocholinesterase.

Pancuronium, atracurium, vecuronium

- Block ACh from binding with cholinergic receptors at the motor end plate. Muscle paralysis occurs because of inhibited nerve depolarization and skeletal muscle contraction.
- Reversal agent is neostigmine.

THERAPEUTIC USES

- Neuromuscular blocking agents are adjuncts to general anesthesia and promote muscle relaxation.
- These medications control spontaneous respiratory movements in clients receiving mechanical ventilation.
- These medications control seizures during electroconvulsive therapy.
- Neuromuscular blocking agents facilitate endotracheal intubation and endoscopy.

COMPLICATIONS

Respiratory arrest

- From paralysis of the intercostal muscles and diaphragm
- Neostigmine can help reverse the action of nondepolarizing neuromuscular blocking agents when necessary.

NURSING ACTIONS
- Maintain continuous cardiac and respiratory monitoring.
- Have equipment ready for resuscitation and mechanical ventilation.
- Monitor for the return of respiratory function after discontinuation of the medication.

ATRACURIUM

Hypotension

Possible with atracurium

NURSING ACTIONS: Monitor for decreased blood pressure. Administer an antihistamine if necessary.

SUCCINYLCHOLINE

Prolonged apnea

Low pseudocholinesterase activity can lead to prolonged apnea.

NURSING ACTIONS
- Test blood or administer a small test dose for clients who might have low levels of pseudocholinesterase.
- Withhold the medication if pseudocholinesterase activity is low.

Malignant hyperthermia

- Manifestations include muscle rigidity with increased temperature, as high as 43° C (109.4° F).
- IV dantrolene helps decrease the metabolic activity of skeletal muscle.

NURSING ACTIONS
- Monitor vital signs.
- Stop succinylcholine and other anesthetics.
- Administer oxygen at 100%.
- Initiate cooling measures (administration of cold 0.9% sodium chloride, applying a cooling blanket, placing ice bags in the groin and other areas). Qᴇʙᴾ
- Have resuscitation and intubation equipment ready.

Muscle pain

Muscle pain in the upper body and back can develop 12 to 24 hr postoperatively and last for hours or days.

NURSING ACTIONS
- Inform clients that this response is not unusual and eventually will subside.
- Ask the provider to consider short-term use of a muscle relaxant.

Hyperkalemia

Succinylcholine can lead to cardiac arrest following hyperkalemia in certain clients.

NURSING ACTIONS
- Monitor potassium levels.
- Observe for manifestations of hyperkalemia.

CONTRAINDICATIONS/PRECAUTIONS

- Pregnancy risk category C
- Clients who have conditions that predispose them to hyperkalemia (major trauma, severe burns, certain types of nerve impairment) should not take succinylcholine.
- Clients who have myasthenia gravis, respiratory dysfunction, or fluid and electrolyte imbalances require caution with this medication.

NOTE: Neuromuscular blocker medications are not anesthetics and therefore have no effect on consciousness, hearing, thinking, or the ability to feel pain.

INTERACTIONS

Clients undergoing surgery often receive general anesthesia concurrently which increases the risk for excessive neuromuscular blockade.
Providers reduce the dosage of the neuromuscular blocker to prevent extreme neuromuscular blockade.

Aminoglycosides and tetracyclines can increase the effects of neuromuscular blockade.
NURSING ACTIONS: Take a complete medication history of clients who are to receive a neuromuscular blockade. Monitor for prolonged neuromuscular blockage.

Neostigmine and other cholinesterase inhibitors increase the effects of depolarizing neuromuscular blockers, such as succinylcholine.
NURSING ACTIONS: Monitor clients during neuromuscular blockade reversal after surgery.

NURSING ADMINISTRATION

- Clients must receive continuous cardiac and respiratory monitoring during therapy. Q̇s
- Monitor clients for respiratory depression following the administration of a neuromuscular blocker. Have life support equipment available.
- Request assistance from the charge nurse and rapid response team if the client demonstrates respiratory depression or cardiac dysrhythmia. Q̇ᴛᴄ
- Continue to monitor carefully for the return of respiratory function.
- Have a cholinesterase inhibitor available to reverse the effects of nondepolarizing neuromuscular blocking agents.

NURSING EVALUATION OF MEDICATION EFFECTIVENESS

Indications of effectiveness include the following.
- Muscle relaxation during surgery
- No spontaneous respiratory movements in clients receiving mechanical ventilation
- Absence of seizures in clients receiving electroconvulsive therapy
- Successful endotracheal intubation

Muscle relaxants and antispasmodics

SELECT PROTOTYPE MEDICATION
- **Centrally acting muscle relaxants:** Diazepam
- **Peripherally acting muscle relaxants:** Dantrolene

OTHER MEDICATIONS: Centrally acting muscle relaxants
- Baclofen
- Cyclobenzaprine
- Tizanidine

PURPOSE

Diazepam

EXPECTED PHARMACOLOGICAL ACTION: Acts in the CNS to enhance GABA, produce sedative effects, and depress spasticity of muscles.

THERAPEUTIC USES
- Muscle spasm due to muscle injury and spasticity
- Anxiety and panic disorders
- Insomnia
- Status epilepticus
- Alcohol withdrawal
- Anesthesia induction

Cyclobenzaprine, tizanidine

EXPECTED PHARMACOLOGICAL ACTIONS: Act in the CNS to enhance GABA, produce sedative effects, and depress spasticity of muscles. They have no direct muscle relaxant action and so do not decrease muscle strength.

THERAPEUTIC USES
- Relief of muscle spasm due to muscle injury
- Relieve pain and tenderness
- Help increase range of motion

Baclofen

EXPECTED PHARMACOLOGICAL ACTION: Acts in the CNS to enhance GABA, produce sedative effects, and depress hyperactive spasticity of muscles. There are no direct effects on skeletal muscles.

THERAPEUTIC USES: Relief of spasticity due to cerebral palsy, spinal cord injury, and multiple sclerosis

Dantrolene

EXPECTED PHARMACOLOGICAL ACTION: A peripherally acting muscle relaxant that acts directly on spastic muscles and inhibits muscle contraction by preventing release of calcium in skeletal muscles

THERAPEUTIC USES
- Relief of spasticity due to cerebral palsy, spinal cord injury, and multiple sclerosis
- Treatment of malignant hyperthermia

COMPLICATIONS

CNS depression

- Sleepiness, lightheadedness, fatigue
- Inform clients of potential adverse effects.
- Can occur with all muscle relaxants and antispasmodic medications.

NURSING ACTIONS
- Providers initially prescribe low doses.
- Advise clients to avoid hazardous activities, such as driving and concurrent use of other CNS depressants, including alcohol.

DIAZEPAM, CYCLOBENZAPRINE, TIZANIDINE

Hepatic toxicity with tizanidine

Anorexia, nausea, vomiting, abdominal pain, jaundice

NURSING ACTIONS
- Document baseline liver function and monitor liver function thereafter.
- Observe for indications of toxicity and notify the provider if they occur.
- Providers initially prescribe low doses.

Physical dependence from chronic long-term use

CLIENT EDUCATION: Do not stop taking the medication abruptly.

BACLOFEN

Nausea, constipation, urinary retention

NURSING ACTIONS
- Inform clients of adverse effects and to notify the provider if they occur.
- Advise clients to take the medication with meals to reduce gastric upset.
- Monitor I&O.
- Advise clients to increase intake of fluids and high-fiber foods.

Seizures

NURSING ACTIONS
- Inform clients of adverse effects and to notify the provider if they occur.
- Monitor for seizure activity

DANTROLENE

Hepatic toxicity

Anorexia, nausea, vomiting, abdominal pain, jaundice

NURSING ACTIONS
- Document baseline liver function studies and monitor liver function thereafter. Q₁
- Observe for indications of toxicity and notify the provider if they occur.
- Providers initially prescribe low doses.

Muscle weakness

NURSING ACTIONS: Monitor effectiveness of the medication.

CONTRAINDICATIONS/PRECAUTIONS

BACLOFEN AND DANTROLENE: Pregnancy risk category C

DIAZEPAM
- Controlled substance (Schedule IV)
- Pregnancy risk category D

  ! Use of these medications by clients who have impairments of liver or kidney function requires caution.

INTERACTIONS

CNS depressants (alcohol, opioids, antihistamines) have additive CNS depressant effects.
CLIENT EDUCATION: Avoid concurrent use.

NURSING ADMINISTRATION

- Instruct clients not to stop taking the medication abruptly to avoid withdrawal.
- Advise clients to avoid CNS depressants while using these medications.
- Provide assistance with self-administration of medication and performance of ADLs. Qpcc

NURSING EVALUATION OF MEDICATION EFFECTIVENESS

Indications of effectiveness include the following.
- Absence of muscle rigidity and spasms
- Adequate or improved range of motion
- Absence of pain
- Increased ability to perform ADLs

Muscarinic agonists

SELECT PROTOTYPE MEDICATION: Bethanechol

OTHER MEDICATIONS
- Cevimeline
- Pilocarpine
- Acetylcholine

PURPOSE

EXPECTED PHARMACOLOGICAL ACTION: Stimulation of muscarinic receptors of the genitourinary (GU) tract, thereby causing relaxation of the trigone and sphincter muscles and contraction of the detrusor muscle to increase bladder pressure and excretion of urine

THERAPEUTIC USES
- Only approved for nonobstructive urinary retention, usually postoperatively or postpartum
- Investigational use: treating gastroesophageal reflux

COMPLICATIONS

Extreme muscarinic stimulation

Can result in increased gastric acid secretion, excessive salivation and sweating, abdominal cramps, diarrhea, tearing, urinary urgency, bradycardia, hypotension, bronchoconstriction

NURSING ACTIONS
- Instruct clients to report adverse effects if they occur.
- Monitor for bradycardia and hypotension.
- Administer on an empty stomach to reduce GI effects.

CONTRAINDICATIONS/PRECAUTIONS

Urinary and gastrointestinal obstruction, peptic ulcer disease, coronary insufficiency, asthma, and hyperthyroidism are contraindications for receiving muscarinic agonists.

NURSING ADMINISTRATION

- Administer by the oral route, 1 hr before or 2 hr after meals to minimize nausea and vomiting.
- Monitor I&O.

NURSING EVALUATION OF MEDICATION EFFECTIVENESS

Indications of effectiveness include relief of urinary retention.

Muscarinic antagonists

SELECT PROTOTYPE MEDICATION: **M3 receptor selective:** oxybutynin

OTHER MEDICATIONS
- **M3 receptor selective:** Darifenacin, solifenacin
- **Nonselective:** Tolterodine, fesoterodine, trospium

PURPOSE

EXPECTED PHARMACOLOGICAL ACTION: Inhibit muscarinic receptors of the detrusor muscle of the bladder, thus preventing contractions of the bladder and the urge to void

THERAPEUTIC USES: Overactive bladder

COMPLICATIONS

Anticholinergic effects

Constipation, dry mouth, blurry vision, photophobia, dry eyes, tachycardia

CLIENT EDUCATION
- Increase dietary fiber. Consume 2 to 3 L/day fluid from beverage and food sources. Sip fluids.
- Avoid driving or other hazardous activities if vision is blurry.

CNS, cardiovascular effects

CNS effects: hallucinations, confusion, insomnia, nervousness

Cardiovascular effects: prolonged QT interval

NURSING ACTIONS
- Instruct clients to report manifestations to the provider and stop taking the medication.
- Monitor ECG.

CONTRAINDICATIONS/PRECAUTIONS

- Glaucoma, myasthenia gravis, paralytic ileus, GI and GU obstruction, and urinary retention are contraindications for receiving muscarinic antagonists.
- Use caution with children and older adults taking these medications.
- Use caution with clients who have gastroesophageal reflux disease, heart failure, or kidney or liver impairment.

INTERACTIONS

Taking antihistamines, tricyclic antidepressants, or phenothiazines concurrently can result in extreme muscarinic blockage.
NURSING ACTIONS: Discourage concurrent use.

NURSING ADMINISTRATION

- Oral formulations are available as syrup, immediate-release tablets, and extended-release (ER) tablets, which minimize anticholinergic effects. Qᴾᶜᶜ
- Advise clients to swallow ER tablets whole and avoid chewing or crushing the tablets.
- Inform clients that the intestines will eliminate the shell of ER tablets whole in the stool.
- Instruct clients to apply transdermal patches twice per week to dry skin on the hip, abdomen, or buttock and to rotate sites.

NURSING EVALUATION OF MEDICATION EFFECTIVENESS

Indications of effectiveness include decreases in urinary urgency, frequency, nocturia, and urge incontinence.

Application Exercises

1. A nurse is assisting with the care of a client who received a dose of succinylcholine prior to endoscopy. During the procedure, the client suddenly develops rigidity, and his body temperature begins to rise. The nurse should anticipate a prescription for which of the following medications?

   A. Neostigmine

   B. Naloxone

   C. Dantrolene

   D. Vecuronium

2. A nurse is assisting with the care of a client who has malignant hyperthermia. Which of the following actions should the nurse expect to be part of the client's plan of care? (Select all that apply.)

   A. Place a cooling blanket on the client.

   B. Administer oxygen at 50%.

   C. Infuse cold 0.9% sodium chloride.

   D. Prepare for endotracheal intubation.

   E. Monitor core body temperature.

3. A nurse is reinforcing teaching with a client who has a new prescription for baclofen to treat muscle spasms. Which of the following statements indicates that the client understands the instructions? (Select all that apply.)

   A. "I will stop taking this medication right away if I develop dizziness."

   B. "I know the doctor will gradually increase my dose of this medication for a while."

   C. "I should eat more fiber to prevent constipation from this medication."

   D. "I shouldn't drink alcohol while I'm taking this medication."

   E. "I should take this medication on an empty stomach each morning."

4. A nurse is reviewing the medical record of a client who reports urinary incontinence and asks about a prescription for oxybutynin. Which of the following conditions is a contraindication for taking oxybutynin?

   A. Peptic ulcer

   B. Peripheral edema

   C. Multiple sclerosis

   D. Angle-closure glaucoma

5. A nurse is collecting data from a client who has a prescription for bethanechol to treat urinary retention. Which of the following findings is a manifestation of muscarinic stimulation?

   A. Dry mouth

   B. Hypertension

   C. Excessive perspiration

   D. Fecal impaction

PRACTICE Active Learning Scenario

A nurse in a surgical center is reviewing nursing responsibilities for clients receiving succinylcholine. Use the ATI Active Learning Template: Medication to complete this item.

THERAPEUTIC USES: Identify two common indications for use.

MEDICATION ADMINISTRATION: Identify two nursing actions for nurses caring for clients receiving succinylcholine.

Application Exercises Key

1. A. Neostigmine is the reversal agent for pancuronium, a nondepolarizing neuromuscular blockers. It can delay inactivation of succinylcholine, prolonging the client's recovery from the complication.

   B. Naloxone reverses the effects of opioids. It does not treat malignant hyperthermia.

   C. **CORRECT:** Muscle rigidity and a sudden rise in temperature are manifestations of malignant hyperthermia. Dantrolene acts on skeletal muscles to reduce metabolic activity and treat malignant hyperthermia.

   D. Vecuronium is an intermediate-acting nondepolarizing neuromuscular blocker. It is not useful for treating malignant hyperthermia.

   (N) *NCLEX® Connection: Pharmacological Therapies, Adverse Effects/ Contraindications/Side Effects/Interactions*

2. A. **CORRECT:** The nurse should expect to place a cooling blanket on the client and apply ice packs to the client's axilla and groin.

   B. The nurse should administer oxygen at 100% to help ensure optimal oxygen saturation.

   C. **CORRECT:** The nurse should assist with monitoring the infusion of cold IV fluids to help decrease the client's body temperature.

   D. **CORRECT:** If initial stabilization is unsuccessful, clients who have malignant hyperthermia might require endotracheal intubation to correct acid-base imbalances.

   E. **CORRECT:** The nurse should monitor core body temperature to help prevent hypothermia and determine progress of treatment measures.

   (N) *NCLEX® Connection: Pharmacological Therapies, Adverse Effects/ Contraindications/Side Effects/Interactions*

3. A. Abrupt cessation of baclofen therapy can result in withdrawal, with a number of adverse effects (visual hallucinations, seizures).

   B. **CORRECT:** The provider prescribes a low dose initially, and then increases it gradually to prevent CNS depression.

   C. **CORRECT:** The client should increase fluids and fiber to reduce the risk for constipation.

   D. **CORRECT:** The intake of alcohol and other CNS depressants can exacerbate the CNS depressant effects of baclofen. Therefore, the client should avoid CNS depressants while taking baclofen.

   E. The client should take baclofen with meals to reduce gastric upset.

   (N) *NCLEX® Connection: Pharmacological Therapies, Expected Actions/Outcomes*

4. A. GI obstruction, not peptic ulcer disease, is a contraindication for taking oxybutynin.

   B. Urinary retention, not peripheral edema, is a contraindication for taking oxybutynin.

   C. Myasthenia gravis, not multiple sclerosis, requires caution when taking oxybutynin.

   D. **CORRECT:** Oxybutynin is an anticholinergic and can increase intraocular pressure. Glaucoma is a contraindication for taking oxybutynin.

   (N) *NCLEX® Connection: Pharmacological Therapies, Adverse Effects/ Contraindications/Side Effects/Interactions*

5. A. Increased salivation is a manifestation of muscarinic stimulation.

   B. Hypotension is a manifestation of muscarinic stimulation.

   C. **CORRECT:** Bethanechol is a muscarinic agonist. Muscarinic stimulation can increase sweating.

   D. Diarrhea is an adverse effect of bethanechol.

   (N) *NCLEX® Connection: Pharmacological Therapies, Adverse Effects/ Contraindications/Side Effects/Interactions*

PRACTICE Answer

Using the Active Learning Template: Medication

THERAPEUTIC USES	MEDICATION ADMINISTRATION
• Endotracheal intubation • Electroconvulsive therapy • Endoscopy • Adjunct to mechanical ventilation • Muscle relaxation during surgery	• Maintain continuous cardiac and respiratory monitoring during therapy. • Monitor clients following administration of a neuromuscular blocker for respiratory depression and have life support equipment available. • Continue to monitor carefully for the return of respiratory function. • Monitor carefully for indications of malignant hyperthermia and have cooling measures available.

(N) *NCLEX® Connection: Pharmacological and Parenteral Therapies, Adverse Effects/ Contraindications/Side Effects/Interactions*

UNIT 2   MEDICATIONS AFFECTING THE NERVOUS SYSTEM

CHAPTER 15 *Sedative-Hypnotics*

Sedatives are CNS depressants that induce a sense of calm and decrease anxiety. Hypnotics are CNS depressants that induce sleep.

The three types of sedative-hypnotics are **benzodiazepines, barbiturates,** and **benzodiazepine-like medications.** The most commonly used are benzodiazepines and benzodiazepine-like medications because barbiturates cause tolerance and dependence, have multiple interactions, and are powerful respiratory depressants.

IV anesthetics usually are administered during induction of general anesthesia. Most have a quick onset of action and short duration. These medications can be nonopioids or opioids.

Benzodiazepines

SELECT PROTOTYPE MEDICATION: Diazepam

OTHER MEDICATIONS
- Alprazolam
- Lorazepam
- Midazolam
- Temazepam
- Triazolam
- Clonazepam
- Oxazepam
- Chlordiazepoxide

PURPOSE

EXPECTED PHARMACOLOGICAL ACTION: Enhance the action of gamma-aminobutyric acid (GABA) in the CNS.

THERAPEUTIC USES Q EBP
- Anxiety disorders (alprazolam, chlordiazepoxide, diazepam, lorazepam, oxazepam)
- Seizure disorders (clonazepam, diazepam, lorazepam)
- Insomnia (triazolam, temazepam)
- Muscle spasm (diazepam)
- Alcohol withdrawal (chlordiazepoxide, diazepam, lorazepam, oxazepam)
- Panic disorder (alprazolam, clonazepam, lorazepam)
- Induction of anesthesia/preoperative sedation (diazepam, midazolam, lorazepam)

COMPLICATIONS

CNS depression

Lightheadedness, drowsiness, incoordination

CLIENT EDUCATION
- Observe for manifestations and notify the provider if they occur.
- Avoid hazardous activities (driving, operating heavy equipment/machinery).

Paradoxical response

Insomnia, excitation, euphoria, anxiety, rage

CLIENT EDUCATION: Observe for manifestations. If manifestations occur, notify the provider and stop the medication.

Nausea, vomiting, anorexia

CLIENT EDUCATION: Medication can be taken with food.

Respiratory depression

Especially with IV administration

NURSING ACTIONS
- Monitor vital signs.
- Have resuscitation equipment available.

Physical dependence

- Benzodiazepines have a lower abuse potential than barbiturates and most other general CNS depressants.
- Withdrawal following short-term therapy manifests as anxiety, insomnia, tremors, and dizziness.
- Withdrawal following long-term therapy manifests as delirium, paranoia, panic, hypertension, and seizures.

NURSING ACTIONS: Discontinue medication slowly by tapering dose over weeks to months.

Acute toxicity

Oral: drowsiness, lethargy, confusion

IV: respiratory depression, cardiac arrest

NURSING ACTIONS
- Oral: Monitor client receiving gastric lavage, followed by activated charcoal administration or saline cathartics.
- IV: Administer flumazenil to counteract sedation and reverse adverse effects.
- Monitor vital signs, maintain patent airway, and provide fluids to maintain blood pressure.
- Have resuscitation equipment available.

TEMAZEPAM, TRIAZOLAM

Anterograde amnesia and sleep-related behaviors

Sleep driving, sleep eating

CLIENT EDUCATION: Observe for manifestations and notify the provider if they occur.

CONTRAINDICATIONS/PRECAUTIONS

- Most benzodiazepines are Pregnancy Risk Category D. Triazolam and temazepam are Pregnancy Risk Category X. Qs
- Contraindicated in clients who have sleep apnea, respiratory depression, and organic brain disease, or who are breastfeeding.
- Use cautiously in clients who have a history of substance use disorder, liver dysfunction, or kidney failure.
- Older adults can require decreased dosages. Precautions should be taken when administering benzodiazepines to older adult clients because memory difficulties can result. Ⓖ

INTERACTIONS

CNS depressants (alcohol, barbiturates, opioids) cause additive CNS depressant effects with concurrent use.

NURSING ACTIONS: Take complete medication history to identify concurrent use of other CNS depressants.

CLIENT EDUCATION: Avoid alcohol and other CNS depressants.

NURSING ADMINISTRATION

- Ensure proper route of administration.
  - All agents may be given by the oral route.
  - IV administration is acceptable with diazepam, midazolam, and lorazepam.
  - Lorazepam is the agent of choice for IM injection.
- Advise clients to take the medication as prescribed and to avoid abrupt discontinuation of treatment to prevent manifestations of medication withdrawal. Qs
- When discontinuing benzodiazepines, taper dose over several weeks.
- Administer medication with meals. Advise clients to swallow and avoid chewing or crushing sustained-release tablets.
- For insomnia, take 15 to 20 min before bedtime. Limit continuous use to 7 to 10 days. Reinforce nonpharmacologic strategies to facilitate sleep. Qpcc
- Inform clients about possible development of dependency during and after treatment, and to notify the provider if manifestations occur.

NURSING EVALUATION OF MEDICATION EFFECTIVENESS

Depending on therapeutic intent, effectiveness can be evidenced by improvement of well-being as evidenced by absence of panic attacks, decrease or absence of anxiety, normal sleep pattern, absence of seizures, absence of withdrawal manifestations from alcohol, and relaxation of muscles.

Nonbenzodiazepines (Benzodiazepine-like medications)

SELECT PROTOTYPE MEDICATION: Zolpidem

OTHER MEDICATIONS
- Zaleplon
- Eszopiclone

PURPOSE

EXPECTED PHARMACOLOGICAL ACTION: Enhance the action of GABA in the CNS. This results in prolonged sleep duration and decreased awakenings. These medications are Schedule IV substances and do not function as antianxiety, muscle relaxant, or antiepileptic agents. There is a low risk of tolerance, substance use disorder, and dependence

THERAPEUTIC USES: Management of insomnia

COMPLICATIONS

Daytime sleepiness and lightheadedness, headache

NURSING ACTIONS: Administer medication at bedtime.

CLIENT EDUCATION
- Take medication allowing for at least 8 hr of sleep.
- More rapid absorption occurs when the medication is taken on an empty stomach.

CONTRAINDICATIONS/PRECAUTIONS

- Pregnancy Risk Category C
- Precautions are necessary for clients who are breastfeeding.
- Zolpidem has been associated with sleep-related complex behaviors similar to benzodiazepines.
- Use cautiously in older adult clients and in clients who have impaired kidney, liver, or respiratory function. Qs

INTERACTIONS

CNS depressants (alcohol, barbiturates, opioids) cause additive CNS depression.
CLIENT EDUCATION: Avoid alcohol and other CNS depressants.

NURSING ADMINISTRATION

- Advise clients to take the medication just before bedtime.
- Administer all agents by oral or sublingual route.

NURSING EVALUATION OF MEDICATION EFFECTIVENESS

Depending on therapeutic intent, effectiveness can be evidenced by an effective sleep pattern.

Melatonin agonist

SELECT PROTOTYPE MEDICATION: Ramelteon

PURPOSE

EXPECTED PHARMACOLOGICAL ACTION: Activation of melatonin receptors

THERAPEUTIC USES: Management of insomnia

COMPLICATIONS

Sleepiness, dizziness, fatigue

CLIENT EDUCATION
- Ramelteon is generally well tolerated. Notify the provider if manifestations occur.
- Avoid activities such as driving if manifestations occur.

Hormonal effects

Amenorrhea, decreased libido, infertility, and galactorrhea caused by increased levels of prolactin

CLIENT EDUCATION: Notify the provider if manifestations occur. Medication may be discontinued.

CONTRAINDICATIONS/PRECAUTIONS

- Pregnancy Risk Category C
- Contraindicated in lactation, severe forms of liver disease, depression, apnea, and COPD
- Use cautiously in older adults and clients who have moderate liver disease. Ⓖ

INTERACTIONS

High-fat meals can prolong absorption of ramelteon.
CLIENT EDUCATION
- Avoid high-fat meals before taking the medication.
- Take medication on an empty stomach for rapid onset.

Concurrent use of fluvoxamine can increase levels of ramelteon.
NURSING ACTIONS: Avoid concurrent use.

CNS depressants such as opioids, alcohol can cause additive CNS depression.
NURSING ACTIONS: Avoid concurrent use.

NURSING ADMINISTRATION

- Administer by oral route.
- Instruct clients to take medication 30 min prior to bedtime.
- Instruct clients to take medication on an empty stomach and to avoid high-fat foods before taking ramelteon.
- Instruct clients that the purpose of ramelteon is to induce sleep; it is not prescribed for sleep maintenance.

NURSING EVALUATION OF MEDICATION EFFECTIVENESS

Depending on therapeutic intent, effectiveness can be evidenced by improvement in sleep patterns.

Intravenous anesthetics

Intravenous nonopioid agents

SELECT PROTOTYPE MEDICATIONS
- **Barbiturates:** Pentobarbital sodium
- **Benzodiazepines** (used for preoperative sedation): Midazolam, diazepam, lorazepam
- **Other medications:** Propofol, ketamine

Intravenous opioid agents

SELECT PROTOTYPE MEDICATION: Fentanyl

OTHER MEDICATIONS
- Alfentanil
- Sufentanil
- Morphine sulfate

PURPOSE

EXPECTED PHARMACOLOGICAL ACTION: Loss of consciousness and elimination of response to painful stimuli

THERAPEUTIC USES
- Induction and maintenance of anesthesia
- Moderate (conscious) sedation (usually an IV nonopioid agent combined with an opioid agent)
- Intubation and mechanical ventilation

COMPLICATIONS

Respiratory and cardiovascular depression with high risk for hypotension and shock

The client will require mechanical ventilation during the procedure.

NURSING ACTIONS
- Provide continuous monitoring of vital signs and ECG.
- Have equipment ready for resuscitation. Ⓠs

PROPOFOL

Bacterial infection

NURSING ACTIONS
- Discard opened vials after 6 hr.
- Monitor for indications of infection (fever, malaise) after surgery.

KETAMINE

Psychological reactions

- Hallucinations, confusion
- Children younger than 15 years and adults older than 65 years are at higher risk.
- Diazepam or midazolam should precede ketamine administration.

NURSING ACTIONS
- Avoid use in clients who have a history of mental illness.
- Maintain a quiet, low-stimulus environment during recovery.

CONTRAINDICATIONS/PRECAUTIONS

- Avoid use in clients who have a history of mental illness.
- Use cautiously in clients who have respiratory and cardiovascular disease.
- Midazolam is contraindicated in clients who have glaucoma. Precautions should be taken in children, older adults, and clients who have kidney or hepatic failure, status asthmaticus, or alcohol intoxication.
- Pentobarbital and midazolam are Pregnancy Risk Category D.

INTERACTIONS

Additive CNS depression
- Created by CNS depressants (alcohol, barbiturates, opioids)
- Clients can require lower dose.
- NURSING ACTIONS
  - Provide continuous monitoring of vital signs and ECG.
  - Have equipment ready for resuscitation.

Additive CNS stimulation
- Created by CNS stimulants (amphetamines, cocaine)
- Clients can require higher doses.
- NURSING ACTIONS
  - Provide continuous monitoring of vital signs and ECG.
  - Have equipment ready for resuscitation.

NURSING ADMINISTRATION

- Slow administration is required for moderate (conscious) sedation or neonatal anesthesia (administer over 2 min).
- Monitor carefully during and after moderate sedation or anesthesia for respiratory arrest or hypotension.
- Injecting propofol into large vein can decrease pain at injection site.
- Instruct clients to arrange for a ride home following outpatient procedure. Qpcc

NURSING EVALUATION OF MEDICATION EFFECTIVENESS

Depending on therapeutic intent, effectiveness can be evidenced by the following.
- Surgical procedure occurs with loss of consciousness and elimination of pain.
- Postoperative recovery as demonstrated by
  - Vital signs return to baseline.
  - Client is oriented to time, place, and person.
  - Bowel sounds return.
  - Voiding occurs within 8 hr.
  - Nausea and vomiting are controlled.

Application Exercises

1. A nurse is reinforcing instructions with a client who has been experiencing insomnia and has a new prescription for temazepam. Which of the following manifestations are adverse effects of temazepam? (Select all that apply.)

   A. Incoordination

   B. Euphoria

   C. Pruritus

   D. Sleep driving

   E. Amnesia

2. A nurse is assisting with the care of a client who becomes oversedated following administration of diazepam IV. The nurse should expect the client to receive which of the following medications?

   A. Ketamine

   B. Naltrexone

   C. Flumazenil

   D. Fluvoxamine

3. A nurse is reinforcing teaching with a client who has a new prescription for ramelteon. The nurse should instruct the client not to take ramelteon with which of the following foods?

   A. Baked potato

   B. Fried chicken

   C. Whole-grain bread

   D. Citrus fruits

4. A nurse is caring for a client who is to undergo a surgical procedure. Which of the following pre-existing conditions can be a contraindication for the use of ketamine as an IV anesthetic?

   A. Peptic ulcer disease

   B. Breast cancer

   C. Diabetes mellitus

   D. Schizophrenia

5. A nurse is reinforcing instructions with a female client who has a new prescription for zolpidem. Which of the following instructions should the nurse include?

   A. "Notify the provider if you plan to become pregnant."

   B. "Take the medication 1 hr before you plan to go to sleep."

   C. "Allow at least 6 hr for sleep when taking zolpidem."

   D. "To increase the effectiveness of zolpidem, take it with a bedtime snack."

PRACTICE Active Learning Scenario

A nurse is helping develop an educational session to review client use of benzodiazepines for other nurses on the unit. What information should the nurse plan to include? Use the ATI Active Learning Template: Medication to complete this item.

THERAPEUTIC USES: Identify five therapeutic uses for benzodiazepines.

CONTRAINDICATIONS/PRECAUTIONS: Identify four contraindications for taking benzodiazepines.

Application Exercises Key

1. A. **CORRECT:** Due to CNS depression, incoordination is an adverse effect of temazepam.

   B. **CORRECT:** Euphoria a paradoxical adverse effect of temazepam.

   C. Pruritus is not an adverse effect of temazepam.

   D. **CORRECT:** Sleep driving (driving after taking the medication without memory of doing so) is an adverse effect of temazepam.

   E. **CORRECT:** Anterograde amnesia, the inability to remember the events that occurred after taking the medication, can occur as an adverse effect of temazepam.

   Ⓝ *NCLEX® Connection: Pharmacological Therapies, Adverse Effects/ Contraindications/Side Effects/Interactions*

2. A. Ketamine is an anesthetic agent.

   B. Naltrexone is an opioid antagonist used to treat opioid overdose and alcohol use disorders.

   C. **CORRECT:** Flumazenil is a competitive benzodiazepine antagonist used to reverse the sedation and other effects of benzodiazepines.

   D. Fluvoxamine is a selective serotonin reuptake inhibitor used to treat depression.

   Ⓝ *NCLEX® Connection: Pharmacological Therapies, Adverse Effects/ Contraindications/Side Effects/Interactions*

3. A. Although any food can affect absorption of ramelteon, a baked potato should not greatly affect the absorption.

   B. **CORRECT:** High-fat foods, such as fried chicken, greatly prolong the absorption of ramelteon. The client should not take ramelteon with or immediately following a high-fat meal.

   C. Although any food can affect absorption of ramelteon, whole-grain breads should not greatly affect the absorption of ramelteon.

   D. Although any food can affect absorption of ramelteon, citrus fruits should not greatly affect the absorption of ramelteon.

   Ⓝ *NCLEX® Connection: Pharmacological Therapies, Adverse Effects/ Contraindications/Side Effects/Interactions*

4. A. Peptic ulcer disease is not a contraindication for the use of ketamine.

   B. Breast cancer is not a contraindication for the use of ketamine.

   C. Diabetes mellitus is not a contraindication for the use of ketamine.

   D. **CORRECT:** Ketamine can produce psychological effects, such as hallucinations. Therefore, mental illness, such as schizophrenia can be a contraindication for the use of ketamine.

   Ⓝ *NCLEX® Connection: Pharmacological Therapies, Adverse Effects/ Contraindications/Side Effects/Interactions*

5. A. **CORRECT:** Zolpidem is Pregnancy Risk Category C. The client should notify the provider if she plans to become pregnant.

   B. Zolpidem should be taken at bedtime.

   C. The client should allow at least 8 hr for sleep when taking zolpidem.

   D. Zolpidem is absorbed best on an empty stomach.

   Ⓝ *NCLEX® Connection: Pharmacological Therapies, Expected Actions/Outcomes*

PRACTICE Answer

Using the ATI Active Learning Template: Medication

THERAPEUTIC USES
- Anxiety disorders
- Seizure disorders
- Insomnia
- Muscle spasms
- Alcohol withdrawal
- Panic disorder
- Induction of anesthesia

CONTRAINDICATIONS/PRECAUTIONS
- Pregnancy: Benzodiazepines are Pregnancy Risk Category D (high risk to the fetus).
- Sleep apnea
- Respiratory depression
- Organic brain disease
- Lactation
- Use caution in clients who have a history of substance use disorders, liver dysfunction, and kidney failure.

Ⓝ *NCLEX® Connection: Pharmacological and Parenteral Therapies, Medication Administration*

ⓝ NCLEX® Connections

When reviewing the following chapters, keep in mind the relevant topics and tasks of the NCLEX outline, in particular:

Pharmacological Therapies

ADVERSE EFFECTS/CONTRAINDICATIONS/SIDE EFFECTS/ INTERACTIONS: Reinforce client teaching on possible effects of medications (common side effects or adverse effects, when to notify the primary health care provider).

EXPECTED ACTIONS/OUTCOMES: Apply knowledge of pathophysiology when addressing the client's pharmacological agents.

MEDICATION ADMINISTRATION: Reinforce client teaching on client self-administration of medications (insulin, subcutaneous insulin pump).

UNIT 3   MEDICATIONS AFFECTING THE
RESPIRATORY SYSTEM

CHAPTER 16 *Airflow Disorders*

Asthma is a chronic inflammatory disorder of the airways. It is an intermittent and reversible airflow obstruction that affects the bronchioles. The obstruction occurs either by inflammation or airway hyper-responsiveness leading to bronchoconstriction. Medication management usually addresses both inflammation and bronchoconstriction. These medications can also be used to treat the manifestations of chronic obstructive pulmonary disease (COPD).

Medications include bronchodilator agents (beta$_2$ adrenergic agonists, methylxanthines, inhaled anticholinergics) and anti-inflammatory agents (glucocorticoids, mast cell stabilizers, leukotriene modifiers).

Bronchodilators

Beta$_2$ adrenergic agonists

SELECT PROTOTYPE MEDICATION: Albuterol

OTHER MEDICATIONS

Short-acting inhalers: Levalbuterol

Long-acting inhalers
- Arformoterol
- Formoterol
- Salmeterol

Long-acting oral medications
- Terbutaline
- Albuterol

PURPOSE

EXPECTED PHARMACOLOGICAL ACTION

Beta$_2$ adrenergic agonists act by selectively activating the beta$_2$ receptors in the bronchial smooth muscle, resulting in bronchodilation. As a result of this:
- Bronchospasm is relieved.
- Histamine release is inhibited.
- Ciliary motility is increased.

THERAPEUTIC USES

Albuterol, levalbuterol

ROUTE
- Inhaled, short-acting
- Oral, long-acting (albuterol)

THERAPEUTIC USES
- Prevention of asthma episode (exercise-induced)
- Inhaled, short-acting, used for prevention of asthma
- Treatment for acute bronchospasm
- Long-term control of asthma

Formoterol, salmeterol

ROUTE: Inhaled, long-acting

THERAPEUTIC USES: Long-term control of asthma (combined with a glucocorticoid)

Terbutaline, albuterol

ROUTE: Oral, long-acting

THERAPEUTIC USES: Long-term control of asthma

COMPLICATIONS

Long-acting beta agonists can increase risk of severe asthma and asthma-related death when used alone for long-term control.

Tachycardia, angina

- Oral agents can cause tachycardia and angina due to activation of alpha$_1$ receptors in the heart.
- Can also occur with short-acting beta agonists but is usually minimal.
- Dosage might need to be reduced.

CLIENT EDUCATION
- Observe for chest, jaw, or arm pain or palpitations. Notify the provider if they occur.
- Check pulse and report changes in pulse rate or rhythm.
- Avoid caffeine.

Tremors

Caused by activation of beta$_2$ receptors in skeletal muscle
- Tremors usually resolve with continued medication use.
- Dosage might need to be reduced.

CONTRAINDICATIONS/PRECAUTIONS

- Pregnancy Risk Category C Qs
- Contraindicated in clients who have tachydysrhythmia
- Use cautiously in clients who have diabetes mellitus, hyperthyroidism, heart disease, hypertension, and angina.

INTERACTIONS

Use of beta adrenergic blockers can negate effects of both medications.
Beta adrenergic blockers should not be used concurrently with beta adrenergic agonists.

MAOIs and tricyclic antidepressants can increase the risk of tachycardia and angina.
CLIENT EDUCATION: Report changes in heart rate and chest pain.

NURSING ADMINISTRATION

- Instruct clients to follow manufacturer's instructions for use of metered-dose inhaler (MDI), dry-powder inhaler (DPI), and nebulizer. **(16.1)**
- When a client has prescriptions for an inhaled beta$_2$ agonist and an inhaled glucocorticoid, advise the client to inhale the beta$_2$ agonist before inhaling the glucocorticoid. The beta$_2$ agonist promotes bronchodilation and enhances absorption of the glucocorticoid. Q$_{EBP}$
- Remind the client to wait at least 1 min between inhalations if more than one is required. This improves medication effectiveness.
- Advise clients not to exceed prescribed dosages.

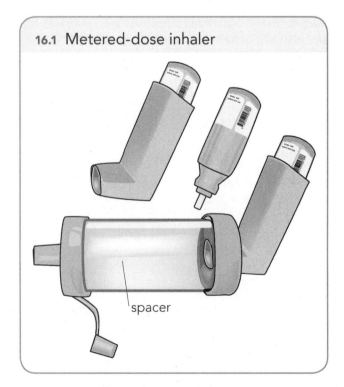

16.1 Metered-dose inhaler

spacer

- Ensure that clients know the dosage schedule (if the medication is to be taken on a fixed or as-needed schedule).
- Formoterol and salmeterol are long-acting beta$_2$ agonist inhalers. These inhalers are used every 12 hr for long-term control and are not used to abort an asthma exacerbation. These long-acting agents are not used alone but are prescribed in combination with an inhaled glucocorticoid.
- A short-acting beta$_2$ agonist is used to treat an acute episode.
- Advise clients to observe for indications of an impending asthma episode and to keep a log of the frequency and intensity of exacerbations.
- Instruct clients to notify the provider if there is an increase in the frequency and intensity of asthma exacerbations.

NURSING EVALUATION OF MEDICATION EFFECTIVENESS

Depending on therapeutic intent, effectiveness is evidenced by the following.
- Long-term control of asthma
- Prevention of exercise-induced asthma
- Resolution of asthma exacerbations as evidenced by absence of shortness of breath, clear breath sounds, absence of wheezing, and return of respiratory rate to baseline
- Some medications can be more effective in nebulizer form if the client does not achieve the desired therapeutic effect.

Methylxanthines

SELECT PROTOTYPE MEDICATION: Theophylline
Aminophylline is a theophylline available in oral and IV preparations

PURPOSE

EXPECTED PHARMACOLOGICAL ACTION
- Relaxation of bronchial smooth muscle, resulting in bronchodilation
- Once the first-line medication for asthma, now used infrequently because newer medications are safer and more effective

THERAPEUTIC USES: Oral theophylline is used for long-term control of chronic asthma or COPD.

ROUTE OF ADMINISTRATION: Oral or IV (emergency use only); aminophylline is the preferred form of theophylline IV

COMPLICATIONS

Toxicity reactions

- More severe reactions (**dysrhythmias, seizures**) can occur with higher therapeutic levels or levels up to 25 mcg/mL.
- Mild reactions include nausea, vomiting, diarrhea, insomnia, and restlessness. These occur typically at levels greater than 30 mcg/mL.

NURSING ACTIONS
- Monitor theophylline serum levels to keep within therapeutic range (5 to 15 mcg/mL). Adverse effects are unlikely to occur at levels less than 20 mcg/mL.
- If manifestations occur, stop the medication. The client can require additional treatment (activated charcoal to decrease absorption, lidocaine to treat dysrhythmias, diazepam to control seizures).

CLIENT EDUCATION: Have blood levels checked periodically. Report nausea, diarrhea, or restlessness, which are indicative of toxicity.

CONTRAINDICATIONS/PRECAUTIONS

- Pregnancy Risk Category C $\mathbf{Q}$**s**
- Use cautiously in clients who have heart disease, hypertension, liver and kidney dysfunction, and diabetes mellitus.
- Use cautiously in children and older adults. ©

INTERACTIONS

Caffeine increases CNS and cardiac effects of theophylline, and can increase theophylline levels.
CLIENT EDUCATION: Avoid consuming caffeinated beverages (coffee, caffeinated colas).

Phenobarbital, phenytoin, and rifampin decrease theophylline levels.
NURSING ACTIONS: When used concurrently, increase the dosage of theophylline.

Cimetidine, ciprofloxacin, and other fluoroquinolone antibiotics increase theophylline levels.
NURSING ACTIONS: When used concurrently, decrease the dosage of theophylline.

NURSING ADMINISTRATION

- Advise clients to take the medication as prescribed. If a dose is missed, the client should not double the next dose.
- Instruct clients to not chew or crush sustained-release preparations. These medications should be swallowed whole.

NURSING EVALUATION OF MEDICATION EFFECTIVENESS

Depending on therapeutic intent, effectiveness is evidenced by long-term control of asthma and COPD.

Inhaled anticholinergics

SELECT PROTOTYPE MEDICATION: Ipratropium

OTHER MEDICATIONS: Tiotropium

PURPOSE

EXPECTED PHARMACOLOGICAL ACTION: Block muscarinic receptors of the bronchi, resulting in bronchodilation

THERAPEUTIC USES
- Relieve bronchospasm associated with COPD
- Allergen-induced and exercise-induced bronchospasm

ROUTE OF ADMINISTRATION: Inhalation

COMPLICATIONS

Local anticholinergic effects

Dry mouth, hoarseness

CLIENT EDUCATION: Sip fluids and suck on sugar-free hard candies to control dry mouth.

CONTRAINDICATIONS/PRECAUTIONS

- Pregnancy Risk Category B $\mathbf{Q}$**s**
- Contraindicated in clients who have an allergy to peanuts because the medication preparations can contain soy lecithin.
- Use cautiously in clients who have narrow-angle glaucoma and benign prostatic hyperplasia (due to anticholinergic effects).

NURSING ADMINISTRATION

- Advise clients to rinse the mouth after inhalation to decrease unpleasant taste.
- Usual adult dosage is 2 puffs. Instruct clients to wait the length of time directed between puffs.
- If two inhaled medications are prescribed, instruct clients to wait at least 5 min between medications.
- Advise clients not to swallow tiotropium capsules. An inhalation device is used for administration of the capsule.

NURSING EVALUATION OF MEDICATION EFFECTIVENESS

Depending on therapeutic intent, effectiveness is evidenced by the following.
- Control of bronchospasm in clients who have COPD
- Prevention of allergen-induced and exercise-induced bronchospasm

Anti-inflammatory agents

Glucocorticoids

SELECT PROTOTYPE MEDICATIONS
- Inhalation: Beclomethasone
- Oral: Prednisone

OTHER MEDICATIONS
- Inhalation
  - Budesonide
  - Budesonide and formoterol
  - Fluticasone and salmeterol
  - Fluticasone
  - Mometasone and formoterol
- Oral: prednisolone
- IV
  - Hydrocortisone
  - Methylprednisolone

PURPOSE

EXPECTED PHARMACOLOGICAL ACTION

- Prevent inflammation, suppress airway mucus production, and promote responsiveness of beta$_2$ receptors in the bronchial tree
- Reduce airway mucosa edema

> The use of glucocorticoids does not provide immediate effects, but rather promotes decreased frequency and severity of acute exacerbations.

THERAPEUTIC USES

- Short-term IV agents are used for status asthmaticus.
- Inhaled agents are used for long-term prophylaxis of asthma.
- Short-term oral therapy is used to treat manifestations following an acute asthma episode.
- Long-term oral therapy is used to treat chronic, severe asthma.
- Promote lung maturity and decrease respiratory distress in fetuses at risk for preterm birth.

COMPLICATIONS

BECLOMETHASONE

- Medication may be administered with metered-dose inhaler, dry-powder inhaler, and nebulizer.
- The use of a spacer can prevent adverse effects.

Difficulty speaking, hoarseness, candidiasis

CLIENT EDUCATION
- Rinse mouth or gargle with water after use.
- Monitor for redness, sores, or white patches and report to provider if they occur.
- Treat candidiasis with nystatin oral suspension.

PREDNISONE

- Preferred glucocorticoid for oral therapy of asthma
- When used for 10 days or more, can result in the following

Suppression of adrenal gland function

Such as a decrease in the ability of the adrenal cortex to produce glucocorticoids (can occur with inhaled agents and oral agents)

NURSING ACTIONS
- Administer oral glucocorticoid on an alternate-day dosing schedule.
- Monitor blood glucose levels.
- Taper the dose. Do not stop abruptly.

Bone loss

Can occur with inhaled agents and oral agents

NURSING ACTIONS
- Advise clients to perform weight-bearing exercises.
- Advise clients to consume a diet with sufficient calcium and vitamin D intake.
- Use the lowest dose possible to control manifestations.
- Give oral medications on an alternate-day dosing schedule.

Hyperglycemia and glycosuria

- Clients who have diabetes should have their blood glucose monitored.
- Clients might need an increase in insulin dosage.

Myopathy

As evidenced by muscle weakness

NURSING ACTIONS
- Instruct clients to report muscle weakness.
- Medication dosage should be decreased.

Peptic ulcer disease

NURSING ACTIONS
- Advise clients to avoid NSAIDs.
- Advise clients to report black, tarry stools. Check stool for occult blood periodically.
- Administer with food or meals.

Infection

CLIENT EDUCATION: Notify the provider if early manifestations of infection occur (sore throat, weakness, malaise).

Disturbances of fluid and electrolytes

- Fluid retention as evidenced by weight gain
- Edema and hypokalemia as evidenced by muscle weakness

CLIENT EDUCATION: Observe for manifestations and report to the provider.

CONTRAINDICATIONS/PRECAUTIONS

- Pregnancy Risk Category C Qs
- Contraindicated in clients who have received a live virus vaccine and those who have systemic fungal infections
- Use cautiously in children and in clients who have diabetes mellitus, hypertension, heart failure, peptic ulcer disease, osteoporosis, or kidney dysfunction.

INTERACTIONS

Prednisone

Concurrent use of potassium-depleting diuretics increases the risk of hypokalemia.
NURSING ACTIONS: Monitor potassium level and administer supplements as needed.

Concurrent use of NSAIDs increases the risk of GI ulceration.
CLIENT EDUCATION: Avoid use of NSAIDs. If GI distress occurs, notify the provider.

Concurrent use of glucocorticoids and hypoglycemic agents (oral and insulin) counteract the effects.
CLIENT EDUCATION: Notify the provider if hyperglycemia occurs. Increased dosage of insulin or oral hypoglycemics might be needed.

NURSING ADMINISTRATION

- Instruct clients to use glucocorticoid inhalers on a regular, fixed schedule for long-term therapy of asthma. Glucocorticoids are not used to treat an acute episode.
- Administer using an MDI device, DPI, or nebulizer.
- Glucocorticoid MDIs using hydrofluoroalkane (HFA) do not require a spacer to increase medication delivery.
- When a client is taking an inhaled beta₂ agonist and an inhaled glucocorticoid, advise the client to inhale the beta₂ agonist before inhaling the glucocorticoid. The beta₂ agonist promotes bronchodilation and enhances absorption of the glucocorticoid.
- Oral glucocorticoids are used short-term, 3 to 10 days following an acute asthma exacerbation.
- If client is on long-term oral therapy, additional dosages of oral glucocorticoids are required in times of stress (infection, trauma).
- Clients who discontinue oral glucocorticoid medications or switch from oral to inhaled agents require additional doses of oral or IV glucocorticoids during periods of stress.
- Inform parents that glucocoriticoids can slow the rate of growth in children; however, it does not affect the adult height. Qpcc

NURSING EVALUATION OF MEDICATION EFFECTIVENESS

Depending on therapeutic intent, effectiveness is evidenced by the following.
- Long-term control of asthma
- Resolution of acute exacerbation as demonstrated by absence of shortness of breath, clear breath sounds, absence of wheezing, and return of respiratory rate to baseline

Leukotriene modifiers

SELECT PROTOTYPE MEDICATION: Montelukast

OTHER MEDICATIONS
- Zileuton
- Zafirlukast

PURPOSE

EXPECTED PHARMACOLOGICAL ACTION: Leukotriene modifiers suppress the effects of leukotrienes, thereby reducing inflammation, bronchoconstriction, airway edema, and mucus production.

THERAPEUTIC USES: Long-term therapy of asthma in adults and children, and to prevent exercise-induced bronchospasm
- Montelukast is used in children as young as 12 months.
- Zafirlukast is used in children 5 years and older.
- Zileuton is used in adolescents and adults.

ROUTE OF ADMINISTRATION: Oral

COMPLICATIONS

Depression, suicidal ideation

NURSING ACTIONS: Monitor for behavior changes and report to the provider.

Liver injury (zileuton, zafirlukast)

NURSING ACTIONS: Obtain baseline liver function tests and monitor periodically.

CLIENT EDUCATION
- Monitor for indications of liver damage (jaundice, fatigue, nausea, anorexia, abdominal pain).
- Notify the provider if manifestations occur.

CONTRAINDICATIONS/PRECAUTIONS

- Montelukast and zafirlukast are Pregnancy Category B.
- Zileuton is Pregnancy Category C. Qs
- Use cautiously in clients who have liver dysfunction.

INTERACTIONS

Zileuton and zafirlukast inhibit metabolism of warfarin, leading to increased warfarin levels.

NURSING ACTIONS

- Advise clients to observe for indications of bleeding and to notify the provider.
- Monitor prothrombin time (PT) and INR levels.

Zileuton and zafirlukast inhibit metabolism of theophylline, leading to increased theophylline levels.

- NURSING ACTIONS: Monitor theophylline levels.
- CLIENT EDUCATION: Observe for manifestations of theophylline toxicity (nausea, vomiting, seizures), and notify the provider.

Montelukast used concurrently with phenytoin can inhibit effects of montelukast.

CLIENT EDUCATION: Observe for therapeutic effects of montelukast.

NURSING ADMINISTRATION

- Advise clients to take zileuton as prescribed, 1 hr before or after a meal.
- Advise clients to take zafirlukast 1 hr before or 2 hr after meals.
- Advise clients to take montelukast once daily at bedtime. For exercise-induced bronchospasm, take 2 hr before exercise. Instruct clients taking daily montelukast to not take an additional dose for exercise induced bronchospasm.

NURSING EVALUATION OF MEDICATION EFFECTIVENESS

Effectiveness is evidenced by long-term control of asthma.

Application Exercises

1. A nurse is reinforcing teaching with a client who has a new prescription for beclomethasone. Which of the following instructions should the nurse include?

    A. "Rinse your mouth after each use of this medication."

    B. "Limit fluid intake while taking this medication."

    C. "Increase your intake of vitamin B$_{12}$ while taking this medication."

    D. "You can take the medication as needed."

2. A nurse is reviewing instructions with a client who has a new prescription for albuterol and beclomethasone inhalers for the control of asthma. Which of the following information should the nurse include?

    A. Take albuterol at the same time each day.

    B. Administer the albuterol inhaler prior to using the beclomethasone inhaler.

    C. Use beclomethasone if experiencing an acute episode.

    D. Avoid shaking the beclomethasone before use.

3. A nurse is talking with an adolescent who has a new prescription for albuterol PO. Which of the following instructions should the nurse include?

    A. "You can take this medication to abort an acute asthma attack."

    B. "Tremors are an adverse effect of this medication."

    C. "Prolonged use of this medication can cause hyperglycemia."

    D. "This medication can slow skeletal growth rate."

4. A nurse is reinforcing teaching with a client who has chronic asthma and a prescription for long-term oral prednisone. The client should monitor for which of the following adverse effects?

    A. Weight gain

    B. Nervousness

    C. Bradycardia

    D. Constipation

PRACTICE Active Learning Scenario

A nurse is instructing a client who has a new prescription for albuterol PO. What should the nurse include in the teaching? Use the ATI Active Learning Template: Medication to complete this item.

THERAPEUTIC USES

COMPLICATIONS: List two adverse effects.

Application Exercises Key

1. A. **CORRECT:** The client should rinse her mouth after each use to reduce the risk of oral fungal infections.

   B. A client who has asthma should increase fluid intake to liquefy respiratory secretions, unless contraindicated by another condition.

   C. Glucocorticoids place the client at risk for bone loss. There is no need for the client to increase intake of vitamin B_{12}. The client should ensure an adequate intake of calcium and vitamin D.

   D. Beclomethasone is an inhaled glucocorticoid; therefore, the client should take it on a fixed schedule.

   Ⓝ *NCLEX® Connection: Pharmacological Therapies, Expected Actions/Outcomes*

2. A. Albuterol is a short-acting inhaled $beta_2$ agonist used for short-term relief of bronchospasm.

   B. **CORRECT:** When a client has prescriptions for an inhaled $beta_2$ agonist (such as albuterol) and an inhaled glucocorticoid (such as beclomethasone), the client should take the $beta_2$ agonist first. The $beta_2$ agonist promotes bronchodilation and enhances absorption of the glucocorticoid.

   C. The nurse should warn the client no to use beclomethasone to treat an acute attack, but to take it on a fixed schedule.

   D. The client should shake the metered dose inhaler well before administration.

   Ⓝ *NCLEX® Connection: Pharmacological Therapies, Expected Actions/Outcomes*

3. A. The nurse should tell the adolescent to use inhaled albuterol to abort an acute asthma episode.

   B. **CORRECT:** Tremors can occur due to excessive stimulation of $beta_2$ receptors of skeletal muscles.

   C. Prolonged use of glucocorticoids can cause hyperglycemia.

   D. Glucocorticoids slow skeletal growth rate in children and adolescents. However, it does not change the overall adulthood height.

   Ⓝ *NCLEX® Connection: Pharmacological Therapies, Adverse Effects/ Contraindications/Side Effects/Interactions*

4. A. **CORRECT:** Weight gain and fluid retention are adverse effects of oral prednisone due to the effect of sodium and water retention.

   B. Nervousness and insomnia are adverse effects of beta agonists, not glucocorticoids.

   C. Tachycardia is an adverse effect of prednisone and beta agonists.

   D. Diarrhea is an adverse effect of prednisone. Constipation is an adverse effect of tiotropium.

   Ⓝ *NCLEX® Connection: Pharmacological Therapies, Adverse Effects/ Contraindications/Side Effects/Interactions*

PRACTICE Answer

Using the ATI Active Learning Template: Medication

THERAPEUTIC USES: $Beta_2$ adrenergic agonists act by selectively activating the $beta_2$ receptors in the bronchial smooth muscle, resulting in bronchodilation. They also suppress histamine release and promote ciliary motility.

COMPLICATIONS
- Oral agents can cause tachycardia and angina due to activation of $alpha_1$ receptors in the heart.
- Activation of $beta_2$ receptors in skeletal muscle causes tremors.

Ⓝ *NCLEX® Connection: Pharmacological and Parenteral Therapies, Medication Administration*

CHAPTER 17   *Upper Respiratory
Disorders*

The medications in this section work on the central nervous system (CNS), nasal passages, or other parts of the respiratory system to treat the effects of allergic or nonallergic rhinitis or coughs from the common cold, influenza, and other disorders.

Antihistamines, often prescribed for allergic rhinitis, can also treat nausea, motion sickness, allergic reactions, and insomnia.

Combining the medications in this section can increase effectiveness. For example, an antitussive combined with an expectorant can result in improved cough reduction.

Antitussives: Opioids

SELECT PROTOTYPE MEDICATION: Codeine

OTHER MEDICATION: Hydrocodone

PURPOSE

EXPECTED PHARMACOLOGICAL ACTION: Codeine suppresses cough through its action on the central nervous system to increase the cough threshold.

THERAPEUTIC USES: Clients who have a chronic nonproductive cough can take codeine to decrease the frequency and intensity of the cough.

COMPLICATIONS

CNS effects

Dizziness, lightheadedness, drowsiness, respiratory depression

NURSING ACTIONS
- Obtain baseline vital signs.
- Monitor clients when ambulating.
- Observe for manifestations of respiratory depression, such as respirations less than 12/min. Stimulate the client to breathe if respiratory depression occurs. It can be necessary to stop the medication and administer naloxone. Qs

CLIENT EDUCATION
- Change position slowly and lie down if feeling lightheaded.
- Avoid activities that require alertness, such as driving, while taking codeine.

GI distress (nausea, vomiting, constipation)

CLIENT EDUCATION
- Take oral codeine with food.
- Increase fluids and dietary fiber.

Opioid use disorder

NURSING ACTIONS
- Advise clients of the potential for physical dependence and misuse.
- Use for a short duration.

CONTRAINDICATIONS/PRECAUTIONS

- Codeine is Pregnancy Risk Category C. Qs
- Codeine used alone is in the Schedule II class of the Controlled Substances Act. Antitussives that contain codeine are in the Schedule V class.
- Contraindications to codeine use include respiratory depression, acute asthma, head trauma, liver and kidney dysfunction, and acute alcohol use disorder.
- Use cautiously in children, older adults, and clients who have a history of substance use disorder. ©
- Children are rarely prescribed codeine.

NURSING ADMINISTRATION

- Advise clients to avoid activities that require alertness, such as driving, while taking codeine.
- Advise clients to change positions slowly and to lie down if feeling dizzy.
- Advise clients to avoid alcohol and other CNS depressants while taking codeine.

Antitussives: Nonopioids

SELECT PROTOTYPE MEDICATION: Dextromethorphan (found in many different products for cough)

OTHER MEDICATIONS
- Benzonatate
- Diphenhydramine

PURPOSE

EXPECTED PHARMACOLOGICAL ACTION:
Dextromethorphan suppresses cough through its action on the CNS. Although not an opioid, it is an opioid-derivative medication.

THERAPEUTIC USES
- Cough suppression
- Reduce pain when combined with an opioid

COMPLICATIONS

- Dextromethorphan has few adverse effects.
- There is some potential for misuse, as the medication can instill euphoria in high doses.
- Avoid the use of alcohol because of the added depressant effect.
- Benzonatate can cause dizziness, sedation and constipation.

CONTRAINDICATIONS/PRECAUTIONS

- Pregnancy Category Risk C Qs
- Benzonatate can be fatal in children even with a single dose; children under 10 years old should not take benzonatate.

INTERACTIONS

Can cause a high fever when used within 2 weeks of MAOI antidepressants.

NURSING ADMINISTRATION

- Some formulations contain alcohol or sucrose.
- Available forms include tablet, chewable tablet, capsules, lozenges (for clients older than 12 years), liquids, and syrups.
- Warn the client that sucking on or chewing benzonatate capsules can result in respiratory distress and circulatory collapse. The client should swallow benzonatate capsules whole. Qs

NURSING EVALUATION OF MEDICATION EFFECTIVENESS

Depending on therapeutic intent, absence or decreased episodes of coughing indicate medication effectiveness.

Expectorants

SELECT PROTOTYPE MEDICATION: Guaifenesin

PURPOSE

EXPECTED PHARMACOLOGICAL ACTION: Guaifenesin promotes increased cough production by increasing and thinning mucous secretions. These actions allow clients to decrease chest congestion by coughing out secretions.

THERAPEUTIC USES: Although guaifenesin is available as an expectorant alone, combining it with antitussives (opioid or nonopioid) or a decongestant reduces manifestations of colds, allergic or nonallergic rhinitis, or cough caused by lower respiratory disorders.

COMPLICATIONS

GI upset

CLIENT EDUCATION: Take with food if GI upset occurs.

Drowsiness, dizziness

CLIENT EDUCATION: If these reactions occur, do not take prior to driving or activities that require alertness.

Allergic reaction (rash)

CLIENT EDUCATION: Stop taking guaifenesin and obtain medical care if rash or other manifestations of allergy occur.

CONTRAINDICATIONS/PRECAUTIONS

- Guaifenesin is Pregnancy Risk Category C. Qs
- Advise clients who are breastfeeding to talk to the provider before taking medications containing guaifenesin.
- Certain formulation and medication combinations of guaifenesin are not indicated for children.

NURSING ADMINISTRATION

- Advise clients to increase fluid intake when taking guaifenesin to promote liquefying secretions.
- This medication is available in tablets and capsules, which can be opened to sprinkle on foods. The client should not crush guaifenesin tablets.
- Advise clients to read over-the-counter labels carefully to discover what medications have been combined in the preparation used. There are many liquid and syrup combinations that include guaifenesin and other medications (antitussives or decongestants, such as pseudoephedrine).
- Report a cough lasting longer than 1 week to the provider.
- Guaifenesin preparations can contain alcohol and sucrose.

NURSING EVALUATION OF MEDICATION EFFECTIVENESS

Depending on therapeutic intent, effectiveness is evidenced by the following.
- Cough that is more productive and mucous is easier to expectorate
- Decreased chest congestion

Mucolytics

SELECT PROTOTYPE MEDICATION: Acetylcysteine

OTHER MEDICATION: Hypertonic saline

PURPOSE

EXPECTED PHARMACOLOGICAL ACTION: Mucolytics thin and enhance the flow of secretions in the respiratory passages.

THERAPEUTIC USES
- Clients who have acute and chronic pulmonary disorders exacerbated by large amounts of secretions, such as cystic fibrosis, can benefit from mucolytic therapy.
- Acetylcysteine is also the antidote for acetaminophen poisoning.

COMPLICATIONS

Aspiration and bronchospasm

When administered orally

NURSING ACTIONS: Monitor for manifestations of aspiration and bronchospasm. Stop medication immediately and notify the provider.

Dizziness, drowsiness, hypotension, tachycardia

NURSING ACTIONS: Monitor vital signs.

CLIENT EDUCATION: Change position slowly, and avoid activities that require alertness.

Hepatotoxicity

NURSING ACTIONS: Monitor liver function tests.

CONTRAINDICATIONS/PRECAUTIONS

- Acetylcysteine is Pregnancy Risk Category B.
- Clients who are hypersensitive to acetylcysteine should not take it.
- Use cautiously in clients who have hypothyroidism, CNS depression, kidney, liver disease, and seizure disorders.
- Due to the potential for bronchospasm, clients who have asthma should use caution when taking acetylcysteine.

NURSING ADMINISTRATION

- Advise clients that acetylcysteine has an odor that smells like rotten eggs.
- Acetylcysteine is administered by inhalation to liquefy nasal and bronchial secretions and facilitate coughing.
- The medication is administered orally or IV for acetaminophen overdose.
- Be prepared to suction clients if aspiration occurs with oral administration. Qs
- Monitor liver function tests, PT, BUN, creatinine, glucose, electrolytes, and acetaminophen levels in clients who have acetaminophen toxicity.

NURSING EVALUATION OF MEDICATION EFFECTIVENESS

Depending on therapeutic intent, effectiveness is evidenced by improvement of manifestations as demonstrated by regular respiratory rate, clear lung sounds, and increased ease of expectoration.

Decongestants

SELECT PROTOTYPE MEDICATION: Phenylephrine

OTHER MEDICATIONS
- Ephedrine
- Naphazoline
- Pseudoephedrine

PURPOSE

EXPECTED PHARMACOLOGICAL ACTION: Sympathomimetic decongestants stimulate the alpha$_1$ adrenergic receptors, causing a reduction in the inflammation of the nasal membranes.

THERAPEUTIC USES
- This medication treats allergic or nonallergic rhinitis by relieving nasal stuffiness.
- The medication acts as a decongestant for clients who have sinusitis and the common cold.

COMPLICATIONS

Rebound congestion

Secondary to prolonged use of topical agents

CLIENT EDUCATION
- Use for short-term therapy, no more than 3 to 5 days.
- Taper use and discontinue medication using one nostril at a time.

CNS stimulation

- Agitation, nervousness, uneasiness
- Rare with the use of topical agents

NURSING ACTIONS

- Advise clients to observe and report manifestations of CNS stimulation.
- Stop medication.

Vasoconstriction (headache, chest pain)

Clients who have hypertension, cerebrovascular disease, dysrhythmias, and coronary artery disease should avoid using these medications.

CONTRAINDICATIONS/PRECAUTIONS

- Closed-angle glaucoma is a contraindication to taking these medications.
- Use cautiously in clients who have coronary artery disease, hypertension, cerebrovascular disease, and dysrhythmias.
- Pseudoephedrine and ephedrine convert easily into amphetamine; therefore, these medications have a high potential for misuse. They are available without a prescription. However, pharmacies must request to see personal identification before selling these medications. Qs

NURSING ADMINISTRATION

- When administering nasal drops, instruct clients to be in the lateral, head-low position to increase the desired effect and prevent swallowing the medication.
- Drops are preferred for children because precise administration reduces the risk of toxicity.
- Educate clients in the differences between topical and oral agents.
  - Topical agents are usually more effective and work faster.
  - Topical agents have a shorter duration.
  - Vasoconstriction and CNS stimulation are uncommon with topical agents, but are a concern with oral agents.
  - Oral agents do not lead to rebound congestion.
- Advise clients to use topical decongestants for no longer than 3 to 5 days to avoid rebound congestion.
- Instruct clients not to exceed recommended doses.

NURSING EVALUATION OF MEDICATION EFFECTIVENESS

Depending on therapeutic intent, effectiveness is evidenced by improvement of manifestations (relief of congestion, increased ease of breathing).

Antihistamines

SELECT PROTOTYPE MEDICATIONS

1st generation H_1 antagonists
- Diphenhydramine
- Promethazine
- Dimenhydrinate

2nd generation H_1 antagonists
- Loratadine
- Cetirizine
- Fexofenadine
- Desloratadine

Intranasal antihistamines
- Azelastine
- Olopatadine

PURPOSE

EXPECTED PHARMACOLOGICAL ACTION

Antihistamine action is on the H_1 receptors, which results in the blocking of histamine release in the small blood vessels, capillaries, and nerves during allergic reactions. These medications relieve itching, sneezing, and rhinorrhea, but not nasal congestion. First-generation antihistamines produce cholinergic effects and drowsiness.

THERAPEUTIC USES

- Mild allergic reactions (seasonal allergic rhinitis, urticaria, mild transfusion reaction)
- Anaphylaxis (hypotension, acute laryngeal edema, bronchospasm)
- Motion sickness
- Insomnia
- Often used in combination with sympathomimetics to provide a nasal decongestant effect

COMPLICATIONS

Sedation

Common with first-generation H_1 antagonists

CLIENT EDUCATION

- Take the medication at night to minimize daytime sedative effect.
- Avoid driving, or other activities that require alertness, consumption of alcohol, and other CNS depressant medications (barbiturates, benzodiazepines, opioids).

Anticholinergic effects

- Dry mouth, constipation
- More common with first-generation agents

CLIENT EDUCATION: Take sips of water, suck on sugarless candies, and maintain 2 to 3 L of water each day from food and beverage sources.

Gastrointestinal discomfort

Nausea, vomiting, constipation

CLIENT EDUCATION: Take antihistamine with meals.

Acute toxicity, excitation, hallucinations, incoordination, and seizures in children

Flushed face, high fever, tachycardia, dry mouth, urinary retention, pupil dilation

NURSING ACTIONS
- Advise clients to notify the provider if effects occur.
- Administer activated charcoal and cathartic to decrease absorption of antihistamine.
- Administer acetaminophen for fever.
- Apply ice packs or administer sponge baths.

Respiratory depression, local tissue injury at IV site

- Occurs with promethazine.
- IM administration is the preferred route. If unavailable, administer through a large-bore IV in concentrations of 25 mg/mL or less.

NURSING ACTIONS
- Monitor for manifestations of respiratory distress, and have resuscitation equipment available.
- Monitor for manifestations of extravasation, and advise clients to report any pain or burning sensations.

CONTRAINDICATIONS/PRECAUTIONS

- Clients in the third trimester of pregnancy, clients who are breastfeeding, and newborns should not take antihistamines. Newborns are sensitive to the adverse effects of these medications, such as sedation. Qs
- Promethazine is Pregnancy Category C.
- Promethazine is also contraindicated in clients younger than 2 years of age; clients who have cardiac dysrhythmias or hepatic diseases; and those on MAOI therapy.
- Use cautiously in children and older adults. Monitor severity of adverse effects, especially respiratory depression. ⑥
- Use cautiously in clients who have asthma, seizure disorder, cardiac disease, kidney disease, urinary retention, open-angle glaucoma, hypertension, and prostate hypertrophy (affect impact of anticholinergic medications).

INTERACTIONS

CNS depressants/alcohol cause additive CNS depression.

CLIENT EDUCATION: Avoid alcohol and medications causing CNS depression (opioids, barbiturates, benzodiazepines).

NURSING ADMINISTRATION

Advise clients taking first-generation medications to be aware of sedating effects.

NURSING EVALUATION OF MEDICATION EFFECTIVENESS

Depending on therapeutic intent, these factors indicate therapeutic effectiveness.
- Improvement of allergic reaction (absence of rhinitis, urticaria)
- Relief of motion sickness (decreased nausea and vomiting)

Nasal glucocorticoids

SELECT PROTOTYPE MEDICATION: Mometasone

OTHER MEDICATIONS
- Fluticasone
- Triamcinolone
- Budesonide

PURPOSE

EXPECTED PHARMACOLOGICAL ACTION: Nasal glucocorticoids decrease the inflammation associated with allergic rhinitis. They are the first-line of treatment for nasal congestion.

THERAPEUTIC USE: Reduce the effects of allergic rhinitis (sneezing, nasal itching, runny nose)

COMPLICATIONS

Sore throat, nosebleed, headache, burning in nose

CLIENT EDUCATION: Contact provider if adverse effects occur.

CONTRAINDICATIONS/PRECAUTIONS

Pregnancy Risk Category C.

CLIENT EDUCATION
- A metered-dose spray device delivers the medication.
- Administer a dose daily, not just when manifestations occur.
- For seasonal allergic rhinitis, it can take 7 days or more to get the maximum relief.
- For perennial allergic rhinitis, it can take as long as 21 days to get the maximum relief.
- Clear blocked nasal passages with a topical decongestant prior to glucocorticoid administration. QEBP

Application Exercises

1. A nurse is caring for a client who states she has been taking phenylephrine nasal drops for the past 10 days for sinusitis. The nurse should monitor for which of the following adverse effects?

   A. Sedation

   B. Nasal congestion

   C. Productive cough

   D. Constipation

2. A nurse is reviewing information with a client who has a new prescription for dextromethorphan to suppress a cough. The nurse should instruct the client to monitor for which of the following adverse effects?

   A. Diarrhea

   B. Anxiety

   C. Sedation

   D. Palpitations

3. A nurse is reinforcing teaching with the family of a child who has cystic fibrosis and a new prescription for acetylcysteine. Which of the following information should the nurse include in the instructions?

   A. "Expect this medication to suppress your cough."

   B. "Expect this medication to smell like rotten eggs."

   C. "Expect this medication to cause euphoria."

   D. "Expect this medication to turn your urine orange."

4. A nurse is reviewing discharge teaching with a client who has a new prescription for diphenhydramine for allergic rhinitis. The nurse should instruct the client to monitor for which of the following adverse reactions? (Select all that apply.)

   A. Dry mouth

   B. Nonproductive cough

   C. Skin rash

   D. Drowsiness

   E. Urinary hesitation

5. A nurse is discussing the use of fluticasone to treat perennial rhinitis with a client at a provider's office. Which of the following statements by the client indicates an understanding of the information?

   A. "I should use the spray every 4 hours while I am awake."

   B. "It can take as long as 3 weeks before the medication takes a maximum effect."

   C. "This medication can also be used to treat motion sickness."

   D. "I can use this medication when my nasal passages are blocked."

PRACTICE Active Learning Scenario

A nurse in a provider's office is reinforcing teaching with a client who has a new prescription for guaifenesin. Use the ATI Active Learning Template: Medication to complete this item.

COMPLICATIONS: Identify two adverse effects of this medication.

EVALUATION OF MEDICATION EFFECTIVENESS: Identify two findings that indicate that the medication is effective.

Application Exercises Key

1. A. Decongestants stimulate the CNS and cause agitation and nervousness.

   B. **CORRECT:** When used for more than 5 days, rebound nasal congestion can occur when taking nasal sympathomimetic medications, such as phenylephrine.

   C. Phenylephrine can cause a headache, but productive cough is not an adverse effect of this medication.

   D. Constipation is an adverse effect of first-generation antihistamines. Sympathomimetic medications such as phenylephrine do not cause constipation.

   Ⓝ NCLEX® Connection: Pharmacological Therapies, Adverse Effects/Contraindications/Side Effects/Interactions

2. A. Dextromethorphan can cause nausea and constipation.

   B. Phenylephrine can cause anxiety and irritability.

   C. **CORRECT:** Dextromethorphan can cause sedation. Advise the client to avoid activities that require alertness.

   D. Phenylephrine can cause tachycardia and palpitations.

   Ⓝ NCLEX® Connection: Pharmacological Therapies, Adverse Effects/Contraindications/Side Effects/Interactions

3. A. Acetylcysteine can stimulate a cough. Dextromethorphan suppresses a cough.

   B. **CORRECT:** Acetylcysteine has a sulfur content that causes a rotten-egg odor.

   C. Dextromethorphan can cause euphoria at high doses. Acetylcysteine can cause drowsiness.

   D. Discoloration of urine is an adverse effect of COMT inhibitors. Acetylcysteine can cause diarrhea.

   Ⓝ NCLEX® Connection: Pharmacological Therapies, Expected Actions/Outcomes

4. A. **CORRECT:** Dry mouth is an anticholinergic manifestation that can occur when a client takes diphenhydramine.

   B. Cough is not an adverse reaction to this medication. Diphenhydramine can treat nonproductive cough.

   C. Skin rash is not an adverse reaction to this medication. Diphenhydramine is effective in treating skin rash caused by allergies.

   D. **CORRECT:** Drowsiness is an adverse reaction of this medication. Diphenhydramine can treat insomnia.

   E. **CORRECT:** Urinary retention is an anticholinergic manifestation that can occur when a client takes diphenhydramine.

   Ⓝ NCLEX® Connection: Pharmacological Therapies, Adverse Effects/Contraindications/Side Effects/Interactions

5. A. The client should use the medication once a day.

   B. **CORRECT:** The client can see some benefits of the medication within a few hours, but the maximum benefits can take up to 3 weeks.

   C. Diphenhydramine is a medication that treats motion sickness.

   D. The client should blow his nose to clear the nasal passages or use a topical decongestant, prior to use of the medication.

   Ⓝ NCLEX® Connection: Pharmacological Therapies, Expected Actions/Outcomes

---

PRACTICE Answer

Using the ATI Active Learning Template: Medication

COMPLICATIONS
- GI upset
- Dizziness
- Drowsiness
- Rash

EVALUATION OF MEDICATION EFFECTIVENESS
- Cough is more productive. Mucous is easier to expectorate.
- Chest congestion is decreased.

Ⓝ NCLEX® Connection: Pharmacological and Parenteral Therapies, Medication Administration

NCLEX® Connections

When reviewing the following chapters, keep in mind the relevant topics and tasks of the NCLEX outline, in particular:

Pharmacological Therapies

ADVERSE EFFECTS/CONTRAINDICATIONS/SIDE EFFECTS/INTERACTIONS: Notify the primary health care provider of actual/potential adverse effects of the client's medications.

DOSAGE CALCULATIONS: Use clinical decision making when calculating dosages.

MEDICATION ADMINISTRATION: Collect required data prior to medication administration.

UNIT 4   MEDICATIONS AFFECTING THE
CARDIOVASCULAR SYSTEM

CHAPTER 18 *Medications Affecting Urinary Output*

Indications for medications that affect urinary output include management of blood pressure, excretion of edematous fluid due to heart failure and kidney and liver disease, and prevention of kidney injury.

Medications include high-ceiling loop diuretics, thiazide diuretics, potassium-sparing diuretics, and osmotic diuretics.

High-ceiling loop diuretics

SELECT PROTOTYPE MEDICATION: Furosemide

OTHER MEDICATIONS
- Ethacrynic acid
- Bumetanide
- Torsemide

PURPOSE

EXPECTED PHARMACOLOGICAL ACTION

High-ceiling loop diuretics work in the ascending limb of the loop of Henle.
- Block reabsorption of sodium and chloride and prevent reabsorption of water
- Cause extensive diuresis even with severe kidney impairment

THERAPEUTIC USES

High-ceiling loop diuretics are useful when there is an emergent need for rapid mobilization of fluid.
- Pulmonary edema due to heart failure
- Conditions that do not respond to other diuretics (edema due to liver, cardiac, or kidney disease; hypertension)

UNLABELED USE: Hypercalcemia

ROUTES OF ADMINISTRATION: Oral, IV, IM

COMPLICATIONS

Dehydration, hyponatremia, hypochloremia

NURSING ACTIONS
- Monitor for manifestations of dehydration (dry mouth, increased thirst, minimal urine output, weight loss).
- Monitor electrolytes.
- Report urine output less than 30 mL/hr. Withhold the medication and notify the provider.
- If headache or chest, calf, or pelvic pain occur, notify the provider. This can indicate thrombosis or embolism.
- Weigh clients daily to detect fluid gains and losses. Qs Initial low doses help minimize the risk for dehydration.

Hypotension

NURSING ACTIONS: Monitor blood pressure.

CLIENT EDUCATION
- Manifestations of postural hypotension include lightheadedness and dizziness.
- Sit or lie down if feeling lightheaded or dizzy.
- Avoid sudden changes of position, and arise slowly from lying down or sitting.
- Elevate the head of the bed slowly before getting out of bed and walking.

Ototoxicity

Transient with furosemide and irreversible with ethacrynic acid

NURSING ACTIONS: Avoid concurrent use of other ototoxic medications, such as aminoglycoside antibiotics (gentamicin).

CLIENT EDUCATION: Notify the provider of tinnitus, which can indicate ototoxicity.

Hypokalemia

Potassium levels below 3.5 mEq/L

NURSING ACTIONS
- Monitor cardiac status and potassium levels.
- Report potassium levels below 3.5 mEq/L.

CLIENT EDUCATION
- Consume high-potassium foods (bananas, potatoes, dried fruits, nuts, spinach, citrus fruit).
- Manifestations of hypokalemia include nausea, vomiting, fatigue, leg cramps, and general weakness.

Other adverse effects

Hyperglycemia, hyperuricemia, hypocalcemia, hypomagnesemia, decreases in HDL levels, increases in LDL levels

NURSING ACTIONS
- Monitor blood glucose, uric acid, calcium, magnesium, and lipid levels.
- Report levels outside of the expected reference range.

CLIENT EDUCATION: Observe for manifestations of low magnesium levels (weakness, muscle twitching, tremors).

CONTRAINDICATIONS/PRECAUTIONS

- Unless absolutely necessary, clients who are pregnant should not take these medications.
- Anuria (no urine output) is a contraindication for taking these medications.
- Clients who have cardiovascular disease, diabetes mellitus, dehydration, electrolyte depletion, or gout require caution when taking these diuretics.
- Clients taking digoxin, lithium, ototoxic medications, NSAIDs, or antihypertensives require caution when taking these diuretics.

INTERACTIONS

Digoxin toxicity (ventricular dysrhythmias) can occur in the presence of hypokalemia.

- Providers sometimes prescribe potassium-sparing diuretics concurrently with loop diuretics to reduce the risk of hypokalemia.
- NURSING ACTIONS
  - Monitor cardiac status and potassium and digoxin levels.
  - Administer potassium supplements when necessary.

Concurrent use of antihypertensives can have an additive hypotensive effect.
NURSING ACTIONS: Monitor blood pressure.

Lithium carbonate levels can increase, which can lead to toxicity, if hyponatremia occurs due to the loop diuretic.
NURSING ACTIONS: Monitor lithium levels. Adjustments in dosage might become necessary.

NSAIDs decrease blood flow to the kidneys, which reduces the diuretic effect.
NURSING ACTIONS: Watch for a decrease in the effectiveness of the diuretic, such as a decrease in urine output.

NURSING ADMINISTRATION

- Obtain baseline data (orthostatic blood pressure, weight, electrolytes, location and extent of edema).
- Weigh clients at the same time each day with same amount of clothing and bed linen (if using a bed scale), usually when they awaken. Q EBP
- Monitor blood pressure and I&O.
- Avoid administering PO diuretics late in the day to prevent nocturia. Usual dosing times are 0800 and 1400.
- If potassium levels drop below 3.5 mEq/L, monitor the ECG, and notify the provider because the client might require a potassium supplement.
- Instruct clients who are taking diuretics to manage hypertension to self-monitor blood pressure and weight and keep a log.
- Advise clients to get up slowly to minimize postural hypotension. Instruct clients to sit or lie down if they feel faint or dizzy.
- Instruct clients to report significant weight loss, lightheadedness, dizziness, GI distress, or general weakness to the provider. These can indicate hypokalemia or hypovolemia.

- Encourage clients to consume foods high in potassium.
- Instruct clients who have diabetes to monitor for elevated blood glucose levels.
- Instruct clients to observe for manifestations of low magnesium levels (weakness, muscle twitching, tremors).
- Instruct clients to observe for manifestations of low calcium levels (muscle twitching, muscle cramps, tingling in hands and feet).
- Instruct clients to report manifestations of ototoxicity (tinnitus, hearing loss).

NURSING EVALUATION OF MEDICATION EFFECTIVENESS

Indications of effectiveness include the following.
- Decrease in pulmonary and peripheral edema
- Weight loss
- Decrease in blood pressure
- Increase in urine output
- Decrease in calcium level

Thiazide diuretics

SELECT PROTOTYPE MEDICATION: Hydrochlorothiazide

OTHER MEDICATIONS
- Chlorothiazide
- Methyclothiazide
- **Thiazide-type diuretics**
  - Indapamide
  - Chlorthalidone
  - Metolazone

PURPOSE

EXPECTED PHARMACOLOGICAL ACTION

Thiazide diuretics work in the early distal convoluted tubule.
- Block the reabsorption of sodium and chloride, and prevent the reabsorption of water at this site
- Promote diuresis when kidney function is adequate

THERAPEUTIC USES

- Thiazide diuretics are often the medication of first choice for essential hypertension.
- These medications treat edema from mild to moderate heart failure and liver and kidney disease.
- Thiazide diuretics with antihypertensive agents increase blood pressure control.
- These medications reduce urine production in clients who have diabetes insipidus.
- These medications promote reabsorption of calcium and can reduce the risk for postmenopausal osteoporosis.

COMPLICATIONS

Dehydration, hyponatremia

NURSING ACTIONS
- Monitor for manifestations of dehydration (dry mouth, increased thirst, minimal urine output, weight loss).
- Monitor electrolytes and weight.
- Report urine output less than 30 mL/hr. Withhold the medication and notify the provider.

Hypokalemia and hypochloremia

NURSING ACTIONS
- Monitor cardiac status and potassium levels, especially for clients taking digoxin.
- Report a decrease in potassium level (less than 3.5 mEq/L).

CLIENT EDUCATION
- Consume foods high in potassium.
- Report manifestations of hypokalemia (nausea, vomiting, general weakness, fatigue, leg cramps).

Hyperglycemia

NURSING ACTIONS: Monitor for an increase in blood glucose levels.

Hyperuricemia, hypomagnesemia, increased LDL

NURSING ACTIONS: Monitor uric acid, magnesium, LDL, and HDL levels.

CLIENT EDUCATION: Observe for manifestations of low magnesium levels (weakness, muscle twitching, tremors).

CONTRAINDICATIONS/PRECAUTIONS

- During pregnancy, thiazide diuretics decrease maternal blood volume and decrease placental perfusion, causing a compromise in the fetal nutrient supply.
- Clients taking a thiazide diuretic should not breastfeed because the diuretic enters the milk and can harm the infant.
- Kidney impairment is a contraindication for taking thiazide diuretics.
- Clients who have cardiovascular disease, diabetes mellitus, hypokalemia, hyperlipidemia, hypomagnesemia, or gout and take thiazide diuretics require caution, as do clients taking digoxin, lithium, or antihypertensives.

INTERACTIONS

- Medication and food interactions are the same as for loop diuretics.
- Thiazide diuretics do not worsen the risk for hearing loss in clients also taking ototoxic medications.

NURSING ADMINISTRATION

- With the exception of chlorothiazide (IV and PO), thiazide diuretics are only for PO administration.
- Obtain baseline data, including orthostatic blood pressure, weight, electrolytes, and the location and extent of edema.
- Monitor potassium levels.
- Instruct clients to take the medication first thing in the morning; for twice-a-day dosing, be sure clients take the second dose by 1400 to prevent nocturia. Q EBP
- Encourage clients to consume foods high in potassium and drink enough fluids.
- If GI upset occurs, clients should take the medication with or after meals.
- Alternate-day dosing can decrease the risk of electrolyte imbalances.
- Weigh clients at the same time each day with same amount of clothing and bed linen (if using a bed scale), usually when they awaken.
- Monitor blood pressure and I&O.
- If potassium levels drop below 3.5 mEq/L, monitor the ECG, and notify the provider because the client might require a potassium supplement.
- Instruct clients who are taking diuretics to manage hypertension to self-monitor blood pressure and weight and keep a log.
- Advise clients to get up slowly to minimize orthostatic hypotension. Instruct clients to sit or lie down if they feel faint or dizzy.
- Instruct clients to report significant weight loss, lightheadedness, dizziness, GI distress, or general weakness to the provider. These can indicate hypokalemia or hypovolemia.
- Instruct clients who have diabetes to monitor for elevated blood glucose levels.
- Instruct clients to observe for manifestations of low magnesium levels (weakness, muscle twitching, tremors).

NURSING EVALUATION OF MEDICATION EFFECTIVENESS

Indications of effectiveness include the following.
- Decrease in blood pressure
- Decrease in edema
- Increase in urine output
- Reduced urine output with diabetes insipidus
- Preservation of bone integrity in women who are postmenopausal

Potassium-sparing diuretics

SELECT PROTOTYPE MEDICATION: Spironolactone

OTHER MEDICATIONS
- Triamterene
- Amiloride

PURPOSE

EXPECTED PHARMACOLOGICAL ACTION

Potassium-sparing diuretics block the action of aldosterone (sodium and water retention), which results in potassium retention and the excretion of sodium and water.

THERAPEUTIC USES

- Potassium-sparing diuretics in combination with other diuretics (loop, thiazide) for potassium-sparing effects treat hypertension and edema.
- Managing heart failure
- Potassium-sparing diuretics block the action of aldosterone in primary hyperaldosteronism by retaining potassium and increasing sodium excretion, causing an opposite effect of the action of aldosterone in the distal nephrons.
- Therapeutic effects can take 12 to 48 hr.

ROUTE OF ADMINISTRATION: Oral

COMPLICATIONS

Hyperkalemia

ACE inhibitors, angiotensin receptor blockers, and direct renin inhibitors require caution in combination with potassium-sparing diuretics because these other medications can elevate potassium levels.

NURSING ACTIONS
- Monitor potassium level. Potassium levels greater than 5 mEq/L require cardiac monitoring.
- Monitor electrolytes and for manifestations of hyperkalemia (weakness, fatigue, dyspnea, dysrhythmias.)
- Treat hyperkalemia by withholding the medication and notifying the provider, and restricting potassium in the diet. If necessary, administer a potassium-excreting diuretic. The provider might also prescribe glucose and insulin IV to drive potassium back into the cell.
- Do not administer potassium supplements or other potassium-sparing diuretics in conjunction with spironolactone.

Endocrine effects

Male clients: Deepened voice, impotence

Female clients: Menstrual irregularities

CLIENT EDUCATION: Observe for adverse effects. Notify the provider if these responses occur.

Drowsiness, metabolic acidosis

NURSING ACTIONS: Monitor for manifestations of metabolic acidosis (drowsiness, restlessness).

CLIENT EDUCATION: Avoid activities that require alertness until they know how these medications affect them.

CONTRAINDICATIONS/PRECAUTIONS

- Do not administer to clients who have hyperkalemia or are taking potassium supplements or another potassium-sparing diuretic. Qs
- Do not administer to clients who have severe kidney failure and anuria.
- Clients who have kidney or liver disease, electrolyte imbalances, or metabolic acidosis require caution when taking potassium-sparing diuretics.

INTERACTIONS

Concurrent use of ACE inhibitors, angiotensin receptor blockers, and direct renin inhibitors increases the risk of hyperkalemia.
NURSING ACTIONS: Monitor the client's potassium levels. Notify the provider if potassium is above 5.0 mEq/L. Avoid concurrent use.

Concurrent use of potassium supplements, salt substitutes, and another potassium-sparing diuretic increases the risk of hyperkalemia.
NURSING ACTIONS: Avoid concurrent use.

NURSING ADMINISTRATION

- Obtain baseline data.
- Weigh clients at the same time each day with same amount of clothing and bed linen (if using a bed scale), usually when they awaken.
- Monitor blood pressure and I&O.
- Monitor the ECG periodically.
- Monitor potassium levels.
- Instruct clients to avoid salt substitutes that contain potassium and reduce their intake of potassium-rich foods (oranges, bananas, dates).
- Instruct clients to self-monitor blood pressure.
- Instruct clients to keep a log of blood pressure and weight.
- Warn clients that triamterene can turn urine a bluish color.
- Instruct clients to report cramps, diarrhea, thirst, menstrual changes, or deepened voice.
- Instruct clients to avoid activities that require alertness until they know how the medication affects them.

NURSING EVALUATION OF MEDICATION EFFECTIVENESS

Indications of effectiveness include the following.
- Potassium levels 3.5 to 5.0 mEq/L
- Weight loss
- Decreases in blood pressure and edema

Osmotic diuretics

SELECT PROTOTYPE MEDICATION: Mannitol

PURPOSE

EXPECTED PHARMACOLOGICAL ACTION

Osmotic diuretics reduce intracranial pressure (ICP) and intraocular pressure (IOP) by raising serum osmolality and drawing fluid back into the vascular and extravascular spaces.

THERAPEUTIC USES

- Prevents kidney failure in specific situations (hypovolemic shock, severe hypotension) because mannitol does not undergo reabsorption. Mannitol remains in the nephron, drawing off water, thus preserving urine flow and preventing kidney failure
- Decreases ICP due to cerebral edema by drawing off fluid from the brain into the bloodstream
- Decreases IOP by drawing ocular fluid into the bloodstream
- Promotes sodium retention and water excretion in clients who have hyponatremia and fluid-volume excess
- Treats the oliguria phase of acute kidney injury

COMPLICATIONS

Heart failure, pulmonary edema
NURSING ACTIONS: If manifestations of heart failure develop (dyspnea, weakness, fatigue, distended neck veins, weight gain), withhold the medication and notify the provider immediately.

Rebound increased intracranial pressure
NURSING ACTIONS: Monitor for increased ICP (change in level of consciousness, change in pupils, headache, nausea, vomiting).

Fluid and electrolyte imbalances, metabolic acidosis
NURSING ACTIONS: Monitor laboratory values. Monitor for manifestations of metabolic acidosis (drowsiness and restlessness).

CONTRAINDICATIONS/PRECAUTIONS

Active intracranial bleeding, anuria, severe pulmonary edema, severe dehydration, and kidney failure are contraindications for receiving mannitol. It requires extreme caution with clients who have heart failure, are pregnant or breastfeeding, have kidney insufficiency, or have electrolyte imbalances. Qs

INTERACTIONS

Increases lithium excretion through the kidneys
NURSING ACTIONS: Monitor lithium levels.

Increases the risk for hypokalemia with cardiac glycosides
NURSING ACTIONS: Monitor potassium and ECG.

NURSING ADMINISTRATION

- Ensure clients receive mannitol by continuous IV infusion.
- Monitor daily weight, I&O, and serum electrolytes.
- Monitor for manifestations of dehydration and increased edema.
- Obtain baseline data (orthostatic blood pressure, weight, electrolytes, location and extent of edema).
- Weigh clients at the same time each day with same amount of clothing and bed linen (if using a bed scale), usually when they awaken.
- Monitor blood pressure
- If potassium levels drop below 3.5 mEq/L, monitor the ECG, and notify the provider because the client might require a potassium supplement. Qrc
- Advise clients to get up slowly to minimize orthostatic hypotension. Instruct clients to sit or lie down if they feel faint or dizzy.
- Instruct clients to report significant lightheadedness, dizziness, GI distress, or general weakness to the provider. These can indicate hypokalemia or hypovolemia.
- Monitor for increased ICP (change in level of consciousness, change in pupils, headache, nausea, vomiting).
- Monitor for manifestations of metabolic acidosis (drowsiness, restlessness).

NURSING EVALUATION OF MEDICATION EFFECTIVENESS

Indications of effectiveness include the following.
- Adequate kidney function
  - Urine output at least 30 mL/hr
  - Creatinine 0.6 to 1.3 mg/dL for male clients and 0.5 to 1.1 mg/dL for female clients
  - BUN levels 10 to 20 mg/dL
- Decrease in intracranial pressure
- Decrease in intraocular pressure

Application Exercises

1. A nurse is contributing to the plan of care for a client who is receiving furosemide to treat peripheral edema. Which of the following interventions should the nurse suggest for inclusion in the plan of care? (Select all that apply.)

   A. Monitor for tinnitus.

   B. Report urine output 50 mL/hr.

   C. Monitor potassium levels.

   D. Elevate the head of the bed slowly before ambulation.

   E. Recommend eating a banana daily.

2. A nurse is reinforcing teaching with a client who has a new prescription for hydrochlorothiazide. Which of the following information should the nurse include?

   A. Take the medication with food.

   B. Plan to take the medication at bedtime.

   C. Expect increased swelling of the ankles.

   D. Limit fluid intake in the morning.

3. A nurse is monitoring a client who is receiving spironolactone. Which of the following findings should the nurse report to the provider?

   A. Sodium 144 mEq/L

   B. Urine output 120 mL in 4 hr

   C. Potassium 5.2 mEq/L

   D. Weight loss of 1 kg (2.2 lb)

4. A nurse is assisting with the care of a client who has increased intracranial pressure and is receiving mannitol. Which of the following findings should the nurse report to the provider?

   A. Blood glucose 120 mg/dL

   B. Urine output 40 mL/hr

   C. Dyspnea

   D. Bilateral equal pupil size

5. A nurse is contributing to the plan of care for a client who is has a new prescription for torsemide. The nurse should suggest monitoring for which of the following as adverse effects of this medication? (Select all that apply.)

   A. Hypernatremia

   B. Hypokalemia

   C. Hypotension

   D. Ototoxicity

   E. Dehydration

PRACTICE Active Learning Scenario

A nurse is reviewing the use of loop diuretics. Use the ATI Active Learning Template: Medication to complete this item.

THERAPEUTIC USES: Identify two.

COMPLICATIONS: Describe three adverse effects.

NURSING INTERVENTIONS: Describe two interventions for each of the three adverse effects.

Application Exercises Key

1. A. **CORRECT:** An adverse effect of furosemide is ototoxicity. The nurse should report tinnitus to the provider.

   B. Urine output of 50 mL/hr is within the expected reference range. A urine output less than 30 mL/hr is a manifestation of dehydration; the nurse should notify the provider if that occurs.

   C. **CORRECT:** A decrease in potassium levels is an adverse effect of furosemide, and the nurse should notify the provider.

   D. **CORRECT:** Slowly elevating the head of the bed will prevent the client from developing orthostatic hypotension, which is a manifestation of hypovolemia.

   E. **CORRECT:** Bananas are high in potassium. The nurse should encourage the client to eat foods high in potassium to prevent hypokalemia.

   Ⓝ *NCLEX® Connection: Pharmacological Therapies, Expected Actions/Outcomes*

2. A. **CORRECT:** The client should take hydrochlorothiazide with or after meals to prevent gastrointestinal upset.

   B. The client should take hydrochlorothiazide in the morning or no later than 1400 (not at bedtime) to prevent nocturia.

   C. The client should expect decreased swelling of the ankles.

   D. The client should maintain an adequate fluid intake throughout the day unless the provider prescribes fluid restriction.

   Ⓝ *NCLEX® Connection: Pharmacological Therapies, Expected Actions/Outcomes*

3. A. A sodium level of 144 mEq/L is within the expected reference range.

   B. Urine output of 30 mL/hr or 120 mL in 4 hr is adequate.

   C. **CORRECT:** A potassium level of 5.2 mEq/L indicates hyperkalemia. Because spironolactone causes potassium retention, the nurse should withhold the medication and notify the provider.

   D. With diuretic therapy, weight loss is an expected finding.

   Ⓝ *NCLEX® Connection: Pharmacological Therapies, Expected Actions/Outcomes*

4. A. This blood glucose level is within the expected reference range.

   B. A urine output of 40 mL/hr is within the expected reference range.

   C. **CORRECT:** Dyspnea is a manifestation of heart failure, an adverse effect of mannitol. The nurse should notify the provider immediately.

   D. Bilateral equal pupil size is an expected finding and can indicate a reduction in intracranial pressure.

   Ⓝ *NCLEX® Connection: Pharmacological Therapies, Adverse Effects/ Contraindications/Side Effects/Interactions*

5. A. Loop diuretics can cause hyponatremia, not hypernatremia.

   B. **CORRECT:** Loop diuretics can cause hypokalemia and hypomagnesemia.

   C. **CORRECT:** Loop diuretics can cause hypotension and hyperglycemia.

   D. **CORRECT:** Loop diuretics can cause ototoxicity and hypocalcemia.

   E. **CORRECT:** Loop diuretics can cause dehydration and hypochloremia.

   Ⓝ *NCLEX® Connection: Pharmacological Therapies, Adverse Effects/ Contraindications/Side Effects/Interactions*

PRACTICE Answer

Using the ATI Active Learning Template: Medication

THERAPEUTIC USES
- When there is an emergent need for rapid mobilization of fluid
- Pulmonary edema due to heart failure
- Liver, cardiac, or kidney disease
- Hypertension
- Unlabeled use: Hypercalcemia

COMPLICATIONS
- Dehydration
- Hypotension
- Ototoxicity
- Hypokalemia

NURSING INTERVENTIONS
- Dehydration: Monitor for dry mouth, increased thirst, low urine output, weight loss.
- Hypotension: Monitor orthostatic blood pressure and heart rate. Monitor for manifestations of postural hypotension.
- Ototoxicity: Monitor for tinnitus. Avoid administering ototoxic medications.
- Hypokalemia: Monitor laboratory values. Offer potassium-rich foods. Observe for general weakness, nausea, and vomiting.

Ⓝ *NCLEX® Connection: Pharmacological and Parenteral Therapies, Medication Administration*

UNIT 4   MEDICATIONS AFFECTING THE
CARDIOVASCULAR SYSTEM

CHAPTER 19   *Medications*
Affecting Blood
Pressure

Many medications, alone or in combination, help control blood pressure. The U.S. Department of Health and Human Services offers guidelines for pharmacological management of hypertension in its *Evidence-Based Guideline for the Management of High Blood Pressure in Adults.*

Angiotensin-converting enzyme inhibitors

SELECT PROTOTYPE MEDICATION: Captopril

OTHER MEDICATIONS
- Enalapril
- Enalaprilat
- Fosinopril
- Lisinopril
- Ramipril
- Moexipril
- Benazepril

PURPOSE

EXPECTED PHARMACOLOGICAL ACTION: Angiotensin-converting enzyme (ACE) inhibitors reduce the production of angiotensin II by blocking the conversion of angiotensin I to angiotensin II and increasing levels of bradykinin, leading to the following.
- Vasodilation (mostly arterioles)
- Excretion of sodium and water and retention of potassium by actions in the kidneys
- Reduction in pathological changes in the blood vessels and heart that result from the presence of angiotensin II and aldosterone

THERAPEUTIC USES
- Hypertension
- Heart failure
- Myocardial infarction (to decrease mortality; to decrease the risks of heart failure and left ventricular dysfunction)
- Diabetic and nondiabetic nephropathy (treatment, not prevention)
- Prevention of myocardial infarction (MI), stroke, and death (ramipril) for clients at high risk for a cardiovascular event

COMPLICATIONS

First-dose orthostatic hypotension

- For clients already taking a diuretic, the provider should stop the medication temporarily for 2 to 3 days prior to starting ACE inhibitor therapy.
- Taking another type of antihypertensive medication increases the hypotensive effects of an ACE inhibitor.
- Providers usually start treatment with a low dosage of the medication.

NURSING ACTIONS: Monitor blood pressure for 2 hr after initiation of treatment. Qs

CLIENT EDUCATION: Change positions slowly and lie down if feeling dizzy, lightheaded, or faint.

Cough

Due to inhibition of kinase II/ACE, which results in an increase in bradykinin

CLIENT EDUCATION: Notify the provider and stop taking the medication if dry cough occurs.

Hyperkalemia

NURSING ACTIONS
- Monitor potassium levels to maintain a level within the expected reference range of 3.5 to 5 mEq/L.
- Monitor for manifestations of hyperkalemia (numbness, tingling, paresthesia in hands and feet).

CLIENT EDUCATION: Avoid the use of salt substitutes containing potassium.

Rash, dysgeusia (taste alterations)

Primarily with captopril

CLIENT EDUCATION
- Inform the provider if these effects occur.
- Adverse effects will stop with discontinuation of the medication.

Angioedema

Potentially fatal swelling of the tongue, oropharynx, lips, eyes, and glottis

NURSING ACTIONS
- Treat severe effects with subcutaneous injection of epinephrine.
- Do not administer further doses of any ACE inhibitor.

Neutropenia

- A rare but serious complication of captopril
- Reversible with early detection

NURSING ACTIONS: Monitor WBC counts every 2 weeks for 3 months, then periodically.

CLIENT EDUCATION: Stop taking the medication and notify the provider at the first indications of infection (fever, sore throat).

CONTRAINDICATIONS/PRECAUTIONS

- Pregnancy Risk Category D; the second and third trimesters are contraindications due to the risk of fetal injury. Qs
- Allergy/angioedema to ACE inhibitors, bilateral renal artery stenosis, and having a single kidney are contraindications.
- Clients who have kidney impairment or collagen vascular disease require caution because they are at greater risk for developing neutropenia. Closely monitor for manifestations of infection.

INTERACTIONS

Diuretics can contribute to first-dose hypotension.
CLIENT EDUCATION: Stop taking diuretics temporarily 2 to 3 days before the start of therapy with an ACE inhibitor.

Antihypertensive medications can have an additive hypotensive effect.
CLIENT EDUCATION: The medication dosage might require adjustment if starting therapy with an ACE inhibitor.

Potassium supplements and potassium-sparing diuretics increase the risk of hyperkalemia.
CLIENT EDUCATION: Only take potassium supplements if prescribed. Avoid salt substitutes that contain potassium.

ACE inhibitors can increase levels of lithium.
NURSING ACTIONS: Monitor lithium levels and report increases so the provider can adjust the dosage and avoid toxicity.

NSAIDs can decrease the antihypertensive effect of ACE inhibitors.
NURSING ACTIONS: Avoid concurrent use.

NURSING ADMINISTRATION

- Administer ACE inhibitors orally except enalaprilat, which is the only ACE inhibitor for IV use. QEBP
- Explain whether clients will take a single formulation or a combination with hydrochlorothiazide (a thiazide diuretic).
- Monitor blood pressure after the first dose for at least 2 hr to detect hypotension.
- Instruct clients to take captopril and moexipril at least 1 hr before meals. They may take other ACE inhibitors with or without food.
- Advise clients to notify the provider if cough, rash, dysgeusia, or indications of infection occur.
- Advise clients to rise slowly from sitting.
- Advise clients to avoid activities that require alertness until they know how the medication affects them.
- Advise clients to inform the provider if they suspect pregnancy.

Angiotensin II receptor blockers

SELECT PROTOTYPE MEDICATION: Losartan

OTHER MEDICATIONS
- Valsartan
- Irbesartan
- Candesartan
- Olmesartan
- Telmisartan

PURPOSE

EXPECTED PHARMACOLOGICAL ACTION: Block the action of angiotensin II in the body, resulting in the following
- Vasodilation (arterioles, veins)
- Excretion of sodium and water (by decreasing the release of aldosterone)

THERAPEUTIC USES
- Hypertension
- Heart failure (valsartan, candesartan)
- Stroke prevention (losartan)
- Delay progression of diabetic nephropathy (irbesartan, losartan)
- Protect against MI, stroke, and death from cardiac causes in clients who cannot tolerate ACE inhibitors (telmisartan)
- Reduce mortality following an acute MI (valsartan)
- Slow the development of diabetic retinopathy (losartan)

COMPLICATIONS

The major difference between angiotensin II receptor blockers (ARBs) and ACE inhibitors is that cough and hyperkalemia are not adverse effects of ARBs.

Angioedema

NURSING ACTIONS: Treat severe effects with subcutaneous injection of epinephrine. Do not administer further doses of any ARB.

CLIENT EDUCATION: Observe for manifestations (skin wheals, swelling of the tongue, pharynx, lips, eyes) and notify the provider immediately if these occur.

Fetal injury

CLIENT EDUCATION
- There is a risk of fetal injury during the second and third trimesters of pregnancy.
- Use contraception while taking this medication.

Hypotension

NURSING ACTIONS: Monitor blood pressure.

CLIENT EDUCATION: Rise slowly from a sitting position.

Dizziness, lightheadedness

CLIENT EDUCATION: Avoid activities that require alertness until the effects of the medication on the body are understood.

CONTRAINDICATIONS/PRECAUTIONS

- Pregnancy Risk Category D. ARBs cause fetal damage in the second and third trimesters. Providers discontinue them as early in pregnancy as possible. Qs
- Renal stenosis is a contraindication because of the risk for kidney injury.
- Clients who had angioedema due to an ACE inhibitor require caution when taking an ARB.

INTERACTIONS

Antihypertensive medications can have an additive effect when clients take them with an ARB.
CLIENT EDUCATION: The medication dosage might require adjustment if starting therapy with an ARB.

Increased risk for lithium toxicity
NURSING ACTIONS: Monitor lithium levels and report increases so the provider can adjust the dosage and avoid toxicity.

NURSING ADMINISTRATION

- Administer medications orally. QEBP
- Explain whether clients will take a single formulation or a combination with hydrochlorothiazide.
- Inform clients that they may take ARBs with or without food.
- Advise clients who have heart failure to monitor weight and edema.

Aldosterone antagonists

SELECT PROTOTYPE MEDICATION: Eplerenone

OTHER MEDICATION: Spironolactone

PURPOSE

EXPECTED PHARMACOLOGICAL ACTION: Reduce blood volume by blocking aldosterone receptors in the kidney, thus promoting excretion of sodium and water and retention of potassium

THERAPEUTIC USES
- Hypertension
- Heart failure

COMPLICATIONS

Hyperkalemia, hyponatremia

NURSING ACTIONS: Monitor potassium and sodium levels periodically.

CLIENT EDUCATION
- Do not use potassium supplements or salt substitutes containing potassium.
- Monitor and report manifestations of hyperkalemia (paresthesia, tingling of hands and feet).

Flu-like manifestations

Fatigue, headache, diarrhea, abdominal pain, cough

CLIENT EDUCATION: Report severe manifestations to the provider.

Gynecomastia

Enlargement, tenderness of breast tissue in males

CLIENT EDUCATION: Report severe manifestations to the provider.

Dizziness, fatigue

CLIENT EDUCATION: Avoid activities that require alertness until the effects of the medication on the body are understood.

CONTRAINDICATIONS/PRECAUTIONS

- High potassium levels, kidney impairment, hepatic disease, and type 2 diabetes mellitus with microalbuminuria are contraindications. Qs
- Clients who have liver impairment require caution when taking an ARB.

INTERACTIONS

Verapamil, ACE inhibitors, ARBs, erythromycin, potassium-sparing diuretics, NSAIDs, and ketoconazole can increase the risk for hyperkalemia.
NURSING ACTIONS
- Monitor potassium levels more often for clients who must take these medications concurrently.
- Reinforce teaching about the manifestations of hyperkalemia.

Aldosterone antagonists can increase levels of lithium.
NURSING ACTIONS: Monitor clients taking lithium for lithium toxicity.

Grapefruit and grapefruit juice inhibit the metabolism of eplerenone.
CLIENT EDUCATION: Avoid grapefruit or grapefruit juice.

Concurrent use with diuretics increases the risk for orthostatic hypotension.
- NURSING ACTIONS: Monitor blood pressure.
- CLIENT EDUCATION: Rise slowly from sitting.

NURSING ADMINISTRATION

- Administer orally with or without food. Q EBP
- Do not administer with potassium supplements.

Direct renin inhibitors

SELECT PROTOTYPE MEDICATION: Aliskiren

PURPOSE

EXPECTED PHARMACOLOGICAL ACTION: Bind with renin to inhibit the production of angiotensin I, thus decreasing the production of both angiotensin II and aldosterone

THERAPEUTIC USE: Treat hypertension alone or with another antihypertensive medication

COMPLICATIONS

Angioedema, rash, cough

Angioedema is a potentially fatal swelling of the tongue, oropharynx, lips, eyes, glottis.

CLIENT EDUCATION: Monitor for rash and angioedema. For angioedema, stop taking the medication and notify the provider or call emergency services.

Hyperkalemia

NURSING ACTIONS: Monitor potassium levels periodically during treatment.

CLIENT EDUCATION
- Do not to use potassium supplements or salt substitutes containing potassium.
- Monitor and report manifestations of hyperkalemia (paresthesia, tingling of hands and feet).

Diarrhea

- Dose-related
- More common in female and older adult clients

NURSING ACTIONS: Monitor for dehydration, especially in older adults. G

CLIENT EDUCATION: Notify the provider for severe diarrhea.

Hypotension

NURSING ACTIONS: Monitor blood pressure.

CLIENT EDUCATION
- Rise slowly from sitting.
- Avoid activities that require alertness until the effects of the medication on the body are understood.

CONTRAINDICATIONS/PRECAUTIONS

- Pregnancy Risk Category D Qs
- Advise clients of childbearing age to use contraception and if pregnancy occurs to stop taking the medication and notify the provider.
- Hyperkalemia is a contraindication.
- Older adults and clients who have asthma, other respiratory disorders, a history of angioedema, diabetes mellitus, renal stenosis, hypotension, or kidney or hepatic disease require caution.

INTERACTIONS

Decreases levels of furosemide
Furosemide dosage can need to be increased.

Increases the effect of other antihypertensive medications
NURSING ACTIONS: Monitor blood pressure for hypotension when clients take combination antihypertensives.

Atorvastatin and ketoconazole increase levels of aliskiren.
NURSING ACTIONS: Monitor for hypotension in clients who use these medications concurrently.

High-fat foods reduce absorption.
CLIENT EDUCATION: Do not to take the medication with foods high in fat.

Increased hyperkalemia with ACE inhibitors, potassium supplements, and potassium-sparing diuretics
NURSING ACTIONS: Monitor potassium levels and for manifestations of hyperkalemia. Avoid concurrent use.

NURSING ADMINISTRATION

- High-fat meals interfere with absorption. Instruct clients to take the medication at the same time daily, away from foods high in fat. Q EBP
- Available alone or in combination tablets with a variety of other antihypertensives (hydrochlorothiazide, a diuretic; valsartan, an ARB)

Calcium channel blockers

SELECT PROTOTYPE MEDICATIONS
- Nifedipine
- Verapamil
- Diltiazem

OTHER MEDICATIONS
- Amlodipine
- Felodipine
- Nicardipine

PURPOSE

EXPECTED PHARMACOLOGICAL ACTION

Nifedipine

- Blocking of calcium channels in blood vessels leads to vasodilation of vascular smooth muscle (peripheral arterioles) and arteries and arterioles of the heart.
- Nifedipine acts primarily on arterioles and does not significantly affect veins.

Verapamil, diltiazem

- Blocking of calcium channels in blood vessels leads to vasodilation of peripheral arterioles and arteries of the heart.
- Blocking of calcium channels in the myocardium, sinoatrial (SA) node, and atrioventricular (AV) node decreases the force of contraction and the heart rate, and slows the rate of conduction through the AV node.
- These medications act on arterioles and the heart at therapeutic doses and do not significantly affect veins.

THERAPEUTIC USES

	NIFEDIPINE	AMLODIPINE	NICARDIPINE	FELODIPINE	VERAPAMIL, DILTIAZEM
Angina pectoris	✓	✓	✓		✓
Hypertension	✓	✓	✓	✓	✓
Cardiac dysrhythmias (atrial fibrillation, atrial flutter, SVT)					✓

COMPLICATIONS

NIFEDIPINE

Reflex tachycardia

NURSING ACTIONS
- Monitor clients for increases in heart rate.
- Administer a beta blocker (metoprolol) to counteract tachycardia.

Acute toxicity

- Excessive doses affect the heart and blood vessels.
- Clients might require additional medications (norepinephrine, calcium, isoproterenol, lidocaine) and IV fluids.

NURSING ACTIONS
- Monitor vital signs. Provide gastric lavage and a cathartic if necessary.
- Have equipment for cardioversion and a cardiac pacer available.

Orthostatic hypotension and peripheral edema

A diuretic can help control edema.

NURSING ACTIONS: Monitor blood pressure, edema, and daily weight.

CLIENT EDUCATION
- Observe for swelling in the lower extremities, and notify the provider if it occurs.
- Manifestations of orthostatic hypotension include lightheadedness and dizziness. Sit or lie down if they occur. Getting up slowly can minimize these effects.

VERAPAMIL, DILTIAZEM

Orthostatic hypotension, peripheral edema

A diuretic can help control edema.

NURSING ACTIONS: Monitor blood pressure, edema, and daily weight.

CLIENT EDUCATION
- Observe for swelling in the lower extremities, and notify the provider if it occurs.
- Manifestations of orthostatic hypotension include lightheadedness and dizziness. Sit or lie down if they occur. Getting up slowly can minimize these effects.

Constipation (primarily verapamil)

CLIENT EDUCATION: Increase intake of high fiber food and oral fluids, if no fluid restrictions are prescribed.

Suppression of cardiac function

Bradycardia, heart failure

NURSING ACTIONS: Monitor ECG, pulse rate, and rhythm.

CLIENT EDUCATION: Monitor for indications of suppressed cardiac function (slow pulse, activity tolerance). The provider might need to lower the medication dose, so notify the provider if these occur

Dysrhythmias

NURSING ACTIONS: Monitor vital signs and the ECG.

Acute toxicity

Resulting in hypotension, bradycardia, AV block, and ventricular tachydysrhythmias

NURSING ACTIONS
- Monitor vital signs and the ECG. Provide gastric lavage and a cathartic if necessary.
- Clients might require additional medications (norepinephrine, calcium, isoproterenol, lidocaine) and IV fluids.
- Have equipment for cardioversion and a cardiac pacer available.

CONTRAINDICATIONS/PRECAUTIONS

- Pregnancy Risk Category C Qs
- Cardiogenic shock is a contraindication for receiving nifedipine.
- Clients who have acute MI, unstable angina, aortic stenosis, hypotension, sick sinus syndrome, or second- or third-degree AV block require caution when taking nifedipine.
- Hypotension, heart block, digoxin toxicity, severe heart failure, and lactation are contraindications for receiving nifedipine.
- Older adults and clients who have kidney or liver disorders, mild to moderate heart failure, or GERD require caution. Ⓖ

INTERACTIONS

NIFEDIPINE

Beta blockers, such as metoprolol, decrease reflex tachycardia.
NURSING ACTIONS: Monitor for excessive slowing of the heart rate.

Cimetidine, ranitidine, and grapefruit juice can lead to toxicity.
- NURSING ACTIONS
  - Monitor for indications of toxicity (decrease in blood pressure, increase in heart rate, flushing).
  - Avoid concurrent use with cimetidine or ranitidine.
- CLIENT EDUCATION: Avoid drinking grapefruit juice.

VERAPAMIL, DILTIAZEM

Verapamil can increase digoxin levels, increasing the risk of digoxin toxicity. Digoxin can cause an additive effect and intensify AV conduction suppression.
NURSING ACTIONS
- Monitor digoxin levels to help keep clients in the therapeutic range.
- Monitor vital signs for bradycardia and for manifestations of AV block, such as a reduced ventricular rate.

Concurrent use of beta blockers can lead to heart failure, AV block, and bradycardia.
NURSING ACTIONS: Monitor the ECG and heart rate.

Consuming grapefruit juice and verapamil or diltiazem can lead to toxicity.
- NURSING ACTIONS: Monitor for indications of toxicity (decreased blood pressure, decreased heart rate, AV block).
- CLIENT EDUCATION: Avoid drinking grapefruit juice.

NURSING ADMINISTRATION

- Advise clients not to chew or crush sustained-release tablets.
- Advise clients who have angina to record their pain frequency, intensity, duration, and location and to notify the provider if attacks increase in frequency, intensity, or duration.
- Instruct clients to monitor blood pressure and heart rate and keep a blood-pressure record. They should withhold the medication and notify the provider for a heart rate less than 50/min or a systolic blood pressure less than 90 mm Hg. Q EBP
- Advise clients to change positions slowly and avoid activities that require alertness until they know how the medication affects them

Alpha adrenergic blockers (sympatholytics)

SELECT PROTOTYPE MEDICATION: Prazosin

OTHER MEDICATIONS
- Doxazosin
- Terazosin

PURPOSE

EXPECTED PHARMACOLOGICAL ACTION

Selective $alpha_1$ blockade results in the following.
- Venous and arterial dilation
- Smooth muscle relaxation of the prostatic capsule and bladder neck

THERAPEUTIC USES

- Primary hypertension
- Doxazosin and terazosin decrease the manifestations of benign prostatic hyperplasia (BPH), which include urgency, frequency, and dysuria.

COMPLICATIONS

First-dose orthostatic hypotension

Providers usually start treatment with a low dosage.

NURSING ACTIONS: Monitor blood pressure for 2 to 6 hr after initiation of treatment.

CLIENT EDUCATION
- Taking the initial dose at bedtime is optimal due to the first-pass effect.
- Avoid activities requiring mental alertness for the first 12 to 24 hr.
- Change positions slowly and lie down if feeling dizzy, lightheaded, or faint.

CONTRAINDICATIONS/PRECAUTIONS

- Pregnancy Risk Category C **Qs**
- Hypotension is a contraindication.
- Clients who have angina pectoris or kidney insufficiency and older adults require caution. **©**

INTERACTIONS

Antihypertensive medications can have an additive hypotensive effect.
CLIENT EDUCATION
- Observe for indications of hypotension (dizziness, lightheadedness, faintness).
- Lie down if these manifestations occur, and change positions slowly.

NURSING ADMINISTRATION

- Inform clients that they may take the medication with food.
- Recommend that clients take the initial dose at bedtime to avoid feeling the "first-dose" hypotensive effect.
- Reinforce teaching about safety measures to minimize the effects of orthostatic hypotension.

Centrally acting alpha₂ agonists

SELECT PROTOTYPE MEDICATION: Clonidine

OTHER MEDICATIONS
- Guanfacine
- Methyldopa

PURPOSE

EXPECTED PHARMACOLOGICAL ACTION

These medications act within the CNS to decrease sympathetic outflow, resulting in decreased stimulation of the adrenergic receptors (both alpha and beta receptors) of the heart and peripheral vascular system.
- A decrease in sympathetic outflow to the myocardium results in bradycardia and decreased cardiac output.
- A decrease in sympathetic outflow to the peripheral vasculature results in vasodilation, which leads to decreases in blood pressure.

THERAPEUTIC USES

- Primary hypertension (alone, with a diuretic, or with another antihypertensive agent)
- Severe cancer pain (parenterally by epidural infusion)

INVESTIGATIONAL USE
- Migraine headache
- Flushing from menopause
- Management of ADHD, Tourette syndrome
- Management of withdrawal from alcohol, tobacco, opioids

COMPLICATIONS

Drowsiness, sedation

Drowsiness will diminish as medication therapy continues.

CLIENT EDUCATION: Avoid activities that require alertness until manifestations subside.

Dry mouth

CLIENT EDUCATION
- Adhere to the medication regimen.
- Dry mouth usually resolves in 2 to 4 weeks.
- Chew gum or suck on hard candy, and take small amounts of water or ice chips.

Rebound hypertension

Providers taper clonidine gradually over 2 to 4 days.

CLIENT EDUCATION: Do not discontinue treatment abruptly or without consulting the provider.

CONTRAINDICATIONS/PRECAUTIONS

- Clonidine is in Pregnancy Risk Category C. Methyldopa and guanfacine are in Pregnancy Risk Category B.
- Avoid use during lactation. Qs
- Avoid use of the transdermal patch on affected skin from scleroderma or systemic lupus erythematosus.
- Bleeding disorders and anticoagulant therapy are contraindications.
- Stroke, asthma, COPD, recent MI, diabetes mellitus, major depressive disorder, and chronic kidney disease require caution.

INTERACTIONS

Antihypertensive medications can have an additive hypotensive effect.
CLIENT EDUCATION
- Observe for manifestations of hypotension (dizziness, lightheadedness, faintness).
- Lie down if feeling dizzy, lightheaded, or faint, and change positions slowly.

Concurrent use of prazosin, MAOIs, and tricyclic antidepressants can counteract the antihypertensive effect of clonidine.
NURSING ACTIONS: Monitor clients for therapeutic effects. Monitor blood pressure. Discourage concurrent use.

Additive CNS depression can occur with concurrent use of other CNS depressants, such as alcohol.
CLIENT EDUCATION: Additive CNS depression occurs with alcohol. Avoid its use.

NURSING ADMINISTRATION

- For hypertension, administer medication by oral or transdermal routes. Epidural administration is also an option for some clients.
- Administer twice a day, or give a larger dose at bedtime to decrease the occurrence of daytime sleepiness. QEBP
- Apply transdermal patches every 7 days. Advise clients to apply patches on hairless, intact skin on their torso or upper arm.

Beta adrenergic blockers (sympatholytics)

SELECT PROTOTYPE MEDICATIONS

Cardioselective: $Beta_1$ (affects only the heart)
- Metoprolol
- Atenolol
- Esmolol

Nonselective: $Beta_1$ and $beta_2$ (affecting both the heart and lungs)
- Propranolol
- Nadolol

Alpha and beta blockers
- Carvedilol
- Labetalol

PURPOSE

EXPECTED PHARMACOLOGICAL ACTION

For cardiac disorders, the primary effects of beta adrenergic blockers are a result of $beta_1$ adrenergic blockade in the myocardium and in the electrical conduction system of the heart.
- Decrease heart rate (negative chronotropic [rate] action)
- Decrease myocardial contractility (negative inotropic [force] action); decrease cardiac output
- Decrease the rate of conduction through the AV node (negative dromotropic action)
- Add vasodilation with medications such as carvedilol and labetalol (due to alpha blockade)
- Reduce the release of renin, which decreases angiotensin II, causes vasodilation, and promotes the excretion of sodium and water

THERAPEUTIC USES

- Primary hypertension (exact mechanism unknown; long-term use: reduction in peripheral vascular resistance)
- Angina, tachydysrhythmias, heart failure, MI
- Suppress reflex tachycardia due to vasodilators
- Treatment of hyperthyroidism, migraine headache, pheochromocytoma, and glaucoma

COMPLICATIONS

BETA₁ BLOCKADE: METOPROLOL, PROPRANOLOL

Bradycardia

NURSING ACTIONS: Monitor pulse. If less than 50/min, withhold the medication and notify the provider.

Hypoglycemia

Clients who have diabetes mellitus require caution. This medication can mask tachycardia, diaphoresis, and perspiration, early manifestations of low blood glucose.

CLIENT EDUCATION: Monitor blood glucose to detect hypoglycemia.

Decreased cardiac output

Clients who have heart failure require caution. Providers start therapy with very low doses and titrate as necessary.

CLIENT EDUCATION: Observe for manifestations of worsening heart failure (shortness of breath, edema, weight gain, fatigue). Notify the provider if manifestations occur.

AV block

NURSING ACTIONS: Obtain a baseline ECG and monitor.

Orthostatic hypotension

CLIENT EDUCATION
- Sit or lie down if dizzy or faint.
- Avoid sudden changes of position and rise slowly.

Rebound myocardium excitation

- Long-term use of beta blockers causes sensitization of the myocardium to catecholamines.
- Providers discontinue beta blockers over 1 to 2 weeks.

CLIENT EDUCATION: Do not stop taking beta blockers abruptly, but follow the provider's instructions.

BETA₂ BLOCKADE: PROPRANOLOL

Bronchoconstriction

Clients who have asthma should receive a beta₁ selective agent, not a beta₂ blocker.

Inhibition of glycogenolysis

- Clients who have diabetes mellitus rely on the breakdown of glycogen into glucose to manage low blood glucose (can happen with insulin overdose).
- In addition, a decreased heart rate can further mask manifestations of impending low blood glucose level. Clients who have diabetes mellitus receive a beta₁ selective agent.

CONTRAINDICATIONS/PRECAUTIONS

- AV block and sinus bradycardia are contraindications. Qs
- Asthma, bronchospasm, and heart failure are contraindications for receiving nonselective beta adrenergic blockers.
- Clients who have asthma require caution when receiving cardioselective beta adrenergic blockers.
- Clients who have myasthenia gravis, hypotension, peripheral vascular disease, diabetes mellitus, depression, or a history of severe allergies, and older adults require caution when receiving beta adrenergic blockers. ©

INTERACTIONS

BETA₁ BLOCKADE: METOPROLOL, PROPRANOLOL

Calcium channel blockers (CCBs) verapamil and diltiazem intensify the effects of beta blockers
- Decreased heart rate
- Decreased myocardial contractility
- Decreased rate of conduction through the AV node
- NURSING ACTIONS
  - Monitor ECG and blood pressure.
  - Monitor clients taking a CCB and a beta blocker concurrently. They might require a dosage reduction.

Concurrent use of antihypertensive medications with beta blockers can intensify the hypotensive effect of both medications.
NURSING ACTIONS: Monitor for a drop in blood pressure.

BETA₂ BLOCKADE: PROPRANOLOL

Propranolol can mask the hypoglycemic effect of insulin and prevent the breakdown of fat in response to hypoglycemia.
NURSING ACTIONS: Monitor blood glucose levels.

NURSING ADMINISTRATION

- Administer medications orally, usually once or twice per day.
- IV administration of atenolol, metoprolol, labetalol, or propranolol is an option for some clients.
- Advise clients not to stop taking the medication without consulting the provider.
- Advise clients to avoid sudden changes in position to minimize the effects of orthostatic hypotension.
- Instruct clients not to crush or chew extended-release tablets.
- Remind clients to self-monitor heart rate and blood pressure at home on a daily basis.
- Advise clients to take the medication with food to increase absorption.

NURSING EVALUATION OF MEDICATION EFFECTIVENESS

Indications of effectiveness include the following.
- Absence of chest pain
- Absence of cardiac dysrhythmias
- Normotensive blood pressure readings
- Control of heart-failure manifestations

Medications for hypertensive crisis

SELECT PROTOTYPE MEDICATION: Nitroprusside (centrally acting vasodilator)

OTHER MEDICATIONS
- Nitroglycerin (vasodilator)
- Nicardipine (calcium channel blocker)
- Clevidipine (calcium channel blocker)
- Enalaprilat (ACE inhibitor)
- Esmolol (beta blocker)

PURPOSE

EXPECTED PHARMACOLOGICAL ACTION: Direct vasodilation of arteries and veins resulting in rapid reduction of blood pressure (decreased preload and afterload)

THERAPEUTIC USES: Hypertensive crisis (a potentially fatal emergency with blood pressure greater than 180/120 mm Hg and target organ damage)

COMPLICATIONS

Excessive hypotension

- IV administration of nitroprusside requires an IV infusion pump.
- Rapid administration will cause blood pressure to drop rapidly.
- Clients must remain supine during administration. Q𝐄𝐁𝐏

NURSING ACTIONS: Monitor blood pressure and ECG continuously.

Cyanide poisoning/thiocyanate toxicity

Headache, drowsiness, cardiac arrest (nitroprusside only)
- Clients who have liver dysfunction are at increased risk.
- Receiving the medication for no longer than 3 days, and at a rate of 5 mcg/kg/min or less, reduces the risk of cyanide poisoning
- Manifestations include weakness, disorientation, and delirium. Thiosulfate reverses these effects.
- Providers will discontinue the medication if cyanide toxicity occurs.

NURSING ACTIONS: Monitor plasma levels of clients who received nitroprusside for more than 3 days. They should be less than 10 mg/dL.

Bradycardia, tachycardia, ECG changes

NURSING ACTIONS: Monitor ECG for changes.

CONTRAINDICATIONS/PRECAUTIONS

- Pregnancy Risk Category C
- Heart failure with reduced peripheral vascular resistance and AV shunt are contraindications.
- Clients who have liver and kidney disease, hypothyroidism, hypovolemia, or fluid and electrolyte imbalances, and older adults require caution. Q𝐏𝐂𝐂

INTERACTIONS

- Other hypotensive medications increase the hypotensive effects.
- Estrogens decrease the therapeutic effects.

NURSING ADMINISTRATION

Protect the IV container and tubing from light. Q𝐄𝐁𝐏

NURSING EVALUATION OF MEDICATION EFFECTIVENESS

Indications of effectiveness include the following.
- Decrease in blood pressure
- Maintenance of normotensive blood pressure
- Improvement of heart failure (ability to perform activities of daily living, improved breath sounds, absence of edema)

Application Exercises

1. A nurse is reviewing the health record of a client who asks about taking propranolol to treat hypertension. Which of the following is a contraindication for taking propranolol?

   A. Asthma

   B. Glaucoma

   C. Hypertension

   D. Tachycardia

2. A nurse is reinforcing teaching with a client who has a new prescription for verapamil to control hypertension. Which of the following instructions should the nurse include?

   A. Increase the amount of dietary fiber in the diet.

   B. Drink grapefruit juice daily to increase vitamin C intake.

   C. Decrease the amount of calcium in the diet.

   D. Withhold food for 1 hr after taking the medication.

3. A nurse is caring for a client who has a new prescription for captopril for hypertension. The nurse should monitor the client for which of the following adverse effects?

   A. Hypokalemia

   B. Hypernatremia

   C. Neutropenia

   D. Bradycardia

4. A nurse in an acute care facility is caring for a client who is receiving IV nitroprusside for hypertensive crisis. The nurse should monitor the client for which of the following adverse reactions?

   A. Intestinal ileus

   B. Neutropenia

   C. Delirium

   D. Hyperthermia

5. A nurse is planning to administer a first dose of captopril to a client who has hypertension. The nurse should monitor the client for an intensification of first-dose hypotension if the client is also taking which of the following medications? (Select all that apply.)

   A. Simvastatin

   B. Hydrochlorothiazide

   C. Phenytoin

   D. Clonidine

   E. Aliskiren

PRACTICE Active Learning Scenario

A nurse in an outpatient facility is reinforcing teaching with a client who has a new prescription for aliskiren to treat hypertension. What should the nurse include about this medication? Use the ATI Active Learning Template: Medication to complete this item.

THERAPEUTIC USES: Identify the therapeutic use for aliskiren.

COMPLICATIONS: List two adverse effects of this medication.

NURSING INTERVENTIONS: Name one test to monitor.

CLIENT EDUCATION: Identify two instructional points.

Application Exercises Key

1. A. **CORRECT:** Propranolol is a nonselective beta adrenergic blocker that blocks both beta$_1$ and beta$_2$ receptors. Blockade of beta$_2$ receptors in the lungs causes bronchoconstriction, so asthma is a contraindication for receiving this medication.

   B. Clients who have glaucoma may take propranolol. Pheochromocytoma and pulmonary edema contraindications for receiving this medication.

   C. Propranolol treats hypertension. Cardiogenic shock is a contraindication for receiving this medication.

   D. Propranolol treats tachydysrhythmias, such as tachycardia. Bradycardia and AV block are contraindications for receiving this medication.

   Ⓝ *NCLEX® Connection: Pharmacological Therapies, Adverse Effects/Contraindications/Side Effects/Interactions*

2. A. **CORRECT:** Increasing dietary fiber intake can help prevent constipation, an adverse effect of verapamil.

   B. Clients should avoid drinking grapefruit juice when taking verapamil because concurrent use can lead to toxicity. It is not necessary to take extra vitamin C when taking verapamil.

   C. There is no restriction on dietary calcium intake for clients taking verapamil. However, verapamil can boost caffeine levels when clients who take it drink coffee or tea that contains caffeine.

   D. There is no restriction on food when taking verapamil. Clients can take verapamil with food to prevent gastrointestinal upset.

   Ⓝ *NCLEX® Connection: Pharmacological Therapies, Expected Actions/Outcomes*

3. A. Hyperkalemia, rather than hypokalemia, is a risk for clients taking ACE inhibitors.

   B. ACE inhibitors cause excretion of sodium and water. Hypernatremia is not a risk for taking an ACE inhibitor.

   C. **CORRECT:** Neutropenia is a serious adverse effect that can occur in clients taking an ACE inhibitor. The nurse should monitor the client's CBC and instruct the client to report indications of infection to the provider.

   D. Tachycardia, not bradycardia, is an adverse effect of ACE inhibitors.

   Ⓝ *NCLEX® Connection: Pharmacological Therapies, Expected Actions/Outcomes*

4. A. Headache, not intestinal ileus, is an adverse effect of nitroprusside.

   B. Bradycardia, not neutropenia, is an adverse effect of nitroprusside.

   C. **CORRECT:** Delirium and other mental status changes can occur with thiocyanate toxicity when clients receive nitroprusside IV at a high dosage. It is essential to monitor thiocyanate level during therapy and make sure it remains below 10 mg/dL.

   D. Hypotension, not hyperthermia, is an adverse effect of nitroprusside.

   Ⓝ *NCLEX® Connection: Pharmacological Therapies, Expected Actions/Outcomes*

5. A. Simvastatin, an antilipemic medication that lowers cholesterol, does not interact with captopril and does not intensify first-dose hypotension.

   B. **CORRECT:** Hydrochlorothiazide, a thiazide diuretic, treats hypertension. Diuretics can intensify the first-dose orthostatic hypotension captopril causes and can continue to interact with antihypertensive medications to cause hypotension. The nurse should monitor clients carefully for hypotension, especially after the first dose of captopril, and keep the client safe from injury.

   C. Phenytoin, an antiseizure medication, does not interact with captopril and does not intensify first-dose hypotension.

   D. **CORRECT:** Clonidine, a centrally acting alpha$_2$ agonist, is an antihypertensive medication that can interact with captopril to intensify first-dose orthostatic hypotension.

   E. **CORRECT:** Aliskiren, a direct renin inhibitor, is an antihypertensive medication that can interact with captopril to intensify its first-dose orthostatic hypotension.

   Ⓝ *NCLEX® Connection: Pharmacological Therapies, Adverse Effects/Contraindications/Side Effects/Interactions*

PRACTICE Answer

Using the ATI Active Learning Template: Medication

THERAPEUTIC USES:
Aliskiren binds with renin to inhibit the production of angiotensin I, thus decreasing the production of both angiotensin II and aldosterone. Aliskiren treats hypertension alone or in combination with other antihypertensives.

COMPLICATIONS
• Diarrhea: dose-related, most common in females and older adults
• Risk for angioedema and rash from allergy to the medication
• Hyperkalemia
• Hypotension

NURSING INTERVENTIONS: Monitor serum electrolytes, paying close attention to potassium levels, because the client is at risk for hyperkalemia. This is especially important when the client takes an ACE inhibitor concurrently, because these medications also raise potassium levels.

CLIENT EDUCATION
• Do not take aliskiren with foods high in fat, because they decrease the absorption of the medication.
• Do not take potassium supplements or salt substitutes containing potassium.
• Do not take aliskiren during pregnancy.
• Stop taking the medication and notify the provider if a rash or angioedema occurs, and call emergency services for severe allergy manifestations.

Ⓝ *NCLEX® Connection: Pharmacological and Parenteral Therapies, Medication Administration*

UNIT 4 MEDICATIONS AFFECTING THE
CARDIOVASCULAR SYSTEM

CHAPTER 20 *Cardiac Glycosides*
and Heart Failure

Heart failure results from inadequate pumping of the heart muscle. The heart's inability to meet all of the body's circulation needs causes manifestations of heart failure. Decreased tissue perfusion results in fatigue, shortness of breath, weakness, and activity intolerance.

Heart failure causes a reduction in cardiac output (CO) and affects heart rate, stroke volume (SV), preload, and afterload. There are two types of heart failure: left-sided (with pulmonary manifestations: dyspnea, cough, oliguria) and right-sided (with systemic congestion: peripheral edema, jugular vein distention, weight gain).

Diuretics, angiotensin-converting enzyme (ACE) inhibitors, angiotensin II receptor blockers (ARBs), and beta adrenergic blockers are the medications of choice for treating heart failure. If these medications do not control the manifestations, cardiac glycosides are the next treatment option.

Cardiac glycosides

SELECT PROTOTYPE MEDICATION: Digoxin

PURPOSE

EXPECTED PHARMACOLOGICAL ACTION

Positive inotropic effect: increased force of myocardial contraction
- Increased force and efficiency of myocardial contraction improves the heart's effectiveness as a pump, improving SV and CO.

Negative chronotropic effect: decreased heart rate
- At therapeutic levels, digoxin slows the rate of sinoatrial (SA) node depolarization and the rate of impulses through the conduction system of the heart.
- A decreased heart rate gives the ventricles more time to fill with blood coming from the atria, which increases SV and CO.

THERAPEUTIC USES

As a second-line medication
- Heart failure
- Dysrhythmias (atrial fibrillation)
- Can reduce manifestations, but does not prolong life

COMPLICATIONS

Dysrhythmias, cardiotoxicity

- Dysrhythmias due to interfering with the electrical conduction in the myocardium
- Cardiotoxicity leading to bradycardia
- Conditions that increase the risk for developing digoxin-induced dysrhythmias include hypokalemia, increased digoxin levels, and cardiovascular disease. Older adult clients are particularly at risk. ⊚
- Providers base dosages on digoxin levels and on how clients respond to the medication.

NURSING ACTIONS
- Monitor potassium levels to maintain a level between 3.5 and 5.0 mEq/L.
- Therapeutic serum levels can vary between conditions and clients. Consider manifestations and digoxin level when toxicity is suspected.

CLIENT EDUCATION
- Report manifestations of hypokalemia (nausea, vomiting, general weakness). Providers prescribe potassium supplements for clients who also take a potassium-wasting diuretic.
- Consume high-potassium foods (green leafy vegetables, bananas, potatoes).
- Monitor heart rate and recognize and report changes, such as an irregular rate with early or extra beats.

Gastrointestinal (GI) effects

Anorexia (usually the first manifestation of toxicity), nausea, vomiting, abdominal pain

CLIENT EDUCATION: Monitor for these effects and report them to the provider if they occur.

CNS effects

Fatigue, weakness, vision changes (blurred vision, yellow-green vision, or white halos around objects)

CLIENT EDUCATION: Monitor for these effects and report them to the provider if they occur.

CONTRAINDICATIONS/PRECAUTIONS

- Pregnancy Risk Category C ⊚s
- Disturbances in ventricular rhythm (ventricular fibrillation, ventricular tachycardia, second- and third-degree heart block) are contraindications for receiving digoxin.
- Clients who have hypokalemia, partial AV block, advanced heart failure, or impaired kidney function require caution with digoxin therapy.

INTERACTIONS

Thiazide diuretics (such as hydrochlorothiazide) and loop diuretics (such as furosemide) can lead to hypokalemia, which increases the risk for developing dysrhythmias.
NURSING ACTIONS
- Monitor potassium levels to maintain a level between 3.5 and 5.0 mEq/L.
- Treat hypokalemia with potassium supplements or a potassium-sparing diuretic.

ACE inhibitors and ARBs increase the risk of hyperkalemia, which can reduce the therapeutic effects of digoxin.
NURSING ACTIONS
- Use caution in clients who take digoxin with potassium supplements or a potassium-sparing diuretic.
- Monitor potassium levels to maintain a level between 3.5 and 5.0 mEq/L.

Sympathomimetic medications such as dopamine complement the inotropic action of digoxin and increase the rate and force of heart muscle contraction. These medications can increase the risk of tachydysrhythmias.
NURSING ACTIONS: Monitor the ECG. Instruct clients to measure their heart rate and report palpitations.

Quinidine increases the risk of digoxin toxicity by displacing digoxin from its binding site and reducing kidney excretion.
NURSING ACTIONS: Avoid concurrent use.

Verapamil increases plasma levels of digoxin.
Providers prescribe a lower dosage for clients who also take verapamil, but generally avoid concurrent use because verapamil's cardiosuppressive action counteracts digoxin's therapeutic effects.

Antacids decrease the absorption of digoxin and can decrease its effectiveness.
CLIENT EDUCATION: Talk to the provider before taking any antacids.

NURSING ADMINISTRATION

- Advise clients not to double the dose if they miss a dose. Q_EBP
- Check pulse rate and rhythm before administering digoxin and document it. Notify the provider if the heart rate is less than 60/min in adults, 70/min in children, or 90/min in infants.
- Administer digoxin at the same time each day.
- Evaluate manifestations and the client's digoxin level when toxicity is suspected.
- Advise clients against taking over-the-counter medications to prevent adverse effects and medication interactions.
- Instruct clients to observe for manifestations of hypokalemia (such as muscle weakness) and to notify the provider if they occur.
- Instruct clients to observe for indications of digoxin toxicity (fatigue, weakness, vision changes, GI effects), and to notify the provider if they occur.
- When caring for clients who receive IV digoxin, monitor for dysrhythmias. Q_EBP

MANAGEMENT OF DIGOXIN TOXICITY
- Withhold digoxin and potassium-sparing medications and notify the provider immediately.
- Monitor potassium levels. Clients whose levels are less than 3.5 mEq/L require potassium IV or PO. Do not give any more potassium if levels are greater than 5.0 mEq/L.
- Phenytoin and lidocaine treat digoxin-induced dysrhythmias.
- Atropine treats bradycardia.
- For digoxin overdoses, activated charcoal, cholestyramine, or digoxin immune Fab binds digoxin and prevents absorption.

NURSING EVALUATION OF MEDICATION EFFECTIVENESS

Indications of effectiveness include the following.
- Control of heart failure
- Absence of cardiac dysrhythmias

Adrenergic agonists

SELECT PROTOTYPE MEDICATION: Catecholamines
- Epinephrine
- Dopamine
- Dobutamine
- Isoproterenol
- Norepinephrine

OTHER MEDICATIONS
- Albuterol
- Ephedrine

PURPOSE

SITE/RESPONSE

Alpha₁ receptors

- Activation of receptors in the arterioles of skin, viscera, mucous membranes, and veins leads to vasoconstriction.
- Mydriasis (dilation of pupils)

Beta₁ receptors

- Heart stimulation increases the heart rate, myocardial contractility, and the rate of conduction through the AV node.
- Activation of receptors in the kidney leads to the release of renin.

Beta₂ receptors

- Activation of receptors in the arterioles of the heart, lungs, and skeletal muscles leads to vasodilation.
- Bronchial stimulation leads to bronchodilation.
- Activation of receptors in uterine smooth muscle causes relaxation.
- Activation of receptors in the liver causes glycogenolysis.
- Skeletal muscle receptor activation leads to muscle contraction.

Dopamine receptors

Activation of receptors in the kidney dilates the renal blood vessels.

MEDICATIONS

Epinephrine

Alpha$_1$ receptors
- PHARMACOLOGICAL ACTION: Vasoconstriction
- THERAPEUTIC USES
  - Slows the absorption of local anesthetics
  - Manages superficial bleeding
  - Decreases congestion of nasal mucosa
  - Increases blood pressure

Beta$_1$ receptors
- PHARMACOLOGICAL ACTION
  - Increases heart rate
  - Increases myocardial contractility
  - Increases the rate of conduction through the AV node
  - Increases CO
  - Improves tissue perfusion
- THERAPEUTIC USES
  - AV block
  - Heart failure
  - Shock
  - Cardiac arrest

Beta$_2$ receptors
- PHARMACOLOGICAL ACTION: Bronchodilation
- THERAPEUTIC USE: Asthma

Dopamine

Low dose: Dopamine receptor
- PHARMACOLOGICAL ACTION: Renal blood vessel dilation
- THERAPEUTIC USES
  - Shock
  - Heart failure
  - Acute kidney injury

Moderate dose: Beta$_1$ receptor
- PHARMACOLOGICAL ACTION
  - Dilates renal blood vessels
  - Increases heart rate
  - Increases myocardial contractility
  - Increases the rate of conduction through the AV node
- THERAPEUTIC USES
  - Shock
  - Heart failure

High dose: Beta$_1$, alpha$_1$ receptors
- PHARMACOLOGICAL ACTION
  - Constricts renal blood vessels
  - Increases heart rate
  - Increases myocardial contractility
  - Increases the rate of conduction through the AV node
  - Causes vasoconstriction
- THERAPEUTIC USES
  - Shock
  - Heart failure

Dobutamine

Beta$_1$
- PHARMACOLOGICAL ACTION
  - Increases heart rate
  - Increases myocardial contractility and CO
  - Increases the rate of conduction through the AV node
- THERAPEUTIC USE: Heart failure

COMPLICATIONS

EPINEPHRINE

Vasoconstriction

Hypertensive crisis due to activation of alpha$_1$ receptors in the heart

NURSING ACTIONS
- Provide continuous cardiac and blood pressure monitoring.
- Report changes in vital signs to the provider.

Cardiac complications

Dysrhythmias due to activation of beta$_1$ receptors in the heart. Beta$_1$ receptor activation also increases the workload of the heart and increases oxygen demand, leading to angina.

NURSING ACTIONS
- Provide continuous cardiac monitoring.
- Monitor closely for dysrhythmias, changes in heart rate, and chest pain.
- Notify the provider of dysrhythmias, increases in heart rate, and chest pain.

DOPAMINE

Cardiac complications

Beta$_1$ receptor activation in the heart can cause dysrhythmias. Beta$_1$ receptor activation also increases the workload of the heart and increases oxygen demand, leading to angina.

NURSING ACTIONS
- Provide for continuous cardiac monitoring.
- Monitor closely for dysrhythmias, changes in heart rate, and chest pain.
- Notify the provider of dysrhythmias, increases in heart rate, and chest pain.

Necrosis

- Can occur from extravasation of high doses of dopamine
- If extravasation occurs, phentolamine (an alpha blocker) counteracts alpha-mediated vasoconstriction.

NURSING ACTIONS
- Monitor the IV site carefully. If possible, clinicians should infuse dopamine through a central venous access device. **Qs**
- Stop the infusion at the first indication of irritation.

DOBUTAMINE

Tachycardia
NURSING ACTIONS
- Provide continuous cardiac monitoring.
- Report changes in vital signs to the provider.

CONTRAINDICATIONS/PRECAUTIONS

- Epinephrine and dopamine are Pregnancy Risk Category C. Qs
- Dobutamine is Pregnancy Risk Category B.
- Tachydysrhythmias and ventricular fibrillation are contraindications for receiving dopamine.
- Clients who have hyperthyroidism, angina, a history of myocardial infarction, hypertension, or diabetes mellitus require caution when receiving dopamine or dobutamine.
- Clients who have hyperthyroidism, angina, cardiac dysrhythmias, or hypertension require caution when receiving epinephrine.

INTERACTIONS

MAOIs prevent inactivation of epinephrine and therefore prolong the effects of epinephrine. MAOIs in combination with dobutamine and dopamine can cause cardiotoxicity.
Clients receiving epinephrine, dopamine, and dobutamine should not take MAOIs.

Tricyclic antidepressants block the uptake of epinephrine, dopamine, and dobutamine, which will prolong and intensify the effects of epinephrine.
Clients taking these medications concurrently might need lower dosages of epinephrine, dopamine, and dobutamine.

General anesthetics can make the heart hypersensitive to the effects of epinephrine, dopamine, and dobutamine, leading to dysrhythmias.
NURSING ACTIONS
- Perform continuous ECG monitoring.
- Notify the provider of chest pain, dysrhythmias, and increases in heart rate.

Alpha adrenergic blocking agents, such as phentolamine, block action at alpha receptors.
Phentolamine treats epinephrine toxicity and extravasation of epinephrine and dopamine. QEBP

Beta adrenergic blocking agents, such as propranolol, block action at beta receptors.
Propranolol treats chest pain and dysrhythmias.

Diuretics promote the beneficial effects of dopamine.
NURSING ACTIONS: Monitor for therapeutic effects.

NURSING ADMINISTRATION

- Clients receive these medications IV by continuous infusion. QEBP
- An IV pump is essential for controlling the rate of infusion.
- Clinicians titrate dosages according to the blood-pressure response.
- Stop the infusion of dopamine at the first indication of infiltration. Local injection of an alpha adrenergic blocking agent, such as phentolamine, treats extravasation.
- Monitor for chest pain. Notify the provider if chest pain occurs.
- Monitor urine output for indications of decreased kidney perfusion.
- Monitor the ECG and notify the provider of indications of tachycardia or dysrhythmias.
- Monitor perfusion to the extremities.
- Clients receiving these medications also require monitoring of cardiac output, pulmonary capillary wedge pressure, and central venous pressure.

NURSING EVALUATION OF MEDICATION EFFECTIVENESS

Indications of effectiveness include a urine output greater than or equal to 30 mL/hr (with adequate kidney function), improved mental status, and a systolic blood pressure greater than or equal to 90 mm Hg.

Application Exercises

1. A nurse in a provider's office is monitoring the electrolyte levels of four older adult clients who take digoxin. Which of the following electrolyte values should the nurse identify as increasing the risk for developing cardiotoxicity?

   A. Calcium 9.2 mg/dL

   B. Calcium 10.3 mg/dL

   C. Potassium 3.4 mEq/L

   D. Potassium 4.8 mEq/L

2. A nurse is caring for an older adult client who has a new prescription for digoxin and takes several other medications. Concurrent use of which of the following medications places the client at risk for digoxin toxicity?

   A. Phenytoin

   B. Verapamil

   C. Warfarin

   D. Aluminum hydroxide

3. A nurse is collecting data from a client who has severe heart failure and is receiving a low-dose dopamine infusion. Which of the following findings is an adverse effect of dopamine?

   A. Decrease in heart rate

   B. Angina

   C. Increase in urine output

   D. Abdominal pain

4. A nurse is reinforcing teaching with a client who has a new prescription for digoxin. The nurse should instruct the client to monitor and report which of the following adverse effects as a manifestation of digoxin toxicity? (Select all that apply.)

   A. Fatigue

   B. Constipation

   C. Anorexia

   D. Rash

   E. Blurred vision

5. A nurse is reinforcing teaching with a client who has a new prescription for digoxin to treat heart failure. Which of the following instructions should the nurse include?

   A. Contact the provider for heart rate less than 60/min.

   B. Check pulse rate for 30 seconds and multiply the result by 2.

   C. Increase intake of sodium.

   D. Take the medication with food if you develop nausea.

PRACTICE Active Learning Scenario

A nurse is reinforcing teaching with a client who has heart failure and a new prescription for digoxin 0.125 mg PO daily. What should the nurse include? Use the ATI Active Learning Template: Medication to complete this item.

THERAPEUTIC USES

COMPLICATIONS: Identify two adverse effects.

NURSING INTERVENTIONS: Describe two diagnostic tests to monitor.

CLIENT EDUCATION: Include three instructional points.

Application Exercises Key

1. A. Calcium 9.2 mg/dL is within the expected reference range and does not put a client at risk for cardiotoxicity.

   B. Calcium 10.3 mg/dL is within the expected reference range and does not put a client at risk for cardiotoxicity.

   C. **CORRECT:** Potassium 3.4 mEq/L is below the expected reference range and puts a client at risk for cardiotoxicity. Low potassium can cause fatal dysrhythmias, especially in older clients who take digoxin. The nurse should notify the provider, who might prescribe a potassium supplement or a potassium-sparing diuretic for the client.

   D. A potassium level of 4.8 mEq/L is within the expected reference range and does not put a client at risk for cardiotoxicity.

   (N) NCLEX® Connection: Pharmacological Therapies, Expected Actions/Outcomes

2. A. Phenytoin, an antiseizure and antidysrhythmic medication, does not increase a client's risk for digoxin toxicity. As an antidysrhythmic, phenytoin can treat dysrhythmias due to digoxin toxicity.

   B. **CORRECT:** Verapamil, a calcium-channel blocker, can increase digoxin levels. When clients receive these two medications concurrently, the effectiveness of digoxin decreases, and the nurse should monitor digoxin levels carefully.

   C. Warfarin does not interact with digoxin to increase digoxin levels. Medications that interact adversely with digoxin include thiazide and loop diuretics.

   D. Antacids, such as aluminum hydroxide, decrease the absorption of digoxin and can decrease digoxin levels and its effectiveness.

   (N) NCLEX® Connection: Pharmacological Therapies, Adverse Effects/ Contraindications/Side Effects/Interactions

3. A. Dopamine stimulates beta₁ receptors, which increases the heart rate.

   B. **CORRECT:** Common adverse effects of dopamine include angina, palpitations, and ECG changes.

   C. Dopamine is administered in low doses to increase renal perfusion, which results in increased urinary output. This is a desired effect.

   D. Dopamine is more likely to cause headache than abdominal pain.

   (N) NCLEX® Connection: Pharmacological Therapies, Adverse Effects/ Contraindications/Side Effects/Interactions

4. A. **CORRECT:** Fatigue and weakness are early CNS findings that can indicate digoxin toxicity.

   B. Nausea, vomiting, and diarrhea are GI manifestations of digoxin toxicity.

   C. **CORRECT:** GI disturbances, such as anorexia, are manifestations of digoxin toxicity.

   D. Rash is not a manifestation of digoxin toxicity.

   E. **CORRECT:** Visual changes, such as blurred and yellow-tinged vision, are manifestations of digoxin toxicity.

   (N) NCLEX® Connection: Pharmacological Therapies, Adverse Effects/ Contraindications/Side Effects/Interactions

5. A. **CORRECT:** The client should contact the provider for a heart rate less than 60/min.

   B. The client should check her pulse rate for 1 full minute before each dose.

   C. The client should reduce her intake of sodium and avoid excess fluids.

   D. The client should report nausea to the provider because it is a manifestation of digoxin toxicity.

   (N) NCLEX® Connection: Pharmacological Therapies, Expected Actions/Outcomes

PRACTICE Answer

Using the ATI Active Learning Template: Medication

THERAPEUTIC USES: Digoxin improves the heart's pumping effectiveness and increases cardiac output and stroke volume. It decreases the heart rate by slowing depolarization through the SA node, thus allowing more time for the ventricles to fill with blood. Due to these effects, digoxin treats heart failure, atrial fibrillation, and some other tachydysrhythmias.

COMPLICATIONS: The nurse should monitor for manifestations of digoxin toxicity, which include GI effects (nausea, vomiting, diarrhea), CNS effects (fatigue, weakness), visual effects (yellow-tinged vision, halos around lights, diplopia), heart rate less than 60/min in adults, and skipped beats when checking the pulse.

NURSING INTERVENTIONS
- Monitor digoxin levels periodically during treatment. The expected reference range is 0.5 to 0.8 ng/mL.
- Monitor serum potassium levels because hypokalemia can cause cardiac dysrhythmias, especially in older adult clients. Monitoring the ECG to check for dysrhythmias.

CLIENT EDUCATION
- Take digoxin at the same time each day. The client should not skip a dose or take more than the dose the prescribed each day.
- Monitor for manifestations of toxicity.
- Report any new prescriptions and contact the provider before taking over-the-counter medications, because digoxin interacts with many other substances.

(N) NCLEX® Connection: Pharmacological and Parenteral Therapies, Medication Administration

CHAPTER 21 *Angina and
Antilipemic Agents*

Angina

Anginal pain often manifests as a sudden pain beneath the sternum radiating to the left shoulder, arm, and jaw. It is a result of too little oxygen to meet myocardial demands. Pharmacological management focuses on prevention of myocardial ischemia, pain, myocardial infarction (MI), and death.

Organic nitrates, beta adrenergic blocking agents, calcium channel blockers, and ranolazine help manage anginal pain. Clients who have chronic stable angina should concurrently take an antiplatelet agent (aspirin, clopidogrel), a cholesterol-lowering agent, and an ACE inhibitor to prevent MI and death.

Organic nitrates

SELECT PROTOTYPE MEDICATION: Nitroglycerin
- Oral extended–release capsules
- Sublingual tablets
- Translingual spray
- Topical ointment
- Transdermal patches
- Intravenous solution

OTHER MEDICATIONS
- Isosorbide dinitrate (sublingual)
- Isosorbide mononitrate (oral)

PURPOSE

EXPECTED PHARMACOLOGICAL ACTION
- With chronic stable exertional angina, nitroglycerin dilates veins and decreases venous return (preload), which decreases cardiac oxygen demand.
- With variant (Prinzmetal's or vasospastic) angina, nitroglycerin prevents or reduces coronary artery spasm, thus increasing the oxygen supply.

THERAPEUTIC USES
- Treatment of acute angina attacks
- Prevention of chronic stable angina or variant angina

COMPLICATIONS

Headache

CLIENT EDUCATION
- Use aspirin, acetaminophen, or other mild analgesics to relieve pain.
- Notify the provider if the headache does not resolve within a few weeks. The provider can reduce the dosage.

Orthostatic hypotension

CLIENT EDUCATION
- Sit or lie down if feeling dizzy or faint.
- Avoid sudden changes of position and rise slowly.

Reflex tachycardia

NURSING ACTIONS
- Monitor vital signs.
- Administer a beta blocker, such as metoprolol, if necessary.

Tolerance

Providers prescribe the lowest effective dose.

NURSING ACTIONS: Administer all long-acting forms of nitroglycerin with a medication–free period each day. This action reduces the risk of tolerance.

CONTRAINDICATIONS/PRECAUTIONS

- Nitroglycerin is Pregnancy Risk Category B for tablets, Category C for the other formulations.
- Hypersensitivity to nitrates is a contraindication for receiving nitroglycerin.
- Severe anemia, closed-angle glaucoma, and traumatic head injury are contraindications because nitroglycerin can increase intracranial pressure.
- Clients taking antihypertensive medications and those who have hyperthyroidism or kidney or liver dysfunction require caution when taking nitroglycerin.

INTERACTIONS

Drinking alcohol can contribute to the hypotensive effect of nitroglycerin.
CLIENT EDUCATION: Avoid drinking alcohol.

Antihypertensive medications (beta blockers, calcium channel blockers, diuretics) can contribute to the hypotensive effect.
Clients receiving these medications require caution when taking nitroglycerin.

Taking PDE5 inhibitors (sildenafil, tadalafil, vardenafil) concurrently with nitroglycerin can result in life-threatening hypotension.
CLIENT EDUCATION: Do not take these medications if also taking nitroglycerin.

NURSING ADMINISTRATION

Sublingual tablet and translingual spray

TYPES
- Rapid onset
- Short duration

USE
- Treatment of an acute attack
- Prevention of acute attacks

CLIENT EDUCATION
- Take this rapid-acting nitrate at the first indication of chest pain. Do not wait until pain is severe. Qs
- Take the medication prior to an activity known to cause chest pain, such as climbing a flight of stairs.

For sublingual tablets
CLIENT EDUCATION
- Place the tablet under the tongue and allow it to dissolve.
- Store tablets in their original bottles in a cool, dark place.
- Spray the translingual spray against the oral mucosa and do not inhale it.

Sustained-release oral capsules

TYPES
- Slow onset
- Long duration

USE: Long-term prevention of anginal attacks

CLIENT EDUCATION
- Swallow capsules without crushing or chewing them.
- Take capsules on an empty stomach with at least 8 oz water.

Transdermal

TYPES
- Slow onset
- Long duration

USE: Long-term prevention of anginal attacks

NURSING ACTIONS
- Place the patch on a hairless area of skin (chest, back, abdomen, thighs) and rotate sites to prevent skin irritation.
- Remove the old patch. Wash the new application site with soap and water and dry it thoroughly before applying a new patch.
- Remove the patch at night to reduce the risk of developing tolerance to nitroglycerin. Clients should be medication-free between 10 and 12 hr/day. QEBP

CLIENT EDUCATION: To self-administer the correct dosage, do not cut the patches.

Topical ointment

TYPES
- Slow onset
- Long duration

USE: Long-term prevention of anginal attacks

NURSING ACTIONS
- Remove the prior dose before applying a new dose. Measure the specific dosage with applicator paper and spread the medication over 6.4 to 8.9 cm (2.5 to 3.5 in) of the paper.
- Apply to a clean, hairless area of the body, and cover with clear plastic wrap.
- Follow the same guidelines for site selection as for transdermal patches.
- Avoid touching the ointment with the hands.

TREATING AN ANGINAL ATTACK USING SUBLINGUAL TABLETS OR TRANSLINGUAL SPRAY

CLIENT EDUCATION
- Stop activity. Sit or lie down. QEBP
- Immediately put one sublingual tablet under the tongue and let it dissolve. Rest for 5 min.
- If the first tablet does not relieve the pain, call 911, then take a second tablet.
- After another 5 min, take a third tablet if still in pain. Do not take more than three sublingual tablets.
- If using nitroglycerin translingual spray, one spray substitutes for one sublingual tablet when treating an anginal attack.
- Do not stop taking long-acting nitroglycerin abruptly.
- Record pain frequency, intensity, duration, and location. Notify the provider if attacks increase in frequency, intensity, or duration.
- Do not crush or chew oral nitroglycerin or isosorbide tablets.

NURSING EVALUATION OF MEDICATION EFFECTIVENESS

Indications of effectiveness include the following.
- Prevention and termination of acute anginal attacks
- Long-term management of stable angina
- Control of perioperative blood pressure
- Control of heart failure following acute MI

Antianginal agent

SELECT PROTOTYPE MEDICATION: Ranolazine

PURPOSE

EXPECTED PHARMACOLOGICAL ACTION: Lower cardiac oxygen demand and thereby improve exercise tolerance and decrease pain

THERAPEUTIC USES: Chronic stable angina in combination with amlodipine, a beta adrenergic blocker, or an organic nitrate

COMPLICATIONS

QT prolongation

Can increase the risk for torsades de pointes

NURSING ACTIONS: Monitor the ECG.

CLIENT EDUCATION: Report palpitations, chest pain, or dyspnea.

Elevated blood pressure

NURSING ACTIONS: Monitor blood pressure.

CONTRAINDICATIONS/PRECAUTIONS

- Pregnancy Risk Category C **Qs**
- QT prolongation, hepatic impairment, ventricular tachycardia, ventricular dysrhythmias, and hypokalemia are contraindications for receiving ranolazine.
- Older adult clients and those who have hypotension or kidney impairment require caution when receiving ranolazine. **Ⓖ**

INTERACTIONS

Inhibitors of CYP3A4 can increase levels of ranolazine and lead to torsades de pointes.
- These include grapefruit juice, HIV protease inhibitors, macrolide antibiotics, azole antifungals, and verapamil.
- NURSING ACTIONS: Discourage concurrent use.

Quinidine and sotalol can further prolong the QT interval.
NURSING ACTIONS: Discourage concurrent use.

Concurrent use of ranolazine with digoxin or simvastatin increases levels of digoxin or simvastatin.
- NURSING ACTIONS: Monitor digoxin levels.
- CLIENT EDUCATION: Report muscle weakness.

NURSING ADMINISTRATION

- Administer as an extended-release oral tablet, twice daily with or without food. Tell clients not to crush or chew the tablets. **Q**EBP
- Obtain a baseline ECG.
- Document a baseline digoxin level with concurrent use and monitor thereafter.
- Clients may take ranolazine concurrently with other antianginal medications, such as nitroglycerin.
- Monitor blood pressure and pulse periodically.
- Inform clients that ranolazine does not treat an acute anginal attack.

NURSING EVALUATION OF MEDICATION EFFECTIVENESS

Indications of effectiveness include the following.
- Prevention of acute anginal attacks
- Long-term management of stable angina

Antilipemic agents

Antilipemic agents work in different ways to help lower low-density lipoprotein (LDL) levels, raise high-density lipoprotein (HDL) levels, and possibly decrease very low-density lipoprotein (VLDL) levels. These medications are an adjunct to lifestyle modifications (regular activity, healthy diet, weight control).

Prior to starting to take these medications, clients should have laboratory tests, including baseline levels of total cholesterol, LDL, HDL, and triglycerides. Monitor blood values periodically throughout the course of therapy. Document baseline liver and kidney function test results and monitor them thereafter.

Medications are not first-line therapy for coronary artery disease and should only follow lifestyle changes if they do not reduce LDL to an acceptable level.

Medication classifications include HMG-CoA reductase inhibitors (statins), cholesterol absorption inhibitors, bile-acid sequestrants, nicotinic acid, fibrates, and antisense oligonucleotide.

HMG-CoA reductase inhibitors (statins)

SELECT PROTOTYPE MEDICATION: Atorvastatin

OTHER MEDICATIONS
- Simvastatin
- Lovastatin
- Pravastatin
- Rosuvastatin
- Fluvastatin
- Pitavastatin

COMBINATION MEDICATIONS
- Simvastatin and ezetimibe
- Simvastatin and niacin
- Lovastatin and niacin

PURPOSE

EXPECTED PHARMACOLOGICAL ACTIONS
- Decrease the synthesis of LDL and VLDL
- Increase the synthesis of HDL
- Other beneficial effects include promotion of vasodilation and decreases in plaque site inflammation, thromboembolism, and risk of atrial fibrillation.

THERAPEUTIC USES
- Primary hypercholesterolemia
- Prevention of coronary events (primary and secondary)
- Protection against myocardial infarction (MI) and stroke for clients who have diabetes mellitus
- Increase in levels of HDL in clients who have primary hypercholesterolemia
- Primary prevention in clients whose LDL is within the expected reference range

COMPLICATIONS

Hepatotoxicity

Increases in aspartate transaminase (AST)

NURSING ACTIONS
- Document baseline liver function.
- Monitor liver function tests after 12 weeks and then every 6 months.

CLIENT EDUCATION
- Observe for indications of liver dysfunction (anorexia, vomiting, nausea, jaundice), and notify the provider if these manifestations occur.
- Avoid drinking alcohol.
- If liver function test results are above the expected reference range, the provider might discontinue statin therapy.

Myopathy
- Muscle aches, pain, and tenderness
- Can progress to myositis or rhabdomyolysis

NURSING ACTIONS
- Document a baseline creatine kinase (CK) level.
- Monitor CK levels periodically during treatment.

CLIENT EDUCATION
- Report muscle aches, pain, and tenderness.
- If CK levels rise, the provider might discontinue statin therapy.

CONTRAINDICATIONS/PRECAUTIONS
- Pregnancy Risk Category X Qs
- Liver disorders and breastfeeding are contraindications for receiving statins.
- Clients of Asian descent should avoid rosuvastatin or take lower dosages.
- Clients who have previously had liver disease, acute infections, electrolyte imbalance, or severe metabolic disorders require caution when receiving statins. Providers should prescribe lower dosages of several statins (lovastatin, pitavastatin, pravastatin, rosuvastatin, simvastatin) for clients who have severe kidney impairment.

INTERACTIONS

Fibrates (gemfibrozil, fenofibrate) and ezetimibe increase the risk of myopathy.
- NURSING ACTIONS
  - Document a baseline CK level.
  - Monitor CK levels periodically during treatment.
- CLIENT EDUCATION
  - Report muscle aches and pain.
  - If CK levels rise, the provider might discontinue statin therapy.

Medications that suppress CYP3A4 (erythromycin, ketoconazole), as well as HIV protease inhibitors, amiodarone, and cyclosporine, can increase levels of some statins when taken concurrently.
- Providers might have to decrease statin dosages for clients who must take medications that suppress CYP3A4.
- CLIENT EDUCATION
  - Do not take atorvastatin, lovastatin, and simvastatin concurrently with medications that suppress CYP3A4.
  - Inform the provider of all medications currently taken.

Grapefruit juice suppresses CYP3A4 and can increase levels of statins.
NURSING ACTIONS: Clients taking statins should avoid grapefruit and grapefruit juice.

NURSING ADMINISTRATION

- Administer statins PO.
- Administer lovastatin with the evening meal. Clients may take other statins without food, but evening dosing is best because most cholesterol synthesis takes place during the night. QEBP
- Atorvastatin and fluvastatin are preferable choices for clients who have impaired kidney function. For other statins, providers reduce the dosage.
- Inform clients about the importance of baseline cholesterol, HDL, LDL, and triglyceride levels, as well as liver and kidney function tests, and monitoring them periodically during treatment.

Cholesterol absorption inhibitor

SELECT PROTOTYPE MEDICATION: Ezetimibe

PURPOSE

EXPECTED PHARMACOLOGICAL ACTION

Ezetimibe inhibits the absorption of cholesterol in bile and from food.

THERAPEUTIC USES

Clients who have diet modifications can take this medication, alone or as an adjunct in combination with a statin to help lower LDL.

COMPLICATIONS

Hepatitis

NURSING ACTIONS: Document baseline liver function.

CLIENT EDUCATION
- Observe for liver dysfunction (anorexia, vomiting, nausea, jaundice) and notify the provider if these effects occur.
- Avoid drinking alcohol.
- If liver function tests are outside the expected reference range, the provider might discontinue ezetimibe therapy.

Myopathy

NURSING ACTIONS
- Document a baseline CK level.
- Monitor CK levels periodically during treatment.

CLIENT EDUCATION
- Notify the provider if manifestations (muscle aches, pains) occur.
- If CK levels rise, the provider might discontinue the medication.

CONTRAINDICATIONS/PRECAUTIONS

- Ezetimibe alone: Pregnancy Risk Category C; in combination with simvastatin: Pregnancy Risk Category X Qs
- Active moderate-to-severe liver disorders, especially in clients taking a statin concurrently, and breastfeeding are contraindications.
- Older adults and clients who have mild liver disorders require caution when receiving ezetimibe. QG

INTERACTIONS

Bile acid sequestrants, such as cholestyramine, interfere with absorption.
CLIENT EDUCATION: Take ezetimibe 1 hr before or 4 hr after taking bile sequestrants.

Statins, such as atorvastatin, can increase the risk of liver dysfunction and myopathy.
- NURSING ACTIONS: Document baseline liver function tests and monitor them periodically.
- CLIENT EDUCATION
  ○ Observe for indications of liver damage (anorexia, vomiting, nausea) and report them. The provider might discontinue the medication.
  ○ Notify the provider of manifestations, such as muscle aches and pains.
  ○ If CK levels rise, the provider might discontinue the medication.

Concurrent use with fibrates, such as gemfibrozil, increases the risks of cholelithiasis and myopathy.
CLIENT EDUCATION: Do not take ezetimibe with fibrates.

Cyclosporine can increase ezetimibe levels.
NURSING ACTIONS: Monitor for adverse effects (liver damage, myopathy).

NURSING ADMINISTRATION

- Advise clients to report muscle aches and pain.
- If CK levels rise, the provider might discontinue the medication.
- Inform clients about the importance of baseline cholesterol, HDL, LDL, and triglyceride levels, as well as liver and kidney function tests, and monitoring them periodically during treatment.
- Advise clients to follow a low-fat, low-cholesterol diet and to follow a regular exercise regimen. QPCC
- Clients can take this medication in a fixed-dose combination with simvastatin.

Bile acid sequestrants

SELECT PROTOTYPE MEDICATION: Colesevelam

OTHER MEDICATION: Colestipol

PURPOSE

EXPECTED PHARMACOLOGICAL ACTION: Decrease in LDL

THERAPEUTIC USE: Alone or as an adjunct with an HMG-CoA reductase inhibitor, such as atorvastatin, and with dietary measures to lower cholesterol levels

COMPLICATIONS

Constipation

CLIENT EDUCATION: Increase intake of high-fiber food and fluids, unless there are fluid restrictions.

CONTRAINDICATIONS/PRECAUTIONS

- Colesevelam is Pregnancy Risk Category B. Colestipol is Pregnancy Risk Category C. Qs
- Bowel obstruction and pancreatitis due to high triglyceride levels are contraindications for receiving colesevelam.
- Clients who have biliary disorders or diabetes mellitus and older adults require caution when receiving bile acid sequestrants. Ⓖ

INTERACTIONS

Bile acid sequestrants interfere with the absorption of many medications, including levothyroxine; second-generation sulfonylureas, such as glipizide; phenytoin; fat-soluble vitamins (A, D, E, K); and oral contraceptives. They also form insoluble complexes with thiazide diuretics, digoxin, and warfarin.

CLIENT EDUCATION
- Take other medications 4 hr before taking bile acid sequestrants.
- Inform the provider of all medications currently taken.

NURSING ADMINISTRATION

- Clients take colesevelam PO in tablet form. They should take it with food and 8 oz of water, and not concurrently with other medications. QEBP
- Colestipol is available as oral tablets that should not be crushed or chewed. Administer tablets 30 min before a meal.
- Colestipol is also available in a powder formulation. Advise clients to use an adequate amount of fluid (90 mL) to dissolve the medication.

Nicotinic acid, niacin

PURPOSE

EXPECTED PHARMACOLOGICAL ACTION

Decrease in LDL and triglyceride levels

THERAPEUTIC USES

- For clients at risk for pancreatitis and elevated triglyceride levels
- Lower elevated LDL and triglycerides, and raise HDL levels

COMPLICATIONS

GI distress

Usually self-limiting

CLIENT EDUCATION: Take the medication with food.

Facial flushing and feeling of warmth, tingling of hands and feet (temporary)

CLIENT EDUCATION: Take aspirin 30 min before each dose.

Hyperglycemia

NURSING ACTIONS: Monitor blood glucose levels.

Hepatotoxicity

NURSING ACTIONS: Document baseline liver function tests and monitor them periodically.

CLIENT EDUCATION
- Observe for indications of liver dysfunction (anorexia, vomiting, nausea, jaundice) and notify the provider if these occur.
- If liver function tests are outside the expected reference range, the provider might discontinue these medications.

Hyperuricemia

NURSING ACTIONS
- Monitor kidney function, BUN, creatinine, and I&O.
- Encourage an adequate fluid intake of 2 to 3 L of water each day from food and beverage sources, unless there are fluid restrictions.
- Administer allopurinol if uric acid levels rise.

CONTRAINDICATIONS/PRECAUTIONS

- Pregnancy Risk Category C Qs
- Liver disease and gout are contraindications for receiving these medications.
- Clients who have diabetes mellitus, asymptomatic hyperuricemia, or peptic ulcer disease require caution when receiving these medications.

NURSING ADMINISTRATION

- Administer PO, either in tablet or liquid form. Tablets are either in the standard form or time-released.
  - Administer the standard form three times per day with or after meals. QEBP
  - Administer time-released formulations once in the evening.
- Advise clients that the dosage is much larger than that of niacin as a vitamin supplement.

Fibrates

SELECT PROTOTYPE MEDICATION: Gemfibrozil

OTHER MEDICATIONS: Fenofibrate

PURPOSE

EXPECTED PHARMACOLOGICAL ACTION

- Decrease in triglyceride levels (increase in VLDL excretion for clients unable to lower triglyceride levels with lifestyle modification or other antilipemic medications)
- Increase in HDL levels by promoting the production of precursors to HDL

THERAPEUTIC USES

- Reduction of plasma triglycerides (VLDL)
- Increased levels of HDL

COMPLICATIONS

GI distress

Usually mild and self-limiting

Gallstones

CLIENT EDUCATION
- Observe for indications of gallbladder disease (right upper quadrant pain, fat intolerance, bloating).
- Notify the provider if these manifestations occur.

Myopathy (muscle tenderness, pain)

- Document baseline CK level.
- Monitor CK levels periodically during treatment.
- Monitor for muscle aches, pain, and tenderness, and notify the provider if these adverse effects occur.
- Withhold the medication if CK levels rise and notify the provider.

Hepatotoxicity

NURSING ACTIONS: Document baseline liver function tests, and monitor them periodically.

CLIENT EDUCATION
- Observe for indications of liver dysfunction (anorexia, vomiting, nausea, jaundice) and notify the provider if these manifestations occur.
- If liver function tests are outside the expected reference range, withhold the medication and notify the provider.

CONTRAINDICATIONS/PRECAUTIONS

- Pregnancy Risk Category C Qs
- Liver disorders, severe kidney dysfunction, and gallbladder disease are contraindications for receiving fibrates.

INTERACTIONS

With concurrent use, warfarin increases the risk of bleeding.
- NURSING ACTIONS: Document baseline prothrombin time (PT) and INR, and monitor periodically.
- CLIENT EDUCATION: Report indications of bleeding (bruising, bleeding gums) and notify the provider if these occur.

Statins increase the risk of myopathy.
CLIENT EDUCATION: Avoid taking statins with fibrates.

NURSING ADMINISTRATION

- Administer via oral route.
- Advise clients to take the medication 30 min prior to breakfast and dinner. QEBP

Antisense oligonucleotide

SELECT PROTOTYPE MEDICATION: Mipomersen

PURPOSE

EXPECTED PHARMACOLOGICAL ACTION: Inhibits the synthesis of apolipoprotein B-100 and thus decreases LDL, non-HDL, total cholesterol, and apolipoprotein B.

THERAPEUTIC USES: Reduces cholesterol levels in clients who have homozygous familial hypercholesterolemia

COMPLICATIONS

Liver toxicity

NURSING ACTIONS: Check baseline ALT, AST, alkaline phosphatase, and total bilirubin before clients start taking the medication and regularly during therapy.

CLIENT EDUCATION: Avoid drinking alcohol while taking this medication.

Flu-like manifestations, nausea, headache

CLIENT EDUCATION: Report these manifestations to the provider.

Hypertension

NURSING ACTIONS: Monitor blood pressure regularly while clients are taking this medication.

Musculoskeletal pain

CLIENT EDUCATION: Report pain to the provider.

CONTRAINDICATIONS/PRECAUTIONS

- Pregnancy Risk Category B
- Older adults require caution when receiving mipomersen due to their increased risks for hypertension and hepatic injury. ⓒ
- Clients who are breastfeeding or have kidney disease require caution when receiving this medication. Qs

INTERACTIONS

Acetaminophen, methotrexate, tetracyclines, and tamoxifen increase levels of mipomersen and can increase the risk for liver damage.
- NURSING ACTIONS: Review clients' medications with the provider.
- CLIENT EDUCATION: Use an alternative to acetaminophen for mild pain relief.

NURSING ADMINISTRATION

- Administer subcutaneously into the abdomen, thigh, or outer arm once weekly on the same day of the week. QEBP
- For missed doses, give the missed dose at least 3 days before the next dose is due.

Application Exercises

1. A nurse is reinforcing teaching with a client who has angina pectoris and is learning how to treat acute anginal attacks. The client asks, "What is my next step if I take one tablet, wait 5 minutes, but still have anginal pain?" Which of the following responses should the nurse make?

   A. "Take two more sublingual tablets at the same time."

   B. "Call the emergency response team."

   C. "Take a sustained-release nitroglycerin capsule."

   D. "Wait another 5 minutes. Then take a second sublingual tablet."

2. A nurse is reinforcing teaching with a client who has a new prescription for nitroglycerin transdermal patches to treat angina pectoris. Which of the following instructions should the nurse include?

   A. Remove the patch each evening.

   B. Cut each patch in half if angina attacks are under control.

   C. Take off the nitroglycerin patch for 30 min if a headache occurs.

   D. Apply a new patch every 48 hr.

3. A nurse is taking a medication history from a client who has angina and a new prescription for ranolazine. Which of the following medications in the client's history can interact with ranolazine? (Select all that apply.)

   A. Digoxin

   B. Simvastatin

   C. Verapamil

   D. Amlodipine

   E. Nitroglycerin transdermal patches

4. A nurse is reinforcing teaching with a client who has a new prescription for simvastatin. Which of the following instructions should the nurse include?

   A. Take this medication in the evening.

   B. Change position slowly when rising from a chair.

   C. Maintain a steady intake of green, leafy vegetables.

   D. Consume no more than 1 L/day of fluid.

5. A nurse is reinforcing teaching with a client who is taking digoxin and has a new prescription for colesevelam. Which of the following instructions should the nurse include?

   A. "Take digoxin with your morning dose of colesevelam."

   B. "Expect monitoring of your sodium and potassium levels while you are taking colesevelam."

   C. "Watch for bleeding or bruising while you are taking colesevelam."

   D. "Take colesevelam with food and at least 8 ounces of water."

PRACTICE Active Learning Scenario

A nurse is caring for a client who has elevated total cholesterol, LDL, and triglycerides, and a new prescription for atorvastatin once daily. The client has type 2 diabetes mellitus and hypertension. What information and instructions should the nurse give the client about atorvastatin? Use the ATI Active Learning Template: Medication to complete this item.

THERAPEUTIC USES: Identify for atorvastatin.

COMPLICATIONS: Identify two adverse effects.

CLIENT EDUCATION: Include two instructional points.

Application Exercises Key

1. A. The client should not take two sublingual doses at once.

   B. **CORRECT:** The next step is to call emergency services and then take a second sublingual tablet. If the first tablet does not work, the client might be having a MI. The client may take a third tablet after another 5 min if the second one has not relieved the pain.

   C. Taking an oral sustained-release capsule will not treat an acute anginal attack.

   D. The client should not wait an additional 5 min before taking a second tablet. The client might be having a MI and should call 911.

   Ⓝ *NCLEX® Connection: Pharmacological Therapies, Expected Actions/Outcomes*

2. A. **CORRECT:** To prevent tolerance to nitroglycerin, the client should remove the patch for 10 to 12 hr during each 24-hr period.

   B. The client should always apply a whole patch to ensure administration of the prescribed dose. Patches are available in several dosages.

   C. The client should not remove patches for a 30-min period if a headache occurs. The client should notify the provider if headaches do not resolve because the provider might have to decrease the dosage of nitroglycerin.

   D. The client should apply a new patch every 24 hr.

   Ⓝ *NCLEX® Connection: Pharmacological Therapies, Expected Actions/Outcomes*

3. A. **CORRECT:** Concurrent use with ranolazine increases digoxin levels, so digoxin toxicity can result.

   B. **CORRECT:** Concurrent use with ranolazine increases simvastatin levels, so liver toxicity can result.

   C. **CORRECT:** Verapamil is an inhibitor of CYP3A4, which can increase ranolazine levels and lead to the dysrhythmia torsades de pointes.

   D. Amlodipine, a calcium channel blocker, treats hypertension and stable angina. Providers prescribe it along with ranolazine to treat angina.

   E. Providers prescribe nitroglycerin transdermal patches along with ranolazine to treat angina.

   Ⓝ *NCLEX® Connection: Pharmacological Therapies, Adverse Effects/ Contraindications/Side Effects/Interactions*

4. A. **CORRECT:** The client should take simvastatin in the evening because nighttime is when the most cholesterol synthesis takes place. Taking statin medications in the evening increases the medication's effectiveness.

   B. Changing positions slowly might be necessary when taking an antihypertensive medication, but not after taking simvastatin.

   C. Consuming a steady intake of green, leafy vegetables is important for clients taking warfarin, but it does not help lower cholesterol for clients who are taking simvastatin.

   D. There is no indication for taking less than 1 L/day of fluid when taking simvastatin.

   Ⓝ *NCLEX® Connection: Pharmacological Therapies, Expected Actions/Outcomes*

5. A. The client should take digoxin 4 hr before taking colesevelam to prevent decreased absorption of digoxin.

   B. It is not necessary to monitor electrolytes during colesevelam therapy. However, the nurse should monitor total cholesterol, LDL, HDL, and triglycerides, as well as blood glucose and HbA1C for clients who have diabetes mellitus.

   C. Bleeding and bruising are not adverse effects of colesevelam. This medication has few adverse effects, primarily the gastrointestinal effects of constipation and dyspepsia.

   D. **CORRECT:** Clients should take colesevelam with food and at least 8 oz water.

   Ⓝ *NCLEX® Connection: Pharmacological Therapies, Expected Actions/Outcomes*

PRACTICE Answer

Using the ATI Active Learning Template: Medication

THERAPEUTIC USES: Atorvastatin decreases LDL and triglycerides and elevates HDL. It reduces the risk for cardiovascular events, such as MI, and also provides secondary prevention for clients who have had a cardiovascular event. For clients who have diabetes mellitus and hypertension, atorvastatin can reduce mortality by controlling cholesterol levels.

COMPLICATIONS
- Muscle pain, tenderness (myopathy)
- Liver toxicity with findings such as jaundice, upper abdominal pain, anorexia, and nausea

CLIENT EDUCATION
- Additional ways to help decrease cholesterol and improve health include exercise, low-fat diet, weight control, and smoking cessation.
- Take atorvastatin in the evening with or without food. (Most cholesterol synthesis takes place during the night.)

Ⓝ *NCLEX® Connection: Pharmacological and Parenteral Therapies, Medication Administration*

ⓝ NCLEX® Connections

When reviewing the following chapters, keep in mind the relevant topics and tasks of the NCLEX outline, in particular:

Pharmacological Therapies

ADVERSE EFFECTS/CONTRAINDICATIONS/SIDE EFFECTS/ INTERACTIONS: Monitor and document the client's response to actions taken to counteract adverse effects of medications.

DOSAGE CALCULATIONS: Perform calculations needed for medication administration.

UNIT 5   MEDICATIONS AFFECTING THE
          HEMATOLOGIC SYSTEM

CHAPTER 22 *Medications*
          Affecting
          Coagulation

Pharmaceutical agents that modify coagulation prevent clot formation or break apart an existing clot. These medications work in the blood to alter the clotting cascade, prevent platelet aggregation, or dissolve a clot. All carry a significant risk of bleeding.

The goal of medications that alter coagulation is to increase circulation and perfusion, decrease pain, and prevent further tissue damage.

These medications include oral and parenteral anticoagulants, direct thrombin inhibitors, direct inhibitors of factor Xa, antiplatelet medications, and thrombolytic agents.

Parenteral anticoagulants

SELECT PROTOTYPE MEDICATION: Heparin

Low molecular weight heparins
- SELECT PROTOTYPE MEDICATION: Enoxaparin
- OTHER MEDICATIONS: Dalteparin

Activated factor Xa inhibitor
- SELECT PROTOTYPE MEDICATION: Fondaparinux

PURPOSE

EXPECTED PHARMACOLOGICAL ACTION

Heparin prevents clotting by activating antithrombin, thus indirectly inactivating both thrombin and factor Xa. This inhibits fibrin formation. Enoxaparin primarily inactivates factor Xa and is much less able to inactivate thrombin. Fondaparinux inactivates factor Xa, thus decreasing thrombin production.

THERAPEUTIC USES

Heparin

- Treats disorders necessitating prompt anticoagulant activity (evolving stroke, pulmonary embolism, massive deep-vein thrombosis [DVT])
- An adjunct for clients having open heart surgery or renal dialysis
- An adjunct to thrombolytic therapy for acute myocardial infarction (MI)
- Low-dose therapy for prophylaxis against postoperative venous thrombosis (hip, knee, or abdominal surgery)
- Treat disseminated intravascular coagulation
- Preferred anticoagulant for use during pregnancy

Low molecular weight heparins

- Prevent DVT in clients who are postoperative
- Treat DVT and pulmonary embolism
- Prevent complications of angina and MI

Activated factor Xa inhibitor (fondaparinux)

- Prevent DVT and pulmonary embolism postoperatively
- Treat acute DVT or pulmonary embolism in conjunction with warfarin

COMPLICATIONS

HEPARIN

Hemorrhage due to heparin overdose

NURSING ACTIONS
- Monitor vital signs.
- Withhold heparin. The client needs protamine IV and should avoid other anticoagulants, including aspirin.
- Monitor activated partial thromboplastin time (aPTT). The usual result is 40 seconds, but a therapeutic response raises the aPTT by 1.5 to 2 times (60 to 80 seconds). Q EBP
- Check the aPTT every 4 to 6 hours during initial therapy and once daily thereafter.

CLIENT EDUCATION: Observe for bleeding (increased heart rate, decreased blood pressure, bruising, petechiae, hematomas, and black tarry stools).

Heparin-induced thrombocytopenia

Low platelet count and increase in thrombus formation

NURSING ACTIONS
- Monitor platelet count periodically throughout treatment, especially in the first month.
- Withhold heparin if platelet count is less than 100,000/mm³. The provider might prescribe a nonheparin anticoagulant, such as argatroban, if anticoagulation is still necessary.

Hypersensitivity reactions (chills, fever, urticaria)

NURSING ACTIONS: Administer a small test dose prior to giving heparin.

Toxicity/overdose

- The client will receive protamine by slow IV injection. It binds with heparin and forms a heparin-protamine complex that has no anticoagulant properties.
- Protamine acts immediately, and its effect lasts for 2 hr.

ENOXAPARIN

Hemorrhage

NURSING ACTIONS: Monitor vital signs and platelet count.

CLIENT EDUCATION
- Observe for bleeding (increased heart rate, decreased blood pressure, bruising, petechiae, hematomas, black tarry stools).
- Avoid aspirin and other anticoagulants.

Neurologic damage

From hematoma formation during spinal or epidural anesthesia

NURSING ACTIONS
- Check the insertion site for indications of hematoma formation (redness, swelling).
- Monitor sensation and movement of lower extremities.
- Notify the provider of any deficiencies.

Thrombocytopenia (low platelet count)

NURSING ACTIONS: Monitor platelets. Withhold the medication and notify the provider for platelet counts less than 100,000/mm³.

Toxicity/overdose

Clients require slow IV injection of protamine (heparin antagonist).

FONDAPARINUX

Hemorrhage

NURSING ACTIONS: Monitor vital signs and platelet count.

CLIENT EDUCATION
- Observe for bleeding (increased heart rate, decreased blood pressure, bruising, petechiae, hematomas, black tarry stools).
- Avoid aspirin and other medications that interfere with hemostasis.

Neurologic damage

From hematoma formation during spinal or epidural anesthesia

NURSING ACTIONS
- Check the insertion site for indications of hematoma formation (redness, swelling).
- Monitor sensation and movement of lower extremities.
- Notify the provider of any deficiencies.

Thrombocytopenia (low platelet count)

NURSING ACTIONS: Monitor platelets. Withhold the medication and notify the provider for platelet counts less than 100,000/mm³.

CONTRAINDICATIONS/PRECAUTIONS

- Thrombocytopenia and uncontrollable bleeding are contraindications for receiving parenteral anticoagulants. Qs
- Surgery of the eye, brain, and spinal cord; lumbar puncture; and regional anesthesia are contraindications.
- Clients who have hemophilia, increased capillary permeability, dissecting aneurysm, peptic ulcer disease, severe hypertension, hepatic or kidney disease, or threatened abortion require caution when receiving parenteral anticoagulants.

INTERACTIONS

Antiplatelet agents (aspirin, NSAIDs, other anticoagulants) can increase the risk for bleeding.
NURSING ACTIONS
- Avoid concurrent use when possible.
- Monitor carefully for evidence of bleeding.
- Take precautionary measures to avoid injury (limiting venipunctures and injections).

NURSING ADMINISTRATION

The intestinal tract cannot absorb these medications. They require subcutaneous injection or IV infusion.

Heparin QEBP

- Document baseline vital signs.
- Document baseline CBC, platelet count, and hematocrit, and monitor thereafter.
- Read labels carefully. Heparin is available in units and in a variety of concentrations.
- Check dosages with another nurse before administration.
- Continuous IV administration requires an infusion pump. Qs
- Monitor aPTT every 4 to 6 hr until the provider determines the appropriate dosage, then monitor daily.

- For subcutaneous injections, use a 20- to 22-gauge needle to withdraw the medication from the vial. Then replace the needle with a smaller one (25- or 26-gauge, ½ to ⅝ inches long).
- Administer deep subcutaneous injections into the abdomen, ensuring a distance of 5 cm (2 in) from the umbilicus. Do not aspirate.
- Apply gentle pressure for 1 to 2 min after the injection. Rotate and record injection sites.
- Instruct clients to monitor for indications of bleeding (bruising, gums bleeding, abdominal pain, nosebleeds, coffee-ground emesis, tarry stools).
- Instruct clients to avoid the use of over-the-counter (OTC) NSAIDs, aspirin, and medications containing salicylates.
- Advise clients to use an electric razor for shaving and to brush their teeth with a soft toothbrush.

Enoxaparin/fondaparinux

- Laboratory monitoring is unnecessary. These medications are acceptable for home use.
- Reinforce teaching about self-administration. Prefilled syringes help simplify the process.
- For subcutaneous injections without a prefilled syringe, use a 20- to 22-gauge needle to withdraw medication from the vial. Then, replace the needle with a smaller one (25- or 26-gauge, ½ to ⅝ inches long). Administer deep subcutaneous injections into the abdomen, ensuring a distance of 5 cm (2 in) from the umbilicus. Do not aspirate.
- Prefilled syringes are available in various dosages for subcutaneous injection. Rotate sites between the right and left anterolateral and posterolateral abdominal wall at least 5 cm (2 in) from the umbilicus. Do not expel the air bubble in the syringe unless adjustments to the dosage are necessary. Pinch up an area of skin, inject at a 90° angle, and insert the needle completely. Do not aspirate. Inject the entire contents of the syringe. Q̇EBP
- Do not rub the site for 1 to 2 min after the injection. Rotate and document injection sites.
- Instruct clients to monitor for indications of bleeding (bruising, gums bleeding, abdominal pain, nosebleeds, coffee-ground emesis, tarry stools).
- Instruct clients to avoid the use of OTC NSAIDs, aspirin, and medications containing salicylates.
- Advise clients to use an electric razor for shaving and to brush their teeth with a soft toothbrush.
- These medications cost more than unfractionated heparin; however, there is a cost savings because there is no need for laboratory monitoring.

NURSING EVALUATION OF MEDICATION EFFECTIVENESS

Indications of effectiveness include the following.

Heparin: aPTT of 60 to 80 seconds

Heparin, enoxaparin, and fondaparinux: No development or no further development of venous thrombi or emboli

Oral anticoagulants

SELECT PROTOTYPE MEDICATION: Warfarin

PURPOSE

EXPECTED PHARMACOLOGICAL ACTION

Oral anticoagulants antagonize vitamin K, thereby preventing the synthesis of four coagulation factors (VII, IX, X, prothrombin). They have no effect on clotting factors already in circulation.

THERAPEUTIC USES

- Prevent venous thrombosis and pulmonary embolism
- Prevent thrombus formation in clients who have atrial fibrillation or prosthetic heart valves
- Prevent recurrent MI, transient ischemic attacks, pulmonary embolus, and DVT

COMPLICATIONS

Hemorrhage

NURSING ACTIONS
- Monitor vital signs.
- Document a baseline prothrombin time (PT), and monitor levels of PT and international normalized ratio (INR) periodically.
- For a warfarin overdose, withhold warfarin and administer vitamin K_1.

CLIENT EDUCATION: Observe for bleeding (increased heart rate, decreased blood pressure, bruising, petechiae, hematomas, black tarry stools, discolored urine, pelvic pain, lumbar pain).

Hepatitis

NURSING ACTIONS: Monitor liver enzymes. Observe for jaundice.

Toxicity/overdose

NURSING ACTIONS
- Administer vitamin K_1 to promote synthesis of coagulation factors VII, IX, X, and prothrombin.
- Administer small doses of vitamin K_1 (2.5 mg PO) to prevent resistance to warfarin. If vitamin K_1 cannot control the bleeding, transfusion of fresh frozen plasma or whole blood might become necessary

CONTRAINDICATIONS/PRECAUTIONS

- Warfarin is Pregnancy Risk Category X due to high risk of fetal hemorrhage, fetal death, and CNS defects. Advise clients to notify the provider if they become pregnant during warfarin therapy. If anticoagulation is necessary during pregnancy, unfractionated or low molecular weight heparin is an option. Qs
- Breastfeeding, thrombocytopenia, and uncontrollable bleeding are contraindications.
- Surgeries of the eye, brain, or spinal cord; lumbar puncture; and regional anesthesia are contraindications.
- Vitamin K deficiencies, liver disorders, and alcohol use disorder are contraindications due to the additive risk of bleeding.
- Clients who have hemophilia, dissecting aneurysm, peptic ulcer disease, severe hypertension, or threatened abortion require caution when receiving warfarin.

INTERACTIONS

Concurrent use of heparin, aspirin, nonaspirin antiplatelet drugs (clopidogrel, dipyridamole, ticlopidine, abciximab), glucocorticoids, sulfonamides, acetaminophen, cimetidine, and parenteral cephalosporins increase the effects of warfarin, which increases the risk for bleeding.

- NURSING ACTIONS
  - Discourage concurrent use if possible.
  - Monitor for indications of bleeding and increased PT, INR, and aPTT levels when clients receive any of these medications concurrently with warfarin. They might require dosage adjustments.
- CLIENT EDUCATION: Check OTC medications to make sure they do not contain aspirin.

Concurrent use of phenobarbital, carbamazepine, rifampin, phenytoin, oral contraceptives, and vitamin K decreases warfarin's anticoagulant effects.
NURSING ACTIONS

- Discourage concurrent use if possible.
- Monitor for reduced PT and INR levels when clients receive any of these medications concurrently. They might require dosage adjustments

Excessive intake of foods high in vitamin K (dark green leafy vegetables [lettuce, cooked spinach], cabbage, broccoli, Brussels sprouts, mayonnaise, canola and soybean oil) can decrease the anticoagulant effects of warfarin.

- NURSING ACTIONS: Provide clients with a list of foods high in vitamin K.
- CLIENT EDUCATION: Maintain a consistent intake of vitamin K to avoid sudden fluctuations that could affect the action of warfarin. Qs

Many medications (OTC medications, herbal supplements) interact with warfarin.
NURSING ACTIONS: Take a complete medication history for clients taking warfarin, and advise clients to inform the provider if they start taking any new medication.

NURSING ADMINISTRATION

- Administration is usually oral, once daily, and at the same time each day.
- Document baseline vital signs.
- Monitor PT levels (therapeutic level: 18 to 24 seconds) and INR levels (therapeutic level: 2 to 3). INR levels are the most accurate. Withhold the dose and notify the provider if these levels exceed therapeutic ranges. QEBP
- It can take 1 week or more to reach a therapeutic INR.
- Frequent monitoring of PT/INR is necessary, initially daily then gradually extending to monthly.
- Document baseline CBC, platelet count, and Hct, and monitor thereafter.
- Inform clients that anticoagulant effects can take 8 to 12 hr, with the full therapeutic effect taking several days. The client might need to continue receiving heparin until warfarin becomes effective.
- Advise clients that anticoagulation effects can persist for up to 5 days following discontinuation of warfarin due to its long half-life.
- Advise clients to avoid alcohol and OTC and nonprescription medications to prevent adverse effects and medication interactions, such as bleeding.
- Advise clients to use nonpharmacological measures to prevent thrombus formation.
  - Avoiding sitting for prolonged periods of time
  - Not wearing constricting clothing
  - Elevating and moving legs when sitting
- Advise clients to wear a medical alert bracelet indicating warfarin use.
- Be prepared to administer vitamin K_1 for a warfarin overdose.
- Instruct clients to self-monitor PT and INR at home. QPCC
- Plan for frequent PT monitoring for clients who take medications that interact with warfarin. Frequent PT monitoring allows for dosage adjustments as necessary.
- Advise clients to record dosage, route, and time of warfarin administration on a daily basis.
- Clients requiring surgery should discontinue warfarin several days prior to the procedure. Emergency surgery might require an injection of vitamin K to suppress bleeding.
- Advise clients to use a soft-bristle toothbrush to prevent gum bleeding and an electric razor for shaving.

NURSING EVALUATION OF MEDICATION EFFECTIVENESS

Indications of effectiveness include the following.
- PT 1.5 to 2 times control
- INR 2 to 3 for treatment of acute MI, atrial fibrillation, pulmonary embolism, venous thrombosis, or tissue heart valves
- INR 3 to 4.5 for mechanical heart valve or recurrent systemic embolism
- No development or no further development of venous thrombi

Direct thrombin inhibitors

SELECT PROTOTYPE MEDICATION: Dabigatran

OTHER MEDICATIONS
- **Hirudin analogs:** Bivalirudin, desirudin
- Argatroban

PURPOSE

EXPECTED PHARMACOLOGICAL ACTION

These medications work by directly inhibiting thrombin, thus preventing a thrombus from developing.

THERAPEUTIC USES

- **Dabigatran** prevents stroke or embolism in clients who have atrial fibrillation without valvular heart disease causing it.
- **Bivalirudin** concurrently with aspirin prevents DVT in clients who undergo coronary angioplasty.
- **Argatroban** prevents or treats thrombosis in clients who cannot take heparin due to heparin-induced thrombocytopenia.
- **Desirudin** prevents DVT in clients having hip arthroplasty.

COMPLICATIONS

Bleeding (gastrointestinal [GI], genitourinary [GU], cranial, other)

- For severe bleeding, no antidote to dabigatran is available. Dialysis or injections of recombinant factor VIIa or factor IX complex can help.
- Clients undergoing elective surgery should stop taking dabigatran before surgery.

CLIENT EDUCATION: Report manifestations of bleeding to the provider.

GI effects

- GI discomfort, nausea, vomiting, esophageal reflux, ulcer formation
- Providers might prescribe a proton pump inhibitor (such as omeprazole) or an H_2 receptor antagonist (such as ranitidine) to prevent or treat these manifestations.

CLIENT EDUCATION: Take dabigatran with food.

Other effects

Bivalirudin can also cause back pain, nausea, hypotension, and headache.

NURSING ACTIONS: Monitor vital signs and evaluate clients receiving this medication for headaches.

CONTRAINDICATIONS/PRECAUTIONS

- Dabigatran and argatroban are Pregnancy Risk Category C. Bivalirudin is Pregnancy Risk Category B.
- Active bleeding and an allergy to the medication are contraindications. Qs
- Clients who have liver or kidney impairment or who are at risk for bleeding require caution when receiving these medications.

INTERACTIONS

Rifampin decreases levels of dabigatran.
NURSING ACTIONS: Use caution when clients take these medications concurrently. Watch for therapeutic effects.

Other thrombolytics and anticoagulants can increase the risk for bleeding with argatroban, desirudin, bivalirudin, and dabigatran.
NURSING ACTIONS: Monitor coagulation studies carefully with concurrent use.

NURSING ADMINISTRATION

- Dabigatran is available in oral capsules that clients should swallow whole and take with or without food. They should use the medication within 30 days of opening the container, and stop taking other anticoagulants when starting dabigatran. Dabigatran has a rapid onset. There is no need to monitor anticoagulation, and it poses a low risk of major bleeding.
- Clients receive bivalirudin IV by direct bolus or continuous infusion.
- Clients receive argatroban IV by continuous infusion to prevent or treat thrombus formation, or as a bolus during percutaneous coronary intervention. Before starting, withhold heparin and check aPTT.
- Administer desirudin by deep subcutaneous injection into the abdomen or thigh.

Direct inhibitor of factor Xa

SELECT PROTOTYPE MEDICATION: Rivaroxaban

OTHER MEDICATION: Apixaban

PURPOSE

EXPECTED PHARMACOLOGICAL ACTION: Provides anticoagulation selectively and directly by inhibiting factor Xa.

THERAPEUTIC USES
- Rivaroxaban treats atrial fibrillation and prevents DVT and pulmonary embolism in clients who are undergoing total hip or knee arthroplasty or who have nonvalvular atrial fibrillation.
- Apixaban prevents stroke and embolism in clients who have nonvalvular atrial fibrillation.

COMPLICATIONS

Bleeding

- GI, GU, cranial, retinal, or epidural bleeding following removal of the epidural catheter
- No antidote is available for severe bleeding, and dialysis is ineffective in removing the medication from the bloodstream. Activated charcoal can help prevent further absorption.

NURSING ACTIONS
- Monitor Hgb and Hct.
- Removal of the epidural catheter should take place at least 18 hr following the last dose. Wait 6 hr after removal before administering rivaroxaban again. Qs

CLIENT EDUCATION: Report bleeding, bruising, headache, or eye pain.

Elevated liver enzymes and bilirubin (rivaroxaban)

- Liver enzymes: ALT, AST, and GGT
- Clients who have moderate or severe hepatic impairment should not take rivaroxaban.

NURSING ACTIONS
- Document baseline liver function and monitor periodically thereafter.
- Report elevated values to the provider.

CONTRAINDICATIONS/PRECAUTIONS

- Rivaroxaban is Pregnancy Risk Category C due to the increased risk of hemorrhage. Qs
- Apixaban is Pregnancy Risk Category B.
- Previous allergy to rivaroxaban, active bleeding, severe kidney impairment, and moderate to severe liver impairment are contraindications.
- Clients taking anticoagulants, antiplatelet medications, or fibrinolytics, and clients who have mild liver or moderate kidney impairment require caution when receiving these medications.

INTERACTIONS

Erythromycin, diltiazem, verapamil, quinidine, and amiodarone increase the risk for bleeding.
NURSING ACTIONS: Monitor for bleeding in clients taking these medications concurrently.

Rifampin, carbamazepine, phenytoin, and St. John's wort can decrease rivaroxaban levels.
NURSING ACTIONS: Monitor for therapeutic effects in clients who take these medications concurrently.

NURSING ADMINISTRATION

- Administer rivaroxaban tablets PO, once or twice daily, with or without food, and at the same time each day. QEBP
- Rivaroxaban has a rapid onset, with a low bleeding risk and no need for INR monitoring.
- Administer apixaban PO twice daily.
- Monitor Hgb, Hct, and liver and kidney function periodically during treatment.

Antiplatelets

Antiplatelet/salicylic
- SELECT PROTOTYPE MEDICATION: Aspirin

Antiplatelet/glycoprotein inhibitors (GP IIa/IIIb inhibitors)
- SELECT PROTOTYPE MEDICATION: Abciximab
- OTHER MEDICATIONS: Eptifibatide, tirofiban

Antiplatelet/ADP inhibitors
- SELECT PROTOTYPE MEDICATIONS: Clopidogrel
- OTHER MEDICATIONS: Ticlopidine, prasugrel, ticagrelor

Other antiplatelets/arterial vasodilator
- SELECT PROTOTYPE MEDICATION: Dipyridamole
- OTHER MEDICATIONS: Cilostazol

PURPOSE

EXPECTED PHARMACOLOGICAL ACTIONS

- Antiplatelets prevent platelets from clumping together by inhibiting enzymes and factors that usually lead to arterial clotting.
- Antiplatelet medications inhibit platelet aggregation at the onset of the clotting process. These medications alter bleeding time.

THERAPEUTIC USES

- Primary prevention of acute MI
- Prevent reinfarction in clients following an acute MI
- Prevent ischemic stroke or transient ischemic attack
- Acute coronary syndromes (abciximab, tirofiban, eptifibatide, clopidogrel)
- Intermittent claudication (cilostazol, pentoxifylline)
- Thromboembolism following heart valve replacement (dipyridamole)

ROUTES OF ADMINISTRATION
- Aspirin: oral
- GP IIb/IIIa inhibitors
  - Eptifibatide: IV
  - Tirofiban: IV
  - Abciximab: IV
- ADP inhibitors
  - Clopidogrel: oral
  - Ticlopidine: oral
  - Ticagrelor: oral
  - Prasugrel: oral
- Dipyridamole: oral
- Cilostazol: oral
- Vorapaxar: oral (with aspirin or clopidogrel)

COMPLICATIONS

ASPIRIN

GI effects (nausea, vomiting, dyspepsia)

Concurrent use of a proton pump inhibitor, such as omeprazole, might decrease GI effects.

CLIENT EDUCATION: Use enteric-coated tablets and to take aspirin with food. Q EBP

Hemorrhagic stroke

CLIENT EDUCATION: Observe for weakness, dizziness, and headache. Notify the provider if these effects occur.

Prolonged bleeding time, gastric bleeding, thrombocytopenia

NURSING ACTIONS
- Monitor bleeding time.
- Monitor for gastric bleeding, such as coffee-ground emesis or bloody, tarry stools.
- Monitor for bruising, petechiae, and bleeding gums.

Tinnitus, hearing loss

NURSING ACTIONS
- Monitor for hearing loss.
- If manifestations occur, withhold the medication and notify the provider.

ABCIXIMAB

Hypotension and bradycardia

NURSING ACTIONS: Monitor heart rate and blood pressure.

Prolonged bleeding time, gastric bleeding, thrombocytopenia, bleeding from cardiac catheterization site

NURSING ACTIONS
- Monitor bleeding time.
- Monitor for gastric bleeding (coffee-ground emesis or bloody, tarry stools).
- Monitor for bruising, petechiae, and bleeding gums.
- Apply pressure to the cardiac catheter access site.

CLOPIDOGREL

Bleeding

Prolonged bleeding time, gastric bleeding, thrombocytopenia

NURSING ACTIONS
- Monitor bleeding time.
- Monitor for gastric bleeding (coffee-ground emesis or bloody, tarry stools).
- Monitor for bruising, petechiae, and bleeding gums.
- Apply pressure to the cardiac catheter access site.

GI effects (diarrhea, dyspepsia, pain)

CLIENT EDUCATION: Monitor for these effects and notify the provider if they occur.

OTHER ANTIPLATELETS/ ARTERIAL VASODILATOR (DIPYRIDAMOLE, CILOSTAZOL)

Headache, dizziness, GI disturbances

Nausea, vomiting, diarrhea, abdominal pain, dyspepsia

Bleeding

Prolonged bleeding time, gastric bleeding, thrombocytopenia

NURSING ACTIONS
- Monitor bleeding time.
- Monitor for gastric bleeding (coffee-ground emesis or bloody, tarry stools).
- Monitor for bruising, petechiae, and bleeding gums.
- Apply pressure to the cardiac catheter access site.

CLIENT EDUCATION: Monitor for these effects and notify the provider if they occur.

CONTRAINDICATIONS/PRECAUTIONS

Aspirin

- Pregnancy Risk Category D
- Bleeding disorders and thrombocytopenia are contraindications. Clients who have peptic ulcer disease or severe kidney or hepatic disorders require caution when taking aspirin. Do not give aspirin to children or adolescents who have influenza or chickenpox due to the risk for Reye's syndrome.
- Older adults require caution when taking aspirin. ⓖ

Abciximab

- Pregnancy Risk Category C
- Bleeding disorders, thrombocytopenia, recent stroke, arteriovenous malformation, aneurysm, uncontrolled hypertension, and recent major surgery are contraindications.
- Clients who have peptic ulcer disease or severe kidney or hepatic disorders require caution when taking abciximab.

Clopidogrel

- Pregnancy Risk Category B
- Bleeding disorders, thrombocytopenia, peptic ulcer disease, and intracranial bleeding are contraindications.
- Clients who have peptic ulcer disease and severe kidney or hepatic disorders require caution when taking clopidogrel.
- Clients who are breastfeeding should not take this medication.

Other antiplatelets/arterial vasodilator (dipyridamole, cilostazol)

- Dipyridamole is Pregnancy Risk Category B. Cilostazol is Pregnancy Risk Category C.
- Bleeding disorders and retinal or cerebral bleeding are contraindications.

INTERACTIONS

Aspirin

Concurrent use of other medications that enhance bleeding (NSAIDs, heparin, warfarin, thrombolytics, antiplatelets) increases the risk for bleeding.
- NURSING ACTIONS: Monitor for indications of bleeding in clients who take these medications concurrently.
- CLIENT EDUCATION Avoid concurrent use.

Urine acidifiers (ammonium chloride) can increase aspirin levels.
NURSING ACTIONS: Monitor for aspirin toxicity (hearing loss, tinnitus).

Concurrent use of aspirin can reduce the hypertensive action of beta blockers.
NURSING ACTIONS: Monitor blood pressure.

Corticosteroids can increase aspirin excretion and decrease aspirin effects. These medications can increase the risk for GI bleeding.
NURSING ACTIONS
- Monitor for decreased aspirin effectiveness.
- Monitor for gastric bleeding (coffee-ground emesis, tarry or bloody stools).

Caffeine can increase aspirin absorption.
NURSING ACTIONS: Monitor for toxicity.

Abciximab

Concurrent use of other medications that enhance bleeding (NSAIDs, heparin, warfarin, thrombolytics, antiplatelets) increases the risk for bleeding.
- NURSING ACTIONS: Monitor for indications of bleeding in clients who take these medications concurrently.
- CLIENT EDUCATION: Avoid concurrent use.

Clopidogrel

Concurrent use of other medications that enhance bleeding (NSAIDs, heparin, warfarin, thrombolytics, antiplatelets) increases the risk for bleeding.
- NURSING ACTIONS: Monitor for indications of bleeding in clients who take these medications concurrently.
- CLIENT EDUCATION: Avoid concurrent use.

Proton pump inhibitors decrease effectiveness.
Pantoprazole interferes the least with platelet inhibition.

Other antiplatelets/arterial vasodilator (dipyridamole, cilostazol)

Concurrent use of other medications that enhance bleeding (NSAIDs, heparin, warfarin, thrombolytics, antiplatelets) increases the risk for bleeding.
- NURSING ACTIONS: Monitor for indications of bleeding in clients who take these medications concurrently.
- CLIENT EDUCATION: Avoid concurrent use.

Omeprazole and CYP3A4 inhibitors, including grapefruit juice, can increase cilostazol levels.
CLIENT EDUCATION: Avoid concurrent use.

NURSING ADMINISTRATION

- Inform clients that low-dose aspirin (81 mg) can help prevent strokes, MI, and reinfarction. Doses greater than 81 mg do not increase benefits but do increase the risk for bleeding.
- Clients should take aspirin 325 mg during an initial acute episode of MI.
- Advise clients to notify the provider about aspirin use. Qs
- Clopidogrel with concurrent aspirin use increases the risk for bleeding. Clients should stop taking clopidogrel 7 days before elective surgery.
- Dipyridamole in combination with warfarin helps prevent thromboembolism; in combination with aspirin, it helps prevent recurrent stroke.
- Cilostazol's full effect of inhibition of platelet aggregation takes up to 12 weeks.

NURSING EVALUATION OF MEDICATION EFFECTIVENESS

Indications of effectiveness include the absence of arterial thrombosis, adequate tissue perfusion, and blood flow without unusual bleeding.

Thrombolytic medications

SELECT PROTOTYPE MEDICATION: Alteplase/tPA (tissue plasminogen activator)

OTHER MEDICATIONS
- Tenecteplase
- Reteplase

PURPOSE

EXPECTED PHARMACOLOGICAL ACTION: Thrombolytic medications dissolve clots that have already formed. Clots dissolve by the conversion of plasminogen to plasmin, which destroys fibrinogen and other clotting factors.

THERAPEUTIC USES
- Treat acute MI (all three medications)
- Treat massive pulmonary emboli (alteplase only)
- Treat acute ischemic stroke (alteplase only)
- Restore patency to central IV catheters (alteplase only)

ROUTE OF ADMINISTRATION: IV only

COMPLICATIONS

ALTEPLASE

Bleeding

Serious risk of bleeding from different sites
- Internal bleeding: GI, GU tracts; cerebral bleeding
- Superficial bleeding: wounds, IV catheter insertion sites

NURSING ACTIONS
- Limit venipuncture, injections, and other invasive procedures.
- Apply pressure dressings to recent wounds.
- Monitor for changes in vital signs, alterations in level of consciousness, weakness, and indications of intracranial bleeding.
- Notify the provider if these manifestations occur.
- Monitor aPTT, PT, Hgb, and Hct.

CONTRAINDICATIONS/PRECAUTIONS

- Pregnancy Risk Category C
- Because of the additive risk for serious bleeding, the following are contraindications. Qs
  - Prior intracranial hemorrhage (hemorrhagic stroke)
  - Structural cerebral vascular lesion (arteriovenous malformation)
  - Active internal bleeding
  - Significant closed head or spinal trauma within the past 2 months
  - Acute pericarditis
  - Bacterial endocarditis
  - Brain tumors
  - Severe hepatic or kidney disorders
- Clients who have severe hypertension, cerebral vascular disorders, recent GU or GI bleeding, or major surgery within past 10 days and older adults require caution when receiving these medications.

INTERACTIONS

Concurrent use of other medications that enhance bleeding (NSAIDs, heparin, warfarin, thrombolytics, antiplatelets) increases the risk for bleeding.

NURSING ACTIONS: Monitor for indications of bleeding in clients who take these medications concurrently.

NURSING ADMINISTRATION

- Identify and report manifestations as soon as possible. Outcomes are improved if thrombolytic agents are administered within 2 to 4 hr after the onset of manifestations. Qebp
- Clients receiving a thrombolytic agent require observation in a setting that provides for close supervision and continuous monitoring during and after administration of the medication.
- Document baseline platelet counts, Hgb, Hct, aPTT, PT, INR, and fibrinogen levels. Monitor periodically.
- Document baseline vital signs (heart rate, blood pressure), and monitor thereafter.
- Clients require continuous monitoring of hemodynamic status to check for therapeutic and adverse effects of the thrombolytic (relief of chest pain, indications of bleeding).
- Minimize bruising or bleeding by limiting venipunctures and subcutaneous/IM injections. Hold direct pressure to the injection site or an ABG site for up to 30 min until oozing stops. Qs
- Following thrombolytic therapy, administer heparin or aspirin to decrease the risk of rethrombosis.
- Following thrombolytic therapy, administer beta blockers to decrease myocardial oxygen consumption and to reduce the incidence and severity of reperfusion arrhythmias.
- Administer H_2 antagonists (such as ranitidine) or proton pump inhibitors (such as omeprazole) to prevent GI bleeding.

NURSING EVALUATION OF MEDICATION EFFECTIVENESS

Indications of effectiveness include evidence of thrombus lysis and restoration of circulation.

Application Exercises

1. A nurse is preparing to administer a prefilled syringe of enoxaparin 40 mg/0.4 mL to an adult client following hip arthroplasty. Which of the following actions should the nurse plan to take?

   A. Expel the air bubble from the prefilled syringe before injecting.

   B. Insert the needle completely into the client's tissue.

   C. Administer the injection into the client's thigh.

   D. Aspirate carefully after inserting the needle through the client's skin.

2. A nurse is caring for a client who is receiving heparin to treat deep-vein thrombosis. The client begins vomiting blood. After stopping the heparin infusion, which of the following medications should the nurse expected the RN to administer?

   A. Vitamin K₁

   B. Atropine

   C. Protamine

   D. Calcium gluconate

3. A nurse is reviewing the current medication list in the medical record of a client who has a new prescription for warfarin. To reduce the risk for hemorrhage, the client should stop taking which of the following medications?

   A. Phenytoin

   B. Acetaminophen

   C. Carbamazepine

   D. Oral contraceptives

4. A nurse is monitoring a client who takes aspirin 81 mg PO daily. The nurse should identify which of the following manifestations as adverse effects of daily aspirin therapy? (Select all that apply.)

   A. Hypertension

   B. Coffee-ground emesis

   C. Tinnitus

   D. Paresthesias of the extremities

   E. Nausea

5. A nurse is caring for a client who has atrial fibrillation and a new prescription for dabigatran to prevent the development of thrombosis. Which of the following medications is the provider likely to prescribe concurrently to treat an adverse effect of dabigatran?

   A. Vitamin K₁

   B. Protamine

   C. Omeprazole

   D. Probenecid

PRACTICE Active Learning Scenario

A nurse is reinforcing teaching with a client who has a new prescription for clopidogrel following a myocardial infarction (MI). What should the nurse include about this medication? Use the ATI Active Learning Template: Medication to complete this item.

THERAPEUTIC USES: Identify for clopidogrel in this client.

COMPLICATIONS: Identify two adverse effects for this medication.

NURSING INTERVENTIONS: Describe three, including one laboratory value the nurse should monitor periodically.

Application Exercises Key

1. A. The nurse should not expel the air bubble in the prefilled syringe prior to injection because expelling the air could result in some loss of the medication.

    B. **CORRECT:** The nurse should inject the needle on the prefilled syringe completely to administer the medication by deep subcutaneous injection.

    C. The nurse should give a deep subcutaneous injection into the abdomen, ensuring a distance of 5 cm (2 in) from the umbilicus.

    D. The nurse should not aspirate when administering enoxaparin or other heparin products subcutaneously. It is an unnecessary step.

    Ⓝ *NCLEX® Connection: Pharmacological Therapies, Medication Administration*

2. A. Vitamin K_1 reverses the effects of warfarin.

    B. Atropine reverses the bradycardia effect of beta adrenergic blockers.

    C. **CORRECT:** Protamine is administered IV and reverses the anticoagulant effect of heparin.

    D. Calcium gluconate treats magnesium sulfate toxicity.

    Ⓝ *NCLEX® Connection: Pharmacological Therapies, Adverse Effects/ Contraindications/Side Effects/Interactions*

3. A. Phenytoin decreases the anticoagulant effects of warfarin, and thus does not increase the client's risk for hemorrhage.

    B. **CORRECT:** Medications that increase the anticoagulant effects of warfarin, and thus increase the client's risk for hemorrhage, include acetaminophen, heparin, aspirin, nonaspirin antiplatelet medications, glucocorticoids, sulfonamides, cimetidine, and parenteral cephalosporins.

    C. Carbamazepine decreases the anticoagulant effects of warfarin, and thus does not increase the client's risk for hemorrhage.

    D. Oral contraceptives decrease the anticoagulant effects of warfarin, and thus do not increase the client's risk for hemorrhage.

    Ⓝ *NCLEX® Connection: Pharmacological Therapies, Adverse Effects/ Contraindications/Side Effects/Interactions*

4. A. Hypotension and shock can result if a severe allergic reaction to aspirin occurs, but hypertension is not an adverse effect of aspirin therapy.

    B. **CORRECT:** GI bleeding with dark stools or coffee-ground emesis is an adverse effect of aspirin therapy.

    C. **CORRECT:** Tinnitus and hearing loss can occur as an adverse effect of aspirin therapy.

    D. Paresthesias of the extremities are not adverse effects of aspirin therapy, although it can cause other CNS effects (headache, dizziness, confusion, seizures).

    E. **CORRECT:** Nausea, vomiting, and abdominal pain can occur as a result of aspirin therapy.

    Ⓝ *NCLEX® Connection: Pharmacological Therapies, Adverse Effects/ Contraindications/Side Effects/Interactions*

5. A. Vitamin K_1 treats hemorrhage or overdose of warfarin, but it is not an antidote for dabigatran.

    B. Protamine treats severe hemorrhage or overdose of heparin, but is not an antidote for dabigatran.

    C. **CORRECT:** Omeprazole or another proton pump inhibitor helps relieve the adverse GI effects of dabigatran. The nurse should advise the client to take dabigatran with food if GI effects occur.

    D. Probenecid treats gout and gouty arthritis, not the adverse effects of dabigatran.

    Ⓝ *NCLEX® Connection: Pharmacological Therapies, Adverse Effects/ Contraindications/Side Effects/Interactions*

PRACTICE Answer

Using the ATI Active Learning Template: Medication

THERAPEUTIC USES: Clopidogrel inhibits platelet aggregation and prolongs bleeding time. It prevents MI or stroke in clients who have already had an MI or stroke.

COMPLICATIONS: Like other platelet inhibitors, clopidogrel can cause bleeding due to thrombocytopenia. It can also cause GI effects (abdominal pain, nausea, diarrhea).

NURSING INTERVENTIONS
*   Monitor platelet count periodically while the client takes clopidogrel.
*   Instruct the client to monitor for bleeding. The client should watch for black stools, coffee-ground emesis, blood in the urine, nosebleeds, unusual bruising, and petechiae. The client should inform the provider if these occur and about GI effects.
*   Identify and document all medications the client is taking, because the risk for bleeding increases if the client takes the medication with anticoagulants or antiplatelet medications. The risk for bleeding increases if the client takes clopidogrel concurrently with aspirin. The client should stop taking the medication 7 days before any elective surgery.

Ⓝ *NCLEX® Connection: Pharmacological and Parenteral Therapies, Medication Administration*

CHAPTER 23 *Growth Factors*

Hematopoiesis is the biologic process that produces the body's blood cells and platelets. Hormones, or hematopoietic growth factors, control this process naturally.

THERAPEUTIC PURPOSES

Genetically engineered products are available for therapeutic purposes.
- Replacement of neutrophils and platelets after chemotherapy
- Hastening of bone marrow function after bone marrow transplant
- Increase in red blood cell production for clients who have chronic kidney disease

HEMATOPOIETIC GROWTH FACTORS

There are three groups of hematopoietic growth factors.

ERYTHROPOIETIC GROWTH FACTORS: erythropoiesis stimulating agents (ESAs)
- Biological name: erythropoietin

LEUKOPOIETIC GROWTH FACTORS
- Biological names
  - Granulocyte colony-stimulating factor
  - Granulocyte-macrophage colony-stimulating factor

THROMBOPOIETIC GROWTH FACTOR: Interleukin-11

Erythropoietic growth factors

SELECT PROTOTYPE MEDICATION: Epoetin alfa: erythropoietin

OTHER MEDICATIONS: Darbepoetin alfa: long-acting erythropoietin

PURPOSE

EXPECTED PHARMACOLOGICAL ACTION

Hematopoietic growth factors act on the bone marrow to increase the production of red blood cells.

THERAPEUTIC USES

Epoetin alfa
- Anemia due to chronic kidney disease
- Anemia resulting from chemotherapy (nonmyeloid cancers)
- Elective surgery: to increase RBC counts preoperatively
- Anemia resulting from taking zidovudine for HIV/AIDS

Darbepoetin alfa: Chronic kidney disease, anemia resulting from palliative chemotherapy (nonmyeloid cancer)

COMPLICATIONS

Cardiac events (hypertension, cardiac arrest, heart failure)

Due to elevations in Hct

NURSING ACTIONS: Monitor Hgb and Hct levels and blood pressure. If elevated, administer antihypertensive medications.

Risk for a thrombotic event

- Myocardial infarction or stroke with a Hgb of 11 g/dL or higher, or an increase of more than 1 g/dL in 2 weeks
- Seizures from a too-rapid rise in the blood counts
- Clotting in the dialysis equipment
- Providers might decrease the dosage and then increase it when the Hct drops to acceptable level.
- If Hgb or blood pressure increases rapidly, clients might require seizure precautions.

Deep-vein thrombosis

- Increased risk preoperatively
- Prophylactic anticoagulants might be necessary preoperatively.

Headache, body aches

NURSING ACTIONS: Report headaches that are frequent or severe to the provider. Hypertension can be the cause.

CONTRAINDICATIONS/PRECAUTIONS

- Pregnancy Risk Category C Qs
- Uncontrolled hypertension is a contraindication.
- Some cancers are contraindications due to the possible increase in tumor growth and shortened survival.

NURSING ADMINISTRATION

- Measure the baseline blood pressure. Clients who have chronic kidney disease require control of hypertension before the start of treatment. QEBP
- Measure blood pressure often, because clients might need adjustments in antihypertensive medication as treatment progresses.
- Clients receive these medications subcutaneously or by IV bolus injection.
- Providers prescribe the lowest dosage that will increase the Hgb concentration gradually and to the lowest level sufficient to reduce the need for RBC transfusion.
- Do not agitate the vial of medication. Use each vial for one dose, and do not put the needle back into the vial when withdrawing the medication.
- Do not dilute or mix the medication with any other medication in the syringe.
- Dosing is usually three times per week, but can be once per week with some types of chemotherapy. Clients receive the longer-acting forms less often.
- Monitor iron levels, and implement measures to ensure an iron level within the expected reference range. RBC growth depends on adequate quantities of iron, folic acid, and vitamin B_{12}. Without adequate levels of these, erythropoietin is significantly less effective.
- Monitor Hgb and Hct once weekly (darbepoetin) and twice per week (erythropoietin) until they reach the target range.
- Monitor CBC and differential routinely.
- Monitor the chemistry panel (BUN, uric acid, creatinine, phosphorus, potassium).
- Ensure that clients receive the FDA's Risk Evaluation and Mitigation Strategy medication guide that explains the risks and benefits of ESAs. The medication guide also discusses ways clients can help minimize the risks of the medication. QPCC

NURSING EVALUATION OF MEDICATION EFFECTIVENESS

Indications of effectiveness include Hgb levels 10 to 11 g/dL and a maximum Hct of 33%.

Leukopoietic growth factors (granulocyte colony-stimulator factors)

SELECT PROTOTYPE MEDICATION: Filgrastim

OTHER MEDICATION: Pegfilgrastim

PURPOSE

EXPECTED PHARMACOLOGICAL ACTION: Leukopoietic growth factors stimulate the bone marrow to increase the production of neutrophils.

THERAPEUTIC USES

- Decrease the risk of infection for clients who have neutropenia from cancer and other disorders, such as congenital neutropenia (Kostmann syndrome)
- Build up the numbers of hematopoietic stem cells prior to harvesting for autologous transplant

COMPLICATIONS

Bone pain

NURSING ACTIONS
- Monitor for bone pain, and notify the provider if it occurs.
- Administer acetaminophen (or an opioid analgesic if acetaminophen is not effective).

Leukocytosis

Providers will reduce the dosage or interrupt treatment if the WBC count is above 100,000/mm³ or the absolute neutrophil count exceeds 10,000/mm³.

NURSING ACTIONS: Monitor CBC two times per week during treatment.

Elevations in uric acid, lactate dehydrogenase, alkaline phosphatase

Elevations are moderate and reversible without intervention.

Splenomegaly, risk of splenic rupture

With long-term use

NURSING ACTIONS: Report left upper quadrant abdominal pain or shoulder tip pain to the provider.

CONTRAINDICATIONS/PRECAUTIONS

- Pregnancy Risk Category C Qs
- Sensitivity to *Escherichia coli* protein is a contraindication. Children or adolescents who weigh less than 45 kg (99 lb) should not receive pegfilgrastim.
- Clients who have cancer of the bone marrow, sickle cell disease, or respiratory disease, and clients who are breastfeeding require caution when receiving these medications.

NURSING ADMINISTRATION

- Clients receive filgrastim via intermittent IV bolus, continuous IV, subcutaneous infusion, or subcutaneous injection.
- Do not agitate the vial of medication. Use each vial for one dose, and do not combine it with other medications. Do not put the needle back into the vial when withdrawing the medication. Qᴱᴮᴾ
- Monitor CBC two times per week during treatment.
- For clients who will self-administer filgrastim subcutaneously at home, reinforce instructions thoroughly.
- Administer pegfilgrastim by subcutaneous injection 24 hr after each round of chemotherapy. The client must then wait at least 14 days before starting the next round of chemotherapy.

NURSING EVALUATION OF MEDICATION EFFECTIVENESS

Indications of effectiveness include the following.
- Absence of infection
- WBC count and differential within the expected reference ranges

Leukopoietic growth factors (granulocyte-macrophage colony-stimulating factor)

SELECT PROTOTYPE MEDICATION: Sargramostim

PURPOSE

EXPECTED PHARMACOLOGICAL ACTION: This medication acts on the bone marrow to increase the production of white blood cells (neutrophils, monocytes, macrophages, eosinophils).

THERAPEUTIC USES
- Hasten bone marrow function after bone marrow transplant
- Treat failed bone marrow transplant
- Treat older adult clients who have acute myelogenous leukemia after induction of chemotherapy to accelerate neutrophil recovery and decrease the incidence of life-threatening infections

COMPLICATIONS

Diarrhea, weakness, rash, malaise, bone pain

NURSING ACTIONS
- Monitor for adverse effects, and notify the provider if they occur.
- Administer acetaminophen.

Leukocytosis, thrombocytosis

Providers will reduce the dosage or interrupt treatment for absolute neutrophil counts of 20,000/mm³ or greater, WBC counts of 50,000/mm³ or greater, or platelet counts of 500,000/mm³ or greater.

NURSING ACTIONS: Monitor CBC two times per week during treatment.

First pass effect

Tachycardia, hypotension, chills, fever, diaphoresis, and dyspnea can occur with the client's first dose.

NURSING ACTIONS: Check carefully for these effects, and notify the provider if they occur.

CLIENT EDUCATION: This effect is not expected with subsequent doses.

CONTRAINDICATIONS/PRECAUTIONS

- Pregnancy Risk Category C
- Allergies to yeast and other substances are contraindications.
- Clients who have lung, cardiac, kidney, or hepatic disease; hypoxia; peripheral edema; bone-marrow cancer; or pleural or pericardial effusion require caution when receiving sargramostim.

NURSING ADMINISTRATION

- Document baseline CBC, differential, and platelet count. Monitor periodically during treatment. Qᴱᴮᴾ
- Clients receive sargramostim by IV infusion. Slow or stop the infusion if clients who have pre-existing heart failure or respiratory disorders have an increase in dyspnea.

NURSING EVALUATION OF MEDICATION EFFECTIVENESS

Indications of effectiveness include the following.
- Absence of infection
- WBC count and differential within the expected reference ranges

Thrombopoietic growth factors

SELECT PROTOTYPE MEDICATION:
Oprelvekin: interleukin-11

PURPOSE

EXPECTED PHARMACOLOGICAL ACTION: Increases the production of platelets

THERAPEUTIC USES: Decrease thrombocytopenia and the need for platelet transfusions for clients receiving chemotherapy

COMPLICATIONS

Fluid retention

Peripheral edema, dyspnea on exertion

NURSING ACTIONS
- Monitor I&O.
- If adverse effects occur, withhold the medication and notify the provider.

Cardiac dysrhythmias

Tachycardia, atrial fibrillation, atrial flutter

NURSING ACTIONS
- Monitor vital signs, heart rate, and heart rhythm.
- If adverse effects occur, withhold the medication and notify the provider.

Eye effects

Conjunctival injection, transient blurring of vision, papilledema (inflammation of the eye and eyelid)

NURSING ACTIONS: Observe for adverse effects. Withhold the medication and notify the provider if these effects occur.

Allergic reactions, possible anaphylaxis

NURSING ACTIONS: Observe carefully for allergic reactions. Withhold the medication and notify the provider if adverse effects occur.

CONTRAINDICATIONS/PRECAUTIONS

- Cancer of the bone marrow is a contraindication because oprelvekin can stimulate tumor growth. Qs
- Clients who have heart failure and pleural effusion or cardiac dysrhythmias require caution when receiving oprelvekin.

NURSING ADMINISTRATION

- Document baseline CBC, platelet count, and electrolyte levels.
- When reconstituting, add sterile water and swirl the vial; do not shake it. Do not combine it with other medications, and use it within 3 hr. Refrigerate it if there is a delay in administering it. QEBP
- Administer oprelvekin once daily by subcutaneous injection.

NURSING EVALUATION OF MEDICATION EFFECTIVENESS

Indications of effectiveness include a platelet count greater than 50,000/mm³.

Application Exercises

1. A nurse is caring for a client who is receiving daily doses of oprelvekin. Which of the following laboratory values should the nurse monitor to determine the effectiveness of this medication?

   A. Hemoglobin

   B. Absolute neutrophil count

   C. Platelet count

   D. Total white blood count

2. A nurse is preparing to administer filgrastim for the first time to a client who has just undergone a bone marrow transplant. Which of the following actions should the nurse take?

   A. Administer the medication IM in a large muscle mass to prevent injury.

   B. Keep the medication in the refrigerator until just prior to administration.

   C. Shake the vial gently to mix it well before withdrawing the dose.

   D. Discard the vial after removing one dose of the medication.

3. A nurse is monitoring a client who is receiving epoetin alfa for adverse effects. Which of the following findings are adverse effects of this medication? (Select all that apply)

   A. Leukocytosis

   B. Hypertension

   C. Edema

   D. Blurred vision

   E. Headache

4. A nurse is collecting data from a client who has chronic neutropenia and who has been receiving filgrastim. Which of the following actions should the nurse take to evaluate the client for an adverse effect of filgrastim?

   A. Ask about bone pain.

   B. Check for right lower quadrant pain.

   C. Auscultate for crackles in the bases of the lungs.

   D. Auscultate the chest for a heart murmur.

PRACTICE Active Learning Scenario

A nurse is reinforcing teaching with a client who has chronic kidney disease and a new prescription for subcutaneous epoetin alfa three times weekly. What should the nurse instruct the client about this medication? Use the ATI Active Learning Template: Medication to complete this item.

THERAPEUTIC USES: Identify for epoetin alfa in this client.

COMPLICATIONS: Identify two adverse effects the client should watch for.

NURSING INTERVENTIONS: Describe four, including two tests the nurse should monitor periodically.

Application Exercises Key

1. A. The nurse should monitor the Hgb levels of clients receiving epoetin alfa.

   B. The nurse should monitor the absolute neutrophil count for clients receiving filgrastim.

   C. **CORRECT:** The expected outcome with oprelvekin is a platelet count greater than 50,000/mm³.

   D. The nurse should monitor the WBC count for clients receiving sargramostim.

   Ⓝ *NCLEX® Connection: Pharmacological Therapies, Expected Actions/Outcomes*

2. A. Administration of filgrastim is IV or subcutaneous.

   B. The nurse should allow the medication to reach room temperature prior to administration.

   C. Before withdrawing a dose of filgrastim, the nurse should not to shake the medication vial.

   D. **CORRECT:** The nurse should withdraw only one dose of filgrastim from the vial and then discard it.

   Ⓝ *NCLEX® Connection: Pharmacological Therapies, Expected Actions/Outcomes*

3. A. Leukocytosis is an adverse effect of filgrastim, rather than for epoetin alfa.

   B. **CORRECT:** Hypertension is an adverse effect of epoetin alfa.

   C. Edema is an adverse effect of oprelvekin due to fluid retention, rather than of epoetin alfa.

   D. Blurry vision is an adverse effect of oprelvekin, rather than of epoetin alfa.

   E. **CORRECT:** Headache, hypertension, seizures, and thromboembolic events are adverse effects of epoetin alfa.

   Ⓝ *NCLEX® Connection: Pharmacological Therapies, Adverse Effects/ Contraindications/Side Effects/Interactions*

4. A. **CORRECT:** Bone pain is a dose-related adverse effect of filgrastim. The nurse should administer acetaminophen if it occurs. If acetaminophen does not relieve the pain, the client might need an opioid analgesic.

   B. The nurse might palpate for abdominal pain as part of data collection, but this will not detect an adverse effect of filgrastim.

   C. The nurse might auscultate for crackles in the bases of the lungs as part of data collection, but this will not detect an adverse effect of filgrastim.

   D. The nurse might auscultate the chest to listen for a heart murmur as part of data collection, but this will not detect an adverse effect of filgrastim.

   Ⓝ *NCLEX® Connection: Pharmacological Therapies, Expected Actions/Outcomes*

PRACTICE Answer

Using the ATI Active Learning Template: Medication

THERAPEUTIC USES: The kidneys produce erythropoietin, a substance that stimulates bone marrow to produce red blood cells. In clients who have chronic kidney disease, erythropoietin is no longer present, and anemia results. Epoetin alfa stimulates the production of RBCs for these clients.

COMPLICATIONS
- Headaches, myalgia (body aches)
- Thrombotic events (myocardial infarction, stroke)
- Hypertension (common, sometimes serious)
- A too-rapid increase (Hgb increases greater than 1 g/dL over 2 weeks, or a Hgb increase greater than 10 g/dL) can worsen hypertension, increase the risk of thrombosis, and cause seizures.

NURSING INTERVENTIONS
- Monitor iron levels, CBC with differential, and platelet counts.
- Monitor Hgb and Hct twice weekly until blood counts stabilize.
- Calculate dosages carefully. Do not shake the epoetin alfa vial. Discard the vial after removing one dose.
- Monitor blood pressure carefully, and report increases to the provider. Question the client about the frequency and severity of headaches, which could be an indication of increasing blood pressure or an adverse effect.

Ⓝ *NCLEX® Connection: Pharmacological and Parenteral Therapies, Medication Administration*

ⓝ NCLEX® Connections

When reviewing the following chapters, keep in mind the relevant topics and tasks of the NCLEX outline, in particular:

Pharmacological Therapies

ADVERSE EFFECTS/CONTRAINDICATIONS/ SIDE EFFECTS/INTERACTIONS: Monitor and document the client side effects of medications.

EXPECTED ACTIONS/OUTCOMES: Evaluate the client's response to medications (adverse reactions, interactions, therapeutic effects).

MEDICATION ADMINISTRATION: Administer medication by gastrointestinal tube (g-tube, nasogastric [NG] tube, g-button, j-tube).

UNIT 6   MEDICATIONS AFFECTING THE
GASTROINTESTINAL SYSTEM AND NUTRITION

CHAPTER 24 *Peptic Ulcer Disease*

Pharmacological management of peptic ulcer disease addresses the imbalance between gastric mucosal defenses (mucus, bicarbonate) and antagonistic factors (*Helicobacter pylori* infection, gastric acid, pepsin, smoking, NSAID use).

For clients who have *H. pylori*, antibiotics eradicate the disease process. Other medications promote healing of the gastrointestinal (GI) tract.

Therapeutic management includes reduction of manifestations, promotion of healing, prevention of complications, and prevention of recurrence.

Antibiotics

SELECT PROTOTYPE MEDICATIONS
- Amoxicillin
- Bismuth
- Clarithromycin
- Metronidazole
- Tetracycline
- Tinidazole

PURPOSE

EXPECTED PHARMACOLOGICAL ACTION: Eradication of *H. pylori* bacteria

THERAPEUTIC USES: Therapy should include a combination of two or three antibiotics along with a proton pump inhibitor or a histamine$_2$ receptor antagonist for 10 to 14 days to increase effectiveness and minimize development of medication resistance. Qpcc

NURSING ADMINISTRATION

- Advise clients to take amoxicillin, clarithromycin, and metronidazole with food to decrease gastric disturbances.
- Inform clients that adverse effects of nausea and diarrhea are common.
- Remind clients to take the full course of the medications prescribed.

Histamine$_2$ receptor antagonists

SELECT PROTOTYPE MEDICATION: Ranitidine

OTHER MEDICATIONS
- Cimetidine
- Nizatidine
- Famotidine

PURPOSE

EXPECTED PHARMACOLOGICAL ACTION: Block H$_2$ receptors, which reduces the volume of gastric acid and lowers the concentration of hydrogen ions in the stomach

THERAPEUTIC USES
- Gastric and duodenal ulcers, GERD, hypersecretory conditions (Zollinger-Ellison syndrome), aspiration pneumonitis, heartburn, acid indigestion
- Ulcers due to *H. pylori* (with antibiotics)

COMPLICATIONS

CIMETIDINE

Blocked androgen receptors

Resulting in decreased libido, gynecomastia, impotence

NURSING ACTIONS: Inform clients of these possible effects.

CNS effects (lethargy, depression, confusion)

More common in older adults who have kidney or liver dysfunction

Pneumonia

CLIENT EDUCATION: Monitor and report manifestations of a respiratory infection.

RANITIDINE

Constipation, diarrhea, nausea

NURSING ACTIONS: Report these effects to the provider.

Pneumonia

CLIENT EDUCATION: Monitor and report manifestations of a respiratory infection.

FAMOTIDINE

Dizziness, drowsiness, constipation

CLIENT EDUCATION: Avoid tasks that require alertness, and take the medication at bedtime.

CONTRAINDICATIONS/PRECAUTIONS

- Pregnancy Risk Category B
- Older adults are at increased risk for CNS effects (confusion). Ⓒ
- H_2 receptor antagonists decrease gastric acidity, which promotes bacterial colonization of the stomach and the respiratory tract. Clients who are at a high risk for pneumonia, including those who have COPD, require caution when taking these medications.

INTERACTIONS

Cimetidine can inhibit medication-metabolizing enzymes and thus increase the levels of warfarin, phenytoin, theophylline, and lidocaine.
NURSING ACTIONS
- For clients taking warfarin, monitor for indications of bleeding.
- Monitor INR and PT levels, and adjust warfarin dosages accordingly. ⒬EBP
- For clients taking phenytoin, theophylline, and lidocaine, monitor serum levels and notify the provider for dosage adjustments.

Concurrent use of antacids can decrease the absorption of histamine₂ receptor antagonists.
CLIENT EDUCATION: Do not take an antacid 1 hr before or after taking a histamine₂ receptor antagonist.

NURSING ADMINISTRATION

- In acute situations, clients receive cimetidine, ranitidine, or famotidine IV.
- Advise clients to eat meals on a regular schedule in a relaxed setting, and to not overeat.
- Instruct clients to avoid foods that promote gastric acid secretion (caffeinated beverages, decaffeinated coffee).
- Inform clients that adequate rest and reduction of stress can promote healing.
- Clients should avoid smoking, which can delay healing.
- Encourage clients to avoid aspirin and other NSAIDs unless taking low-dose aspirin therapy to prevent cardiovascular disease.
- Alcohol can exacerbate peptic ulcer disease. Advise clients to avoid drinking alcohol.
- Availability of these medications over the counter can discourage clients from seeking appropriate health care. Encourage clients to see a provider if manifestations persist.
- The medication regimen can be complex, often requiring clients to take two or three medications for an extended period of time. Encourage clients to adhere to the medication regimen, and provide support.
- Clients may take ranitidine with or without food.
- Treating peptic ulcer disease begins with an oral dose twice a day until the ulcer heals, then a maintenance dose once a day at bedtime.
- Instruct clients to notify the provider for any indication of obvious or occult GI bleeding, such as coffee-ground emesis.

Proton pump inhibitors

SELECT PROTOTYPE MEDICATION: Omeprazole

OTHER MEDICATIONS
- Pantoprazole
- Lansoprazole
- Dexlansoprazole
- Rabeprazole
- Esomeprazole

PURPOSE

EXPECTED PHARMACOLOGICAL ACTION: Block basal and stimulated acid production, and reduce gastric acid secretion by irreversibly inhibiting the enzyme that produces gastric acid

THERAPEUTIC USE: Gastric and duodenal ulcers, erosive esophagitis, GERD, hypersecretory conditions (Zollinger–Ellison syndrome)

COMPLICATIONS

SHORT-TERM TREATMENT

Minor adverse effects include headache, diarrhea, nausea, and vomiting.

LONG-TERM TREATMENT

Pneumonia

CLIENT EDUCATION: Monitor and report manifestations of a respiratory infection.

Osteoporosis, fractures

CLIENT EDUCATION: Increase vitamin D and calcium intake.

Rebound acid hypersecretion

CLIENT EDUCATION: Take a low dose if possible and taper slowly to discontinue it.

Hypomagnesemia

CLIENT EDUCATION: Monitor and report manifestations of hypomagnesemia (tremors, muscle cramps, seizures).

CONTRAINDICATIONS/PRECAUTIONS

- These medications are Pregnancy Risk Category B (except omeprazole, rabeprazole, and esomeprazole, which are Pregnancy Risk Category C).
- Lactation and hypersensitivity to the medications are contraindications.
- Children and clients who have dysphagia or liver disease require caution when taking these medications.
- Clients at high risk for pneumonia, including those who have COPD, require caution when taking these medications.

INTERACTIONS

Digoxin and phenytoin levels can increase when clients take them concurrently with omeprazole.
NURSING ACTIONS: Monitor digoxin and phenytoin levels.

Proton pump inhibitors decrease the absorption of ketoconazole and itraconazole.
NURSING ACTIONS: Discourage concurrent use. When necessary, separate medication administration by 2 to 12 hr.

Proton pump inhibitors decrease absorption of atazanavir, delavirdine, and nelfinavir.
NURSING ACTIONS: Discourage concurrent use.

Beneficial effects of clopidogrel can decrease with concurrent use.
NURSING ACTIONS: Monitor for thrombotic events.

NURSING ADMINISTRATION

- Do not crush or break sustained-release capsules. Tell clients not to chew them.
- Do not open capsules and sprinkle contents over food.
- Clients should take omeprazole once per day prior to eating in the morning.
- Encourage clients to avoid alcohol and irritating medications, such as NSAIDs.
- Active ulcers require treatment for 4 to 6 weeks.
- Clients can receive pantoprazole IV. In addition to headache and diarrhea, there can be irritation at the injection site leading to thrombophlebitis. Monitor the IV catheter insertion site for indications of inflammation (redness, swelling, local pain), and report these findings.
- Instruct clients to notify the provider for any indication of obvious or occult GI bleeding, such as coffee-ground emesis.

Mucosal protectants

SELECT PROTOTYPE MEDICATION: Sucralfate

PURPOSE

EXPECTED PHARMACOLOGICAL ACTION

- The acidic environment of the stomach and duodenum changes sucralfate into a protective barrier that adheres to an ulcer. This protects the ulcer from further injury from acid and pepsin.
- This viscous substance can stick to the ulcer for up to 6 hr.

THERAPEUTIC USES

- Acute duodenal ulcers and for maintenance therapy
- Investigational use: gastric ulcers, GERD

COMPLICATIONS

Constipation (sucralfate)

CLIENT EDUCATION: To prevent constipation, increase dietary fiber and drink 2 to 3 L/day unless there are fluid restrictions.

CONTRAINDICATIONS/PRECAUTIONS

- Pregnancy Risk Category B
- Hypersensitivity to the medication is a contraindication.
- Clients who have chronic kidney disease require caution when taking sucralfate.

INTERACTIONS

Sucralfate can interfere with the absorption of phenytoin, digoxin, warfarin, and ciprofloxacin.
NURSING ACTIONS: Maintain a 2-hr interval between taking these medications and sucralfate to minimize this interaction.

Antacids interfere with the absorption of sucralfate.
NURSING ACTIONS: Administer sucralfate 30 min before or after antacids.

NURSING ADMINISTRATION

- Assist clients with the medication regimen.
- Instruct clients to take sucralfate four times a day, 1 hr before meals, and again at bedtime.
- Clients can break or dissolve the medication in water, but should not crush or chew the tablets.
- Encourage clients to complete the course of treatment.

Antacids

SELECT PROTOTYPE MEDICATION: Aluminum hydroxide

OTHER MEDICATIONS
- Magnesium hydroxide
- Calcium carbonate
- Sodium bicarbonate

PURPOSE

EXPECTED PHARMACOLOGICAL ACTION
- Antacids neutralize gastric acid by producing neutral salts and inactivating pepsin.
- Mucosal protection can occur from stimulation of the production of prostaglandins.

THERAPEUTIC USES: Peptic ulcer disease, GERD (promote healing, relieve pain)

COMPLICATIONS

Constipation, diarrhea

Aluminum and calcium compounds: Constipation

Magnesium compounds: Diarrhea

CLIENT EDUCATION
- Alternate these compounds to offset intestinal effects and keep bowel function regular. Q EBP
- For managing bowel function, a combination product that contains aluminum hydroxide and magnesium hydroxide is recommended.

Fluid retention

Antacids containing sodium can result in fluid retention.

CLIENT EDUCATION: Clients who have hypertension or heart failure should avoid antacids that contain sodium.

Hypophosphatemia, hypomagnesemia

Possible effects of aluminum hydroxide

NURSING ACTIONS: Monitor electrolyte levels.

Toxicity, hypermagnesemia

Magnesium compounds can lead to toxicity and hypermagnesemia in clients who have impaired kidney function.

CLIENT EDUCATION
- Clients who have impaired kidney function should avoid antacids that contain magnesium.
- Monitor for CNS depression.

CONTRAINDICATIONS/PRECAUTIONS

- Aluminum hydroxide is Pregnancy Risk Category C.
- Clients who have GI perforation or obstruction require caution when taking antacids.
- Clients who have abdominal pain require caution when taking antacids.

INTERACTIONS

Aluminum compounds bind to phenytoin, and tetracycline interferes with absorption.
CLIENT EDUCATION: Take these medications 4 to 6 hr apart.

NURSING ADMINISTRATION

- Instruct clients taking tablets to chew them thoroughly and then drink at least 8 oz water or milk.
- Advise clients to shake liquid formulations to ensure even dispersion of the medication.
- Adherence is difficult for clients due to the frequency of administration (seven times per day: 1 hr and 3 hr after meals, and again at bedtime). Encourage adherence by reinforcing the intended effect of the antacid (relief of pain, healing of ulcers). Q PCC
- Instruct clients to take all medications at least 1 hr before or after taking an antacid.

Prostaglandin E analog

SELECT PROTOTYPE MEDICATION: Misoprostol

PURPOSE

EXPECTED PHARMACOLOGICAL ACTION

Acts as an endogenous prostaglandin in the GI tract that decreases acid secretion, increases the secretion of bicarbonate and protective mucus, and promotes vasodilation to maintain submucosal blood flow. These actions help prevent gastric ulcers.

THERAPEUTIC USES

- Prevention of gastric ulcers for clients taking long-term NSAIDs
- Unlabeled use: Induction of labor via cervical ripening

COMPLICATIONS

Diarrhea

With concurrent use of magnesium antacids

CLIENT EDUCATION: Notify the provider of diarrhea or abdominal pain. The provider might reduce the dosage.

Dysmenorrhea, spotting

CLIENT EDUCATION: Notify the provider if dysmenorrhea and spotting occur. The provider might discontinue the medication.

CONTRAINDICATIONS/PRECAUTIONS

- Pregnancy Risk Category X
- If clients of childbearing years take misoprostol, they must comply with birth-control measures, receive oral and written warnings about the adverse effects, have a negative serum pregnancy test 2 weeks prior to initiating therapy, and begin therapy only on the second or third day of the menstrual cycle. Qs

NURSING ADMINISTRATION

Instruct clients to take misoprostol with meals and at bedtime.

NURSING EVALUATION OF MEDICATION EFFECTIVENESS

Indications of effectiveness include the following.
- Reduced frequency or absence of GERD manifestations (heartburn, bloating, belching)
- Absence of GI bleeding
- Healing of gastric and duodenal ulcers
- No reoccurrence of ulcers

PRACTICE Active Learning Scenario

A nurse is caring for a female client who has a prescription for aluminum hydroxide suspension to treat peptic ulcer disease. Use the ATI Active Learning Template: Medication to complete this item.

THERAPEUTIC USES: Identify the therapeutic use of aluminum hydroxide.

CLIENT EDUCATION: Identify three instructions the nurse should include for taking this medication.

Application Exercises

1. A nurse is reinforcing instructions with a client who has a prescription for amoxicillin and clarithromycin to treat a peptic ulcer. Which of the following information should the nurse include?
   - A. "Take these medications with food."
   - B. "These medications can turn your stool black."
   - C. "These medications can cause photosensitivity."
   - D. "These medications decrease the pH of gastric juices in the stomach."

2. A nurse is reinforcing teaching with a client who has a new prescription for omeprazole for heartburn. Which of the following information should the nurse include?
   - A. Take this medication at bedtime.
   - B. This medication decreases the production of gastric acid.
   - C. Take this medication 2 hr after eating.
   - D. This medication can cause hyperkalemia.

3. A nurse is reinforcing teaching with a client who is taking sucralfate PO to treat peptic ulcer disease and has a new prescription for phenytoin to control seizures. Which of the following instructions should the nurse include?
   - A. Take an antacid with sucralfate.
   - B. Take sucralfate with 8 oz milk.
   - C. Allow a 2-hr interval between taking these medications.
   - D. Chew sucralfate thoroughly before swallowing it.

4. A nurse is caring for four clients who have peptic ulcer disease. Which of the following conditions should the nurse identify as a contraindication for taking misoprostol?
   - A. Pregnancy
   - B. Osteoarthritis
   - C. Renal calculi
   - D. Urinary tract infection

5. A nurse is reinforcing teaching with a client who has peptic ulcer disease about managing the disorder. Which of the following instructions should the nurse include? (Select all that apply.)
   - A. "Eat a bedtime snack."
   - B. "Drink decaffeinated coffee."
   - C. "Avoid low-dose aspirin therapy."
   - D. "Seek measures to reduce stress."
   - E. "Avoid drinking alcohol."

Application Exercises Key

1. A. **CORRECT:** The client should take these medications with food to reduce GI disturbances.

   B. Bismuth can cause stool to turn black. Black stool can also be a manifestation of gastric bleeding.

   C. Tetracycline can cause photosensitivity.

   D. Antacids neutralize the pH of the gastric juices in the stomach.

   Ⓝ *NCLEX® Connection: Pharmacological Therapies, Expected Actions/Outcomes*

2. A. The client should take omeprazole in the morning to help manage heartburn.

   B. **CORRECT:** Omeprazole reduces gastric acid secretion by inhibiting the enzyme that produces gastric acid.

   C. The client should take omeprazole before meals and with water.

   D. Omeprazole can cause hypomagnesemia, not hyperkalemia.

   Ⓝ *NCLEX® Connection: Pharmacological Therapies, Expected Actions/Outcomes*

3. A. Antacids can interfere with the effects of sucralfate, so the client should allow at least 30 min between taking sucralfate and the antacid.

   B. The client should take sucralfate on an empty stomach, 1 hr before meals and at bedtime.

   C. **CORRECT:** Sucralfate can interfere with the absorption of phenytoin, so the client should allow 2 hr between taking sucralfate and phenytoin.

   D. The client should swallow sucralfate whole.

   Ⓝ *NCLEX® Connection: Pharmacological Therapies, Expected Actions/Outcomes*

4. A. **CORRECT:** Misoprostol can induce labor; pregnancy is a contraindication for receiving this medication.

   B. Osteoarthritis is not a contraindication for receiving misoprostol.

   C. Renal calculi are not a contraindication for receiving misoprostol.

   D. Urinary tract infection is not a contraindication for receiving misoprostol.

   Ⓝ *NCLEX® Connection: Pharmacological Therapies, Adverse Effects/ Contraindications/Side Effects/Interactions*

5. A. The client should avoid a bedtime snack to reduce gastric acid secretion.

   B. The client should avoid caffeinated and decaffeinated coffee to reduce gastrin release.

   C. Although frequent use of NSAIDs can decrease prostaglandin production, resulting in injury to gastric tissue, low-dose aspirin therapy does not cause this effect.

   D. **CORRECT:** Reducing stress is beneficial for healing of the ulcer and prevention of complications.

   E. **CORRECT:** The client should avoid drinking alcohol to prevent peptic ulcers.

   Ⓝ *NCLEX® Connection: Pharmacological Therapies, Expected Actions/Outcomes*

PRACTICE Answer

Using the ATI Active Learning Template: Medication

THERAPEUTIC USES: Aluminum hydroxide raises the pH of gastric contents, which reduces irritation of stomach mucosa, resulting in relief of pain.

CLIENT EDUCATION
- Aluminum hydroxide is in Pregnancy Risk Category C. Stop taking it and notify the provider if you become pregnant.
- Shake the medication prior to taking each dose to disperse the medication.
- Take other medications at least 1 hr before or after taking aluminum hydroxide.
- Aluminum hydroxide can cause constipation. Notify the provider if it persists. You might need to alternate this antacid with one that is a magnesium compound and has diarrhea as an adverse effect.
- Continue to take the medication even after you no longer have manifestations, so that the ulcer will continue to heal.
- You should take the medication at frequent dosing intervals to promote healing of the ulcer. Seven times a day (1 hr before meals, 3 hr after meals, and at bedtime) is a common dosing schedule.

Ⓝ *NCLEX® Connection: Pharmacological and Parenteral Therapies, Medication Administration*

CHAPTER 25 *Gastrointestinal
Disorders*

These medications affect some aspect of the gastrointestinal (GI) tract to treat or prevent nausea, vomiting, motion sickness, diarrhea, or constipation; treat hiatal hernia by controlling reflux; and treat gastroesophageal reflux disease (GERD) by increasing gastric motility, protecting the stomach lining, and inhibiting the secretion of gastric acid.

Medications include antiemetics, laxatives, antidiarrheals, prokinetic agents, medications for irritable bowel syndrome (IBS), 5-aminosalicylates, probiotics, and medications for hiatal hernia.

Antiemetics

SELECT PROTOTYPE MEDICATIONS
- **Glucocorticoids:** Dexamethasone
- **Substance P/neurokinin₁ antagonists:** Aprepitant
- **Serotonin receptor antagonists:** Ondansetron
- **Dopamine antagonists:** Promethazine
- **Cannabinoids:** Dronabinol
- **Anticholinergics:** Scopolamine
- **Antihistamines:** Dimenhydrinate
- **Benzodiazepines:** Lorazepam
- **Butyrophenones:** Haloperidol

PURPOSE

Glucocorticoids

Dexamethasone, methylprednisolone

EXPECTED PHARMACOLOGICAL ACTION: The antiemetic mechanism is unknown.

THERAPEUTIC USES: Chemotherapy-induced nausea and vomiting (CINV), usually in combination with other antiemetics

ROUTE OF ADMINISTRATION: IV only

Substance P/neurokinin₁ antagonists

Aprepitant, fosaprepitant

EXPECTED PHARMACOLOGICAL ACTION: Inhibit substance P/neurokinin₁ in the brain

THERAPEUTIC USES
- Prevent postoperative nausea and vomiting (PONV) and CINV, ideally in combination with a glucocorticoid or a serotonin antagonist
- Its extended duration of action makes it effective for immediate use and delayed response.

ROUTE OF ADMINISTRATION: PO (aprepitant) or IV (fosaprepitant)

Serotonin antagonist

Ondansetron, granisetron, dolasetron, palonosetron

EXPECTED PHARMACOLOGICAL ACTION: Prevents emesis by blocking the serotonin receptors in the chemoreceptor trigger zone (CTZ), and antagonizing the serotonin receptors on the afferent vagal neurons that travel from the upper GI tract to the CTZ.

THERAPEUTIC USES: Prevent emesis due to chemotherapy, radiation therapy, postoperative recovery

ROUTE OF ADMINISTRATION
- PO, IM, or IV (ondansetron)
- PO, IV, or transdermal (granisetron)
- PO or IV (dolasetron)
- IV only (palonosetron)

Dopamine antagonists

Prochlorperazine (a subset of phenothiazine), chlorpromazine, perphenazine, promethazine

EXPECTED PHARMACOLOGICAL ACTION: Antiemetic effects result from the blockade of dopamine receptors in the CTZ.

THERAPEUTIC USES: Prevent emesis due to chemotherapy, opioids, postoperative recovery

ROUTE OF ADMINISTRATION: PO, IM, or IV

Cannabinoids (dronabinol, nabilone)

EXPECTED PHARMACOLOGICAL ACTION: The antiemetic mechanism is unknown.

THERAPEUTIC USES: Control CINV and increase appetite for clients who have AIDS

ROUTE OF ADMINISTRATION: PO

Anticholinergic (scopolamine)

EXPECTED PHARMACOLOGICAL ACTION: Interferes with the transmission of nerve impulses traveling from the vestibular apparatus of the inner ear to the vomiting center (VC) in the brain

THERAPEUTIC USES: Motion sickness

ROUTE OF ADMINISTRATION: Transdermal, PO, or subcutaneous

Antihistamines

Dimenhydrinate, cyclizine, diphenhydramine, hydroxyzine, meclizine

EXPECTED PHARMACOLOGICAL ACTION: Block muscarinic and histaminergic receptors in nerve pathways that connect the inner ear and the VC

THERAPEUTIC USES: Motion sickness

ROUTE OF ADMINISTRATION
- PO, IM, or IV (dimenhydrinate, diphenhydramine)
- PO (cyclizine, meclizine)
- IM (hydroxyzine)

Benzodiazepines (lorazepam)

EXPECTED PHARMACOLOGICAL ACTION: Depresses nerve function at multiple CNS sites

THERAPEUTIC USES
- CINV, in combination with other medications
- Extrapyramidal reactions due to phenothiazine antiemetics

ROUTE OF ADMINISTRATION: IV prior to chemotherapy

Butyrophenones (haloperidol, droperidol)

EXPECTED PHARMACOLOGICAL ACTION: Antiemetic effects result from the blockade of dopamine receptors in the CTZ.

THERAPEUTIC USES: Prevent emesis due to chemotherapy, radiation therapy, postoperative recovery

ROUTE OF ADMINISTRATION
- PO, IM, or IV (haloperidol)
- IM or IV (droperidol)

COMPLICATIONS

SUBSTANCE P/NEUROKININ$_1$ ANTAGONIST (APREPITANT, FOSAPREPITANT)

Fatigue, diarrhea, dizziness, possible liver damage

NURSING ACTIONS
- Monitor stool pattern.
- Monitor liver function tests periodically

SEROTONIN ANTAGONIST (ONDANSETRON, OTHERS)

Headache, diarrhea, dizziness

NURSING ACTIONS
- Treat headache with nonopioid analgesics.
- Monitor stool pattern.

Prolonged QT interval

Can lead to a serious dysrhythmia (torsades de pointes).

NURSING ACTIONS: Monitor ECG of clients who have cardiac disorders.

DOPAMINE ANTAGONISTS (PROCHLORPERAZINE, OTHERS)

Extrapyramidal symptoms (EPSs)

NURSING ACTIONS: Administer an anticholinergic medication (diphenhydramine, benztropine) to treat EPSs.

CLIENT EDUCATION
- Possible adverse effects include restlessness, anxiety, and spasms of the face and neck.
- Stop taking the medication and inform the provider if EPSs occur.

Hypotension

NURSING ACTIONS: Monitor clients receiving antihypertensive medications for low blood pressure.

CLIENT EDUCATION: Rise slowly from lying to standing to prevent dizziness and falls. Qs

Sedation

CLIENT EDUCATION
- There is a potential for sedation.
- Avoid activities that require alertness, such as driving.

Anticholinergic effects

Dry mouth, urinary retention, constipation

NURSING ACTIONS
- Administer a stimulant laxative (such as senna) to counteract a decrease in bowel motility, or stool softeners (such as docusate sodium) to prevent constipation.
- Monitor I&O, and palpate the lower abdomen every 4 to 6 hr to check the bladder.

CLIENT EDUCATION
- Increase fluid intake.
- Increase physical activity by engaging in regular exercise.
- Suck on hard candy or chew gum to help relieve dry mouth.
- Attempt to urinate every 4 hr.

CANNABINOIDS (DRONABINOL, NABILONE)

Potential for dissociation, dysphoria

NURSING ACTIONS: Discourage use by clients who have mental health disorders.

Drowsiness

CLIENT EDUCATION: Do not to take these medications concurrently with alcohol, sedatives, or CNS depressants.

Hypotension, tachycardia

NURSING ACTIONS: Monitor blood pressure and heart rate for clients who have cardiovascular disorders. Qs

ANTICHOLINERGICS (SCOPOLAMINE) AND ANTIHISTAMINES (DIMENHYDRINATE, OTHERS)

Sedation

CLIENT EDUCATION
- There is a potential for sedation.
- Avoid activities that require alertness, such as driving.

Anticholinergic effects

Dry mouth, urinary retention, constipation

NURSING ACTIONS
- Administer a stimulant laxative (such as senna) to counteract a decrease in bowel motility, or stool softeners (such as docusate sodium) to prevent constipation.
- Monitor I&O, and palpate the lower abdomen every 4 to 6 hr to check the bladder.

CLIENT EDUCATION
- Increase fluid intake.
- Increase physical activity by engaging in regular exercise.
- Suck on hard candy or chew gum to help relieve dry mouth.
- Attempt to urinate every 4 hr.

BUTYROPHENONES (HALOPERIDOL, DROPERIDOL)

Extrapyramidal symptoms

NURSING ACTIONS: Administer an anticholinergic medication (diphenhydramine, benztropine) to treat EPSs.

CLIENT EDUCATION
- Possible adverse effects include restlessness, anxiety, and spasms of the face and neck.
- Stop taking the medication and inform the provider if EPSs occur.

Hypotension

NURSING ACTIONS: Monitor clients receiving antihypertensive medications for low blood pressure.

CLIENT EDUCATION: Rise slowly from lying to standing to prevent dizziness and falls. Qs

Sedation

CLIENT EDUCATION
- There is a potential for sedation.
- Avoid activities that require alertness, such as driving.

CONTRAINDICATIONS/PRECAUTIONS

- Long QT syndrome is a contraindication for receiving ondansetron. Qs
- Children and older adults require caution when receiving dopamine antagonists due to the increased risk of EPSs.
- Clients who have urinary retention or obstruction, asthma, or narrow-angle glaucoma require caution when receiving dopamine antagonists, antihistamines, and anticholinergic antiemetics.
- Children and clients who have severe liver or kidney disease require caution when receiving aprepitant.
- Age younger than 2 years is a contraindication for receiving promethazine; older children require extreme caution when receiving this medication.

INTERACTIONS

CNS depressants (opioids, alcohol) can intensify the CNS depression antiemetics cause.
CLIENT EDUCATION: Avoid activities that require mental alertness.

Concurrent use of antihypertensives can intensify the hypotensive effects of antiemetics.
NURSING ACTIONS: Assist with ambulation as necessary.

CLIENT EDUCATION: Sit or lie down if feeling lightheaded or dizzy. Avoid sudden changes in position by moving slowly from a lying to a sitting or standing position.

Concurrent use of anticholinergic medications (antihistamines) can intensify the anticholinergic effects of antiemetics.
CLIENT EDUCATION: To reduce anticholinergic effects, sip fluids, take laxatives, and urinate on a regular basis.

NURSING ADMINISTRATION

- Antiemetics prevent or treat nausea and vomiting from various causes. Try to identify the underlying related factors and verify that clients receive the appropriate medication.
- Clients receiving a chemotherapy agent can develop CINV. To prevent CINV, clients receive antiemetics prior to chemotherapy because prevention is easier than treating nausea once it occurs. Combining three antiemetics is more effective than use of a single antiemetic. QEBP
- Transdermal scopolamine requires applying a patch behind the ear several hours prior to surgery or 4 hr before travel to prevent motion sickness. The patches require replacement every 3 days.

NURSING EVALUATION OF MEDICATION EFFECTIVENESS

Indications of effectiveness include absence of nausea and vomiting.

Laxatives

SELECT PROTOTYPE MEDICATIONS
- Psyllium
- Docusate sodium
- Bisacodyl
- Magnesium hydroxide

OTHER MEDICATIONS
- Senna
- Lactulose
- Methylcellulose
- Polycarbophil
- Docusate calcium
- Castor oil

PURPOSE

Bulk-forming laxatives (psyllium)

EXPECTED PHARMACOLOGICAL ACTION: Bulk-forming laxatives soften the fecal mass and increase bulk, just as dietary fiber does.

THERAPEUTIC USES
- Decrease diarrhea in clients who have diverticulosis and IBS
- Control stool for clients who have an ileostomy or a colostomy
- Promote defecation for older adults who have a decrease in peristalsis due to age-related changes in the GI tract ⓒ

Surfactant laxatives (docusate sodium)

EXPECTED PHARMACOLOGICAL ACTION: Surfactant laxatives lower the surface tension of the stool to allow penetration of water.

THERAPEUTIC USES
- Relieve constipation due to pregnancy or opioid use
- Prevent painful elimination due to hemorrhoids or following a procedure such as an episiotomy
- Prevent straining by clients who have disorders such as cerebral aneurysm or a myocardial infarction
- Decrease the risk of fecal impaction due to immobility
- Promote defecation by older adults who have decreased peristalsis due to age-related changes in the GI tract

Stimulant laxatives (bisacodyl)

EXPECTED PHARMACOLOGICAL ACTION: Stimulate intestinal peristalsis

THERAPEUTIC USES
- Prepare clients prior to surgery or diagnostic tests, such as a colonoscopy
- Short-term treatment of constipation due to high-dose opioid use

Osmotic laxatives (magnesium hydroxide)

EXPECTED PHARMACOLOGICAL ACTION: Draw water into the intestine to increase the mass of stool, stretching musculature, which results in peristalsis.

THERAPEUTIC USES
- **Low dose:** Prevent painful elimination (episiotomy, hemorrhoids)
- **High dose:** Prepare clients for surgery or diagnostic tests, such as a colonoscopy
- Rapid evacuation of the bowel after ingestion of poisons or following anthelmintic therapy to rid the body of dead parasites

COMPLICATIONS

GI irritation

CLIENT EDUCATION: Do not crush or chew enteric-coated tablets.

Rectal burning sensation, leading to proctitis

CLIENT EDUCATION: Do not use bisacodyl suppositories on a regular basis.

Toxic magnesium levels

Laxatives with magnesium salts, such as magnesium hydroxide, can lead to accumulation of toxic levels of magnesium.

CLIENT EDUCATION: Clients who have impaired kidney function should read labels carefully and avoid laxatives that contain magnesium.

Sodium absorption and fluid retention

Laxatives with sodium salts, such as sodium phosphate, put clients at risk for sodium absorption and fluid retention.

CLIENT EDUCATION
- Clients who have heart failure or coronary heart disease should read labels carefully and avoid laxatives that contain sodium.
- Clients who have kidney disease and who are taking medications that alter kidney function should avoid laxatives that contain sodium. Qs

Dehydration

Osmotic laxatives can cause dehydration.

NURSING ACTIONS
- Monitor I&O.
- Monitor for manifestations of dehydration, such as poor skin turgor.

CLIENT EDUCATION: Increase water intake to prevent dehydration.

CONTRAINDICATIONS/PRECAUTIONS

- Contraindications for receiving laxatives include fecal impaction, bowel obstruction, and acute surgical abdomen to prevent perforation. Qs
- Nausea, cramping, and abdominal pain are contraindications for receiving laxatives.
- Contraindications for receiving laxatives, with the exception of bulk-forming laxatives, include ulcerative colitis and diverticulitis.
- During pregnancy and lactation, clients taking laxatives require caution. Bisacodyl and docusate sodium are Pregnancy Risk Category C.

INTERACTIONS

Milk and antacids can destroy the enteric coating of bisacodyl.
CLIENT EDUCATION: Take bisacodyl at least 1 hr apart from ingesting these substances.

NURSING ADMINISTRATION

- Obtain a complete history of laxative use. Qpcc
- Inform clients that chronic laxative use can lead to fluid and electrolyte imbalances.
- To promote defecation and resumption of normal bowel function, instruct clients to increase intake of fluids and high-fiber foods (bran, fresh fruits and vegetables). Recommend fluid intake of at least 2.2 L/day for women and 3 L/day for men from beverages and food sources.
- Encourage clients to follow a regular exercise regimen to improve bowel function.
- Instruct clients to take bulk-forming and surfactant laxatives with 237 mL (8 oz) water.
- Do not administer castor oil at bedtime; its use is for situations that require rapid evacuation of the bowel.
- Castor oil has an unpleasant taste; chilling it and mixing it with fruit juice can help.
- Administer bisacodyl PO or rectally (suppository).

NURSING EVALUATION OF MEDICATION EFFECTIVENESS

Indications of effectiveness include the following.
- Return to regular bowel function
- Evacuation of the bowel in preparation for surgery or diagnostic tests

Antidiarrheals

SELECT PROTOTYPE MEDICATION: Diphenoxylate plus atropine

OTHER MEDICATIONS
- Loperamide
- Paregoric

PURPOSE

EXPECTED PHARMACOLOGICAL ACTION: Antidiarrheals activate opioid receptors in the GI tract to decrease intestinal motility and increase the absorption of fluid and sodium in the intestine.

THERAPEUTIC USES
- **Specific antidiarrheal agents** treat the underlying cause of diarrhea. For example, antibiotics treat diarrhea resulting from a bacterial infection.
- **Nonspecific antidiarrheal agents** provide treatment of diarrhea manifestations (decreases in the frequency and fluid content of stool). These include opioid preparations such as diphenoxylate, difenoxin, loperamide, paregoric, and opium tincture. They manage diarrhea by adding bulk to make stools more firm and less watery and to relieve cramping.

COMPLICATIONS

Diphenoxylate: At recommended dosages for diarrhea, does not affect the CNS.

Diphenoxylate; difenoxin: At high dosages, clients can have typical opioid effects (euphoria, CNS depression). However, the addition of atropine, which has unpleasant adverse effects (blurry vision, dry mouth, urinary retention, constipation, tachycardia), to diphenoxylate discourages the ingestion of dosages higher than those prescribed and results in a low potential for abuse. Diphenoxylate is in controlled substance schedule V; difenoxin is in schedule IV.

Loperamide: Very large dosages do not cause opioid effects; loperamide has little or no potential for abuse.

Paregoric: It contains morphine but does not cause euphoria nor analgesia at antidiarrheal dosages. Paregoric has a moderate potential for abuse and is in schedule III.

CONTRAINDICATIONS/PRECAUTIONS

- There is an increased risk of megacolon in clients who have inflammatory bowel disorders. This could lead to a serious complication, such as perforation of the bowel.
- Contraindications for diphenoxylate include severe electrolyte imbalance and dehydration. It is in schedule V. Qs
- COPD is a contraindication for receiving paregoric.

INTERACTIONS

Alcohol and other CNS depressants can enhance CNS depression.

NURSING ADMINISTRATION

- Loperamide is an analog of the opioid meperidine. This medication is not a controlled substance, and at high dosages does not cause morphine-like effects.
- Advise clients who have diarrhea to drink small amounts of clear liquids or a commercial oral electrolyte solution to maintain electrolyte balance for the first 24 hr. Qpcc
- Advise clients to avoid drinking plain water because it does not contain electrolytes to replace what has been lost in the stool.
- Advise clients to avoid caffeine. Caffeine exacerbates diarrhea by increasing GI motility.
- Severe cases of diarrhea require hospitalization to manage dehydration.
- For clients who have dehydration, monitor weight, I&O, and vital signs. Clients might require an IV infusion of a hypotonic solution, such as 0.45% sodium chloride.

NURSING EVALUATION OF MEDICATION EFFECTIVENESS

Indications of effectiveness include the return of a normal bowel pattern, with decreases in the frequency and fluid volume of stool.

Prokinetic agents

SELECT PROTOTYPE MEDICATION: Metoclopramide

PURPOSE

EXPECTED PHARMACOLOGICAL ACTION
- The vomiting response occurs when an agent (such as chemotherapy) stimulates the CTZ, which activates the VC to expel gastric contents. Metoclopramide controls nausea and vomiting by blocking dopamine and serotonin receptors in the CTZ.
- Metoclopramide augments the action of acetylcholine, which causes an increase in upper GI motility, thus increasing peristalsis.

THERAPEUTIC USES
- Control PONV and CINV
- Facilitate intubation and examination of the GI tract
- Management of diabetic gastroparesis (delayed stomach emptying with gas and bloating) and GERD through its ability to increase gastric motility

COMPLICATIONS

Extrapyramidal symptoms

Providers prescribe the lowest effective dose for as brief a period as possible.

NURSING ACTIONS: Administer an antihistamine, such as diphenhydramine, to minimize EPSs.

CLIENT EDUCATION: Possible adverse effects include restlessness, anxiety, and spasms of the face and neck.

Sedation

CLIENT EDUCATION
- There is a potential for sedation.
- Avoid activities that require alertness, such as driving.

Diarrhea

NURSING ACTIONS: Monitor bowel function and for indications of dehydration.

CONTRAINDICATIONS/PRECAUTIONS

- Contraindications include GI perforation, GI bleeding, bowel obstruction, and hemorrhage.
- Seizure disorders are a contraindication because this medication increases the risk of seizures.
- Children and older adults require caution when receiving this medication due to the increased risk for EPSs.

INTERACTIONS

Concurrent use of alcohol and other CNS depressants increases the risks of seizures and sedation.
CLIENT EDUCATION: Avoid the use of alcohol and other CNS depressants. Qebp

Opioids and anticholinergics decrease the effects of metoclopramide.
CLIENT EDUCATION: Avoid using opioids and medications with anticholinergic effects.

NURSING ADMINISTRATION

- Monitor for CNS depression and EPSs.
- Administration is PO, IM, or IV.

NURSING EVALUATION OF MEDICATION EFFECTIVENESS

Indications of effectiveness include the absence of nausea and vomiting.

Medications for irritable bowel syndrome with diarrhea (IBS-D)

SELECT PROTOTYPE MEDICATION: Alosetron

PURPOSE

EXPECTED PHARMACOLOGICAL ACTION: Selective blockade of 5-HT3 receptors, which innervate the viscera and result in increased firmness in stool and decreases in the urgency and frequency of defecation

THERAPEUTIC USES: For female clients who have severe IBS-D that has lasted more than 6 months and has been resistant to conventional management

COMPLICATIONS

Constipation

Because of the potentially fatal outcome of GI toxicity (ischemic colitis, bowel obstruction, impaction, perforation), only clients who meet specific criteria and are willing to sign a treatment agreement may receive prescriptions for the medication. Qs

CLIENT EDUCATION: Watch for rectal bleeding, bloody diarrhea, and abdominal pain. Report these to the provider, who will discontinue the medication therapy.

CONTRAINDICATIONS/PRECAUTIONS

Contraindications include chronic constipation, history of bowel obstruction, Crohn's disease, ulcerative colitis, impaired intestinal circulation, diverticulitis, and thrombophlebitis.

INTERACTIONS

Medications that induce cytochrome P450 enzymes, such as phenobarbital, can decrease levels of alosetron.
NURSING ACTIONS: Monitor effectiveness of the medication.

NURSING ADMINISTRATION

Inform clients that manifestations should resolve within 1 to 4 weeks but will return 1 week after discontinuing the medication therapy. If manifestations continue beyond 4 weeks of treatment, the provider will stop the treatment because the medication is not effective.

NURSING EVALUATION OF MEDICATION EFFECTIVENESS

Indications of effectiveness include relief of diarrhea and decreases in the urgency and frequency of defecation.

Medications for irritable bowel syndrome with constipation (IBS-C)

SELECT PROTOTYPE MEDICATION: Lubiprostone

PURPOSE

EXPECTED PHARMACOLOGICAL ACTION

Increases fluid secretion in the intestine to promote intestinal motility

THERAPEUTIC USES

- IBS-C in female clients
- Chronic idiopathic constipation

COMPLICATIONS

Diarrhea

NURSING ACTIONS: Monitor frequency and consistency of stools. Notify the provider if severe diarrhea occurs.

Nausea

CLIENT EDUCATION: Take the medication with food.

CONTRAINDICATIONS/PRECAUTIONS

- Pregnancy Risk Category C
- Bowel obstruction is a contraindication for receiving lubiprostone.

INTERACTIONS

No significant interactions

NURSING ADMINISTRATION

- Instruct clients to take the medication with food to decrease nausea.
- Dosing is twice daily.
- The dosage is lower for IBS-C than for chronic idiopathic constipation, so it causes less nausea, diarrhea, and chest discomfort.

NURSING EVALUATION OF MEDICATION EFFECTIVENESS

Indications of effectiveness include relief of constipation.

Medications for inflammatory bowel disease

SELECT PROTOTYPE MEDICATION: Sulfasalazine

OTHER MEDICATIONS FOR IBD
- **5-aminosalicylates:** Mesalamine, olsalazine, balsalazide
- **Glucocorticoids:** Dexamethasone, budesonide
- **Immunosuppressants:** Thiopurines (azathioprine, mercaptopurine; cyclosporine); methotrexate
- **Immunomodulator:** Infliximab, certolizumab, adalimumab, natalizumab
- **Antibiotics:** Metronidazole, ciprofloxacin

PURPOSE

EXPECTED PHARMACOLOGICAL ACTION

5-aminosalicylates: Decrease inflammation by inhibiting prostaglandin synthesis

Glucocorticoids: Reduce inflammation

Immunosuppressants: Reduce the activity of the immune system that contributes to the inflammation

Immunomodulators
- Neutralize the activity of tumor necrosis factor-alpha in Crohn's disease
- Decrease infiltration of inflammatory cells

Antibiotics: Help control manifestations

THERAPEUTIC USES

- IBS, Crohn's disease, ulcerative colitis
- Control (not cure) of IBD

COMPLICATIONS

5-AMINOSALICYLATES

Blood disorders

Agranulocytosis; hemolytic and macrocytic anemia

NURSING ACTIONS: Monitor CBC.

Nausea, cramps, rash, arthralgia

NURSING ACTIONS: Notify the provider if adverse effects persist.

GLUCOCORTICOIDS AND IMMUNOSUPPRESSANTS

Adrenal insufficiency, osteoporosis, increased susceptibility to infection, cushingoid syndrome

NURSING ACTIONS: Monitor CBC. Report signs of infection (fever, chills, sore throat).

IMMUNOMODULATORS

Infusion reactions

Fever, chills, pruritus, urticaria, cardiopulmonary reactions

NURSING ACTIONS: Monitor vital signs. Notify the provider if adverse effects persist.

Lymphoma

NURSING ACTIONS: Monitor CBC

CONTRAINDICATIONS/PRECAUTIONS

- Clients who are pregnant, plan to become pregnant, or are breastfeeding should consult the provider about continuing to take sulfasalazine.
- Sensitivity to sulfonamides, salicylates, or thiazide diuretics is a contraindication for receiving 5-aminosalicylates.
- Older adults require caution when receiving 5-aminosalicylates. ⓖ
- Clients who have liver or kidney disease or blood dyscrasias require caution when receiving 5-aminosalicylates.

INTERACTIONS

- Iron and antibiotics can alter the absorption of sulfasalazine.
- Mesalamine can decrease the absorption of digoxin.

NURSING ADMINISTRATION

Do not crush and instruct clients not to chew controlled-release and enteric-coated forms of the medications.

NURSING EVALUATION OF MEDICATION EFFECTIVENESS

Indications of effectiveness include the following.
- Decreased bowel inflammation and relief of GI distress
- Return to normal bowel function

Probiotics: Dietary supplements

PURPOSE

EXPECTED PHARMACOLOGICAL ACTION: Various preparations of bacteria and yeast (which are normal flora of the intestine and colon) help metabolize foods, promote nutrient absorption, and reduce colonization by pathogenic bacteria. They also can increase nonspecific cellular and humoral immunity.

THERAPEUTIC USE: Probiotics treat the manifestations of IBS, ulcerative colitis, and diarrhea from *Clostridium difficile* and rotavirus (children).

COMPLICATIONS

Flatulence, bloating

INTERACTIONS

With concurrent use of antibiotics or antifungals, administer them at least 2 hr apart from probiotics. These medications destroy the bacteria and yeast in probiotic supplements. Q EBP

Medications for hiatal hernia

For complications and other information about these medications, refer to CHAPTER 24: PEPTIC ULCER DISEASE.

PROTON PUMP INHIBITORS
- Omeprazole
- Esomeprazole
- Lansoprazole

ANTACIDS
- Aluminum hydroxide
- Sodium bicarbonate
- Calcium carbonate

PURPOSE

EXPECTED PHARMACOLOGICAL ACTION

Proton pump inhibitors block the final step of gastric acid production to prevent reflux from a sliding hiatal hernia.

Antacids neutralize gastric acid to provide relief of manifestations such as heartburn, belching, and dysphagia.

NURSING EVALUATION OF MEDICATION EFFECTIVENESS

Indications of effectiveness include decreased frequency of manifestations of hiatal hernia (heartburn, belching, dysphagia).

Application Exercises

1. A nurse is caring for a client who received prochlorperazine 4 hr ago. The client reports spasms of the muscles in his face. The nurse should anticipate a prescription for which of the following medications?

   A. Fomepizole

   B. Naloxone

   C. Phytonadione

   D. Diphenhydramine

2. A nurse is collecting data from an older adult client who is receiving ondansetron IV, has a history of diabetes mellitus and cardiac myopathy, and is receiving chemotherapy to treat cancer. For which of the following adverse effects of ondansetron should the nurse monitor? (Select all that apply.)

   A. Headache

   B. Diarrhea

   C. Shortened PR interval

   D. Hyperglycemia

   E. Prolonged QT interval

3. A nurse is reinforcing instructions about the use of laxatives with a client who has heart failure. The client should avoid which of the following laxatives?

   A. Sodium phosphate

   B. Psyllium

   C. Bisacodyl

   D. Polyethylene glycol

4. A nurse is caring for a client who has diabetes mellitus and nausea due to gastroparesis. The nurse should anticipate a prescription for which of the following medications?

   A. Lubiprostone

   B. Metoclopramide

   C. Bisacodyl

   D. Loperamide

5. A nurse is reinforcing information about probiotic supplements with a client who is taking an antibiotic to treat a bacterial infection. Which of the following information should the nurse include? (Select all that apply.)

   A. "Probiotics are micro-organisms that inhabit the GI tract."

   B. "Probiotics treat *Clostridium difficile* infections."

   C. "Probiotics treat benign prostatic hyperplasia."

   D. "Expect some bloating while taking probiotic supplements."

   E. "Take your antibiotic at the same time you take your probiotic supplement."

Application Exercises Key

1. A. Fomepizole is an antidote for ethylene glycol poisoning.

    B. Naloxone treats opioid overdoses.

    C. Vitamin K₁ treats warfarin overdoses.

    D. **CORRECT:** An adverse effect of prochlorperazine is acute dystonia, which includes spasms of the muscles in the face, neck, and tongue. Diphenhydramine suppresses the extrapyramidal effects of prochlorperazine.

    Ⓝ NCLEX® Connection: Pharmacological Therapies, Adverse Effects/ Contraindications/Side Effects/Interactions

2. A. **CORRECT:** Headache, dizziness, and fatigue are common adverse effects of ondansetron.

    B. **CORRECT:** Diarrhea and constipation are adverse effects of ondansetron.

    C. A shortened PR interval is not an adverse effect of ondansetron.

    D. Ondansetron does not affect blood glucose, but it can elevate liver enzymes.

    E. **CORRECT:** A prolonged QT interval is a possible adverse effect of ondansetron that can lead to torsades de pointes, a serious dysrhythmia.

    Ⓝ NCLEX® Connection: Pharmacological Therapies, Adverse Effects/ Contraindications/Side Effects/Interactions

3. A. **CORRECT:** Typically, clients who have heart failure follow a sodium-restricted diet. Absorption of sodium from sodium phosphate causes fluid retention; therefore, heart failure is a contraindication for receiving sodium phosphate.

    B. The intestines do not absorb psyllium. Heart failure is not a contraindication for receiving this laxative.

    C. Bisacodyl does not appear to have systemic effects. Heart failure is not a contraindication for receiving this laxative.

    D. Several GI disorders are contraindications for receiving polyethylene glycol, but heart failure is not.

    Ⓝ NCLEX® Connection: Pharmacological Therapies, Expected Actions/Outcomes

4. A. Lubiprostone treats irritable bowel syndrome with constipation in female clients.

    B. **CORRECT:** Metoclopramide is a dopamine antagonist that treats nausea and also increases gastric motility. It can relieve the bloating and nausea of diabetic gastroparesis.

    C. Bisacodyl is a stimulant laxative that provides short-term treatment of constipation.

    D. Loperamide is an antidiarrheal agent that decreases gastrointestinal peristalsis.

    Ⓝ NCLEX® Connection: Pharmacological Therapies, Expected Actions/Outcomes

5. A. **CORRECT:** Probiotics consist of lactobacilli, bifidobacteria, and *Saccharomyces boulardii*, which are normal inhabitants of the digestive tract.

    B. **CORRECT:** Probiotics treat a number of GI disorders, including irritable bowel syndrome, diarrhea due to *Clostridium difficile infections*, and ulcerative colitis.

    C. Saw palmetto is a supplement that clients can use to treat benign prostatic hyperplasia.

    D. **CORRECT:** Flatulence and bloating are adverse effects of probiotic supplements.

    E. The client should take the probiotic supplement at least 2 hr after taking an antibiotic or antifungal medication. Antibiotics and antifungal medications destroy the bacteria and yeast in probiotic supplements.

    Ⓝ NCLEX® Connection: Pharmacological Therapies, Expected Actions/Outcomes

A nurse is caring for a client who has a prescription for sulfasalazine. Use the ATI Active Learning Template: Medication to complete this item to include the following.

THERAPEUTIC USES: Identify two therapeutic uses for sulfasalazine.

COMPLICATIONS: Identify two blood disorders that occur as a complication of the use of sulfasalazine.

INTERACTIONS: Identify two medications that interact adversely with sulfasalazine.

Using the ATI Active Learning Template: Medication

THERAPEUTIC USES: Crohn's disease and ulcerative colitis

COMPLICATIONS: Agranulocytosis, and hemolytic and macrocytic anemia

INTERACTIONS: Iron and antibiotics can alter the absorption of sulfasalazine. Mesalamine can decrease the absorption of digoxin.

Ⓝ NCLEX® Connection: Pharmacological and Parenteral Therapies, Medication Administration

CHAPTER 26 *Vitamins, Minerals, and Supplements*

Vitamins and minerals have important roles in the body, including the production of red blood cells, building bones, making hormones, regulating body fluid volume, and supporting nerve cell function. Vitamin and mineral deficiencies can increase the risk for health problems (anemias, heart disease, cancers, osteoporosis). Supplements of vitamins and minerals can help prevent multiple health conditions.

Iron preparations

SELECT PROTOTYPE MEDICATIONS
- **Oral:** Ferrous sulfate
- **Parenteral:** Iron dextran

OTHER MEDICATIONS
- **Oral:** Ferrous gluconate, ferrous fumarate
- **Parenteral:** Ferumoxytol, iron sucrose, sodium-ferric gluconate complex (SFGC)

PURPOSE

EXPECTED PHARMACOLOGICAL ACTION

Iron preparations provide iron needed for red blood cell (RBC) development and oxygen transport to cells. During times of increased growth (in growing children or during pregnancy) or when RBCs are in high demand (after blood loss), the need for iron can be greatly increased. Iron is poorly absorbed by the body, so relatively large amounts must be ingested orally to increase Hgb and Hct levels.

THERAPEUTIC USES

- Iron preparations are used to treat and prevent iron-deficiency anemia.
  - **Ferumoxytol** is limited to clients who have chronic kidney disease, regardless if on dialysis or receiving erythropoietin. Ferumoxytol requires only two doses over 3 to 8 days compared with SFGC and iron sucrose, which require three to 10 doses over several weeks.
  - **SFGC** is used for clients who are undergoing long-term hemodialysis and are deficient in iron.
  - **Iron sucrose** is used for clients who have chronic kidney disease, are receiving erythropoietin, and are hemodialysis- or peritoneal dialysis-dependent; and clients who have chronic kidney disease, are not receiving erythropoietin, and are not dialysis-dependent.
- Iron preparations are used to prevent iron deficiency anemia for clients who are at an increased risk (infants, children, pregnant clients).
- Parenteral forms should only be used in clients who are unable to take oral medications, or when the client experiences gastrointestinal intolerance to oral iron administration, in which case the IV route is preferred.

COMPLICATIONS

GI distress (nausea, constipation, heartburn)

- Vitamin C increases absorption, but also increases incidence of GI complications.
- Dosage might need to be reduced.

NURSING ACTIONS
- If intolerable, administer medication with food, but this greatly reduces absorption.
- Monitor bowel pattern and intervene as appropriate. This adverse effect usually resolves with continued use.

Teeth staining (liquid form)

CLIENT EDUCATION: Dilute liquid iron with water or juice, drink with a straw, and rinse mouth after swallowing.

Staining of skin and other tissues (IM injections)

NURSING ACTIONS
- Give IM doses deep IM using Z-track technique.
- Avoid this route if possible.

Anaphylaxis

- Risk with parenteral administration of iron dextran.
- Anaphylaxis is triggered by the dextran in iron dextran, not by the iron.
- Anaphylaxis is minimal with SFGC, iron sucrose, and ferumoxytol.
- IV route is safer than IM.

NURSING ACTIONS
- Ask the charge nurse to administer a test dose and observe the client closely. No test dose is needed before administering ferumoxytol and iron sucrose. Q EBP
- Ensure the medication is administered slowly, and use manufacturer's recommendation for specific product.
- Be prepared with life-support equipment and epinephrine.

Hypotension

Can progress to circulatory collapse with parenteral administration

NURSING ACTIONS: Monitor vital signs when the client is receiving parenteral iron.

Fatal iron toxicity in children

Can occur when an overdose of iron (2 to 10 g) is ingested Manifestations of toxicity include severe GI distress, shock, acidosis, and liver and heart failure. The chelating agent deferoxamine, given parenterally, is used to treat toxicity.

NURSING ACTIONS: Avoid using oral and parenteral iron concurrently.

CONTRAINDICATIONS/PRECAUTIONS

- Contraindicated for clients who have previous hypersensitivity to iron, and anemias other than iron-deficiency anemia.
- Use oral preparations cautiously in clients who have peptic ulcer disease, regional enteritis, ulcerative colitis, or severe liver disease.

Concurrent administration of antacids or tetracyclines reduces absorption of iron.
NURSING ACTIONS: Separate use by at least 2 hr.

Caffeine and dairy products can interfere with absorption.
NURSING ACTIONS: Avoid administering the medication with foods containing caffeine or dairy.

Food reduces absorption but reduces gastric distress.
NURSING ACTIONS: Administer with food at the start of therapy if gastric distress occurs.

Vitamin C increases absorption, but also increases incidence of GI complications.
CLIENT EDUCATION: Avoid taking iron with vitamin C supplements or foods that contain high amounts of vitamin C if distress occurs.

NURSING ADMINISTRATION

NURSING CARE

- Instruct clients to take iron on an empty stomach, such as 1 hr before meals, because stomach acid increases absorption.
- Instruct clients to take with food if GI adverse effects occur. This might increase adherence to therapy even though absorption is also decreased.
- Instruct clients to space doses at approximately equal intervals throughout day to most efficiently increase RBC production.
- Inform clients to anticipate a harmless dark green or black color of stool.
- Instruct clients to dilute liquid iron with water or juice, drink with a straw, and rinse the mouth after swallowing.

- Instruct clients to increase water and fiber intake (unless contraindicated) and to maintain an exercise program to counter the constipation effects.
- Advise clients that therapy can last 1 to 2 months. Usually, dietary intake will be sufficient after Hgb has returned to a therapeutic level.
- Encourage concurrent intake of appropriate quantities of foods high in iron (liver, egg yolks, muscle meats, yeast, grains, green leafy vegetables).

NURSING EVALUATION OF MEDICATION EFFECTIVENESS

Depending on therapeutic intent, effectiveness is evidenced by the following.
- Increased reticulocyte count is expected at least 1 week after beginning iron therapy.
- Increase in hemoglobin of 2 g/dL is expected 1 month after beginning therapy.
- Fatigue and pallor (skin, mucous membranes) should subside, and the client reports increased energy level.

Vitamin B_{12}/Cyanocobalamin

SELECT PROTOTYPE MEDICATION: Vitamin B_{12}

OTHER MEDICATIONS: Intranasal cyanocobalamin

PURPOSE

EXPECTED PHARMACOLOGICAL ACTION

- Vitamin B_{12} is necessary to convert folic acid from its inactive form to its active form. All cells rely on folic acid for DNA production.
- Vitamin B_{12} deficiency can result in megaloblastic (macrocytic) anemia and cause dysrhythmias and heart failure if not corrected. Vitamin B_{12} is administered to prevent or correct deficiency. Damage to rapidly multiplying cells can affect the skin and mucous membranes, causing GI disturbances. Neurologic damage (numbness and tingling of extremities) and CNS damage caused by demyelination of neurons can result from deficiency of this vitamin.
- Vitamin B_{12} deficiency affects all blood cells produced in the bone marrow.
  - Loss of erythrocytes leads to heart failure, cerebral vascular insufficiency, and hypoxia.
  - Loss of leukocytes leads to infections.
  - Loss of thrombocytes leads to bleeding and hemorrhage.
- Loss of intrinsic factor within the cells of the stomach causes an inability to absorb vitamin B_{12}, making it necessary to administer parenteral or intranasal vitamin B_{12} or high doses of oral B_{12} for the rest of the client's life.

THERAPEUTIC USES

- Treatment of vitamin B_{12} deficiency
- Megaloblastic (macrocytic) anemia related to vitamin B_{12} deficiency

COMPLICATIONS

Hypokalemia

- Secondary to the increased RBC production effects of vitamin B_{12}
- Clients might require potassium supplements.

NURSING ACTIONS

- Monitor potassium levels during the start of treatment.
- Observe for manifestations of potassium deficiency (muscle weakness, irregular cardiac rhythm).

CONTRAINDICATIONS/PRECAUTIONS

- Vitamin B_{12} deficiency should not be treated only with folic acid. Treatment with folic acid alone can reverse the hematologic effects of the deficiency but can allow neurologic damage to progress. If folic acid is used for a client who has vitamin B_{12} deficiency, ensure that dosage of vitamin B_{12} is adequate.
- Oral and intranasal cyanocobalamin are Pregnancy Risk Category A.
- Parenteral cyanocobalamin is Pregnancy Risk Category C.

INTERACTIONS

Masks manifestations of vitamin B_{12} deficiency with concurrent administration of folic acid
NURSING ACTIONS: Ensure clients receive adequate doses of vitamin B_{12} when using folic acid.

NURSING ADMINISTRATION

NURSING CARE

- Obtain baseline vitamin B_{12}, Hgb, Hct, RBC, reticulocyte counts, and folate levels. Monitor periodically.
- Monitor for manifestations of vitamin B_{12} deficiency (beefy red tongue, pallor, neuropathy).
- Cyanocobalamin is administered intranasally, orally, IM, or subcutaneously. Injections are painful and usually reserved for clients who have significant reduced ability to absorb vitamin B_{12} (lack of intrinsic factor [pernicious anemia], enteritis, partial removal of the stomach).

- Clients who have malabsorption syndrome can use intranasal or parenteral preparations.
- Administer intranasal cyanocobalamin 1 hr before or after eating hot foods, which can cause the medication to be removed from nasal passages without being absorbed (because of increased nasal secretions).
- Clients who have irreversible malabsorption syndrome (parietal cell atrophy or total gastrectomy) will need lifelong treatment, usually parenterally. If oral therapy is used, doses must be very high. Q︎EBP
  - Encourage concurrent intake of foods high in vitamin B_{12}, such as dairy products.
  - Perform a Schilling test to determine vitamin B_{12} absorption in the gastrointestinal tract.
  - Measurement of plasma B_{12} levels helps determine the need for therapy.
  - Advise clients to adhere to prescribed laboratory tests. Monitor blood counts and vitamin B_{12} levels every 3 to 6 months.

NURSING EVALUATION OF MEDICATION EFFECTIVENESS

Depending on therapeutic intent, effectiveness can be evidenced by the following.
- Disappearance of megaloblasts (in 2 to 3 weeks)
- Increased reticulocyte count
- Increase in hematocrit
- Improvement of neurologic injury, such as absence of tingling sensation of hands and feet and numbness of extremities. Improvement can take months, and some clients never attain full recovery.

Folic acid

SELECT PROTOTYPE MEDICATION: Folic acid

PURPOSE

EXPECTED PHARMACOLOGICAL ACTION: Folic acid is essential in the production of DNA and erythropoiesis (RBC, WBC, platelets).

THERAPEUTIC USES
- Treatment of megaloblastic (macrocytic) anemia secondary to folic acid deficiency
- Prevention of neural tube defects that can occur early during pregnancy (thus needed for all clients of childbearing age who might become pregnant)
- Treatment of malabsorption syndrome, such as sprue
- Supplement for alcohol use disorder (due to poor dietary intake of folic acid and injury to the liver)

CONTRAINDICATIONS/PRECAUTIONS

Avoid indiscriminate use of folic acid to reduce the risk of masking manifestations of vitamin B_{12} deficiency.

INTERACTIONS

Folic acid levels are decreased by methotrexate and sulfonamides.
NURSING ACTIONS: Avoid concurrent use of these medications.

Folic acid can decrease phenytoin serum levels because of increased metabolism.
NURSING ACTIONS: Monitor serum phenytoin levels.

NURSING ADMINISTRATION

NURSING CARE

- Monitor for manifestations of megaloblastic anemia (pallor, easy fatigability, palpitations, paresthesias of hands or feet).
- Obtain baseline folic acid, Hgb and Hct levels, and RBC and reticulocyte counts. Monitor periodically.
- Advise clients who have folic acid deficiency to increase intake of food sources of folic acid (liver, green leafy vegetables, citrus fruits, dried peas and beans). Monitor for risk factors indicating that folic acid therapy is needed (heavy alcohol use, childbearing age).

NURSING EVALUATION OF MEDICATION EFFECTIVENESS

Depending on therapeutic intent, effectiveness is evidenced by the following.
- Folate level within expected reference range
- Return of RBC, reticulocyte count, and Hgb and Hct to levels within expected reference range
- Improvement of anemia findings (absence of pallor, dyspnea, easy fatigability)
- Absence of neural tube defects in newborns

Potassium supplements

SELECT PROTOTYPE MEDICATION: Potassium chloride

OTHER MEDICATIONS
- Potassium gluconate
- Potassium phosphate
- Potassium bicarbonate

PURPOSE

EXPECTED PHARMACOLOGICAL ACTION: Potassium is essential for conducting nerve impulses, maintaining electrical excitability of muscle, and regulation of acid/base balance.

THERAPEUTIC USES
- Treating hypokalemia (potassium less than 3.5 mEq/L)
- For clients receiving diuretics resulting in potassium loss, such as furosemide
- For clients who have potassium loss due to excessive or prolonged vomiting, diarrhea, excessive use of laxatives, intestinal drainage, and GI fistula

COMPLICATIONS

Local GI ulceration and distress

Nausea, vomiting, diarrhea, abdominal discomfort, and esophagitis with oral administration

CLIENT EDUCATION
- Take the medication with meals or at least 8 oz water to minimize GI discomfort and prevent ulceration.
- Do not dissolve the tablet in the mouth because oral ulceration will develop.

Hyperkalemia (potassium more than 5.0 mEq/L)

- Hyperkalemia rarely occurs with oral administration.
- Severe hyperkalemia can require treatment (calcium salt, glucose and insulin, sodium bicarbonate, sodium polystyrene sulfonate, peritoneal dialysis, hemodialysis).

NURSING ACTIONS: Monitor clients receiving IV potassium for manifestations of hyperkalemia (bradycardia, ECG changes, vomiting, confusion, anxiety, dyspnea, weakness, numbness, tingling).

CONTRAINDICATIONS/PRECAUTIONS

Contraindicated for clients who have severe kidney disease or hypoaldosteronism.

INTERACTIONS

Concurrent use of potassium-sparing diuretics (such as spironolactone) or ACE inhibitors (lisinopril) increases the risk of hyperkalemia.
NURSING ACTIONS: Avoid concurrent use.

NURSING ADMINISTRATION

Oral formulations

- Mix powdered formulations in at least 120 mL (4 oz) liquid.
- Advise clients to take potassium chloride with a meal or at least 8 oz water to reduce the risk of adverse GI effects.
- Instruct clients not to crush extended-release tablets.
- Instruct clients to notify the provider if they have difficulty swallowing the pills. Medication is supplied as a powder or a sustained-release tablet that is easier to tolerate.

IV administration

- Cardiac monitoring is indicated for serum potassium levels outside of expected reference ranges. ECG changes (prolonged PR interval, peaked T-waves) can indicate potassium toxicity.
- Monitor the IV site for local irritation, phlebitis, and infiltration. Ensure the IV is discontinued immediately if infiltration occurs.
- Monitor I&O to ensure an adequate urine output of at least 30 mL/hr.

NURSING EVALUATION OF MEDICATION EFFECTIVENESS

Depending on therapeutic intent, effectiveness is evidenced by serum potassium level within the expected reference range (3.5 to 5.0 mEq/L).

Magnesium sulfate

SELECT PROTOTYPE MEDICATION
- **Parenteral:** Magnesium sulfate
- **Oral:** Magnesium hydroxide, magnesium oxide, magnesium citrate

! Magnesium hydroxide and magnesium oxide act as antacids when administered in a low dose. Magnesium hydroxide, magnesium oxide, and magnesium citrate act as laxatives.

PURPOSE

EXPECTED PHARMACOLOGICAL ACTION: Magnesium activates many intracellular enzymes, binds the messenger RNA to ribosomes, and plays a role in regulating skeletal muscle contractility and blood coagulation.

THERAPEUTIC USES
- Magnesium supplements are used for clients who have hypomagnesemia (magnesium level less than 1.3 mEq/L).
- Oral preparations of magnesium sulfate are used to prevent or treat low magnesium levels and as laxatives.
- Parenteral magnesium is used for clients who have severe hypomagnesemia.
- IV magnesium sulfate is used to stop preterm labor and as an anticonvulsant during labor and delivery.

COMPLICATIONS

Muscle weakness, flaccid paralysis, painful muscle contractions, suppression of AV conduction through the heart, respiratory depression

NURSING ACTIONS
- Monitor the cardiac and neuromuscular status of the client receiving IV administration.
- Monitor serum magnesium levels.
- Avoid administering with neuromuscular blocking agents, which can potentiate respiratory depression and apnea.
- Ensure IV calcium is available to reverse the effects of magnesium. Qs

Diarrhea

NURSING ACTIONS
- Monitor electrolyte levels for electrolyte loss from diarrhea.
- Monitor I&O, and observe for manifestations of dehydration.

CONTRAINDICATIONS/PRECAUTIONS

- Magnesium is Pregnancy Risk Category A.
- Contraindicated in clients who have AV block, rectal bleeding, nausea, vomiting, and abdominal pain.
- Use cautiously with clients who have kidney or cardiac disease.

INTERACTIONS

Magnesium sulfate can decrease the absorption of tetracyclines and digoxin.
NURSING ACTIONS: Monitor the therapeutic effect to determine if absorption has been affected.

NURSING ADMINISTRATION

NURSING CARE

- Monitor serum magnesium, calcium, and phosphorus.
- Monitor blood pressure, heart rate, and respiratory rate when administered IV.
- Check for depressed or absent deep tendon reflexes as a manifestation of toxicity.
- Calcium gluconate is given for magnesium sulfate toxicity. Always have an injectable form of calcium gluconate available when administering magnesium sulfate by IV. Qs
- Reinforce teaching with clients about dietary sources of magnesium (whole-grain cereals, nuts, legumes, green leafy vegetables, bananas).

NURSING EVALUATION OF MEDICATION EFFECTIVENESS

Depending on therapeutic intent, effectiveness is evidenced by serum magnesium levels within expected reference range (1.3 to 2.1 mEq/L).

Herbal supplements

- Herbal supplements are widely used but less tested and regulated than conventional medications. Dosages are less precise than for more regulated medications. Because different formulations are not standardized, it can be difficult to know which preparations can provide therapeutic effects.
- Supplements are regulated by the FDA for manufacturing devoid of impurities, and for accurate labeling.

Aloe, aloe vera

- Topical anti-inflammatory, analgesic, and cathartic
- Soothes pain
- Heals burns
- Softens skin
- Laxative

ADVERSE EFFECTS AND PRECAUTIONS
- Skin preparations: Possible hypersensitivity
- Laxative: Possible fluid and electrolyte imbalances
- Increases menstrual flow when taken during menses
- Avoid in clients who have kidney disorders.

INTERACTIONS: Interacts with digoxin, diuretics, corticosteroids and antidysrhythmics

CLIENT EDUCATION: Recognize manifestations of fluid and electrolyte imbalance if using as a laxative.

Black cohosh

- Acts as an estrogen substitute
- Mechanism of action is unknown
- Treats manifestations of menopause

ADVERSE EFFECTS AND PRECAUTIONS
- GI distress, lightheadedness, headache, rash, weight gain
- Avoid taking during pregnancy, especially the first two trimesters.
- Limit use to 6 months due to lack of information regarding long-term effects.

INTERACTIONS
- Increases effects of antihypertensive medications
- Can increase effect of estrogen medications
- Increases hypoglycemia in clients taking insulin or other medications for diabetes

NURSING ACTIONS: Question clients who take antihypertensives, insulin, or hypoglycemic agents, or clients who might be pregnant about possible use of black cohosh.

Echinacea

- Stimulates the immune system
- Decreases inflammation
- Topically heals skin disorders, wounds, and burns
- Possibly treats viruses (common cold, herpes simplex)
- Used to increase T-lymphocyte, tumor necrosis factor, and interferon production
- Available in many forms (dried roots, plants, extracts, teas)

ADVERSE EFFECTS
- Bitter taste
- Mild GI distress or fever can occur.
- Allergic reactions, especially in clients who are allergic to plants such as ragweed or others in the daisy family

INTERACTIONS: With long-term use (more than 6 months), echinacea can decrease positive effects of medications for tuberculosis, HIV, or cancer.

NURSING ACTIONS: Question clients who have tuberculosis, cancer, HIV, lupus erythematosus, and rheumatoid arthritis about concurrent use. Advise these clients to talk to the provider.

Feverfew

- Can block platelet aggregation
- Can block a factor that causes migraines
- Can decrease the number and severity of migraine headaches (does not treat an existing migraine)

ADVERSE EFFECTS AND PRECAUTIONS
- Mild GI distress
- Post-feverfew syndrome can occur, causing agitation, tiredness, inability to sleep, headache, and joint discomfort.
- Can cause allergic reactions in clients allergic to ragweed or echinacea

INTERACTIONS
- Can cause increased risk of bleeding in clients taking NSAIDs, heparin, and warfarin
- Discontinue 2 weeks before elective surgery.

NURSING ACTIONS: Question clients about concurrent use of NSAIDs, heparin, and warfarin.

Garlic

- When crushed, forms the enzyme allicin
- Blocks LDL and raises HDL; lowers triglycerides
- Suppresses platelet aggregation and disrupts coagulation
- Acts as a vasodilator (can lower blood pressure)

ADVERSE EFFECTS: GI distress

INTERACTIONS
- Due to antiplatelet qualities, can increase risk of bleeding in clients taking NSAIDs, warfarin, and heparin
- Decreases levels of saquinavir (a medication for HIV treatment) and cyclosporine

NURSING ACTIONS
- Question clients about concurrent use of NSAIDs, heparin, and warfarin.
- Caution clients who are taking antiplatelet or anticoagulant medication, cyclosporine, or saquinavir to contact their provider.

Ginger root

- Relieves vertigo and nausea
- Increases intestinal motility
- Increases gastric mucous production
- Decreases GI spasms
- Produces an anti-inflammatory effect
- Suppresses platelet aggregation
- Used to treat morning sickness, motion sickness, and nausea from surgery
- Can decrease pain and stiffness of rheumatoid arthritis

ADVERSE EFFECTS AND PRECAUTIONS

- Use cautiously in clients who are pregnant because high doses can cause uterine contractions.
- Adverse effects are unknown, with potential CNS depression and cardiac dysrhythmias with very large overdose.

INTERACTIONS

- Interacts with medications that interfere with coagulation (NSAIDS, warfarin, and heparin)
- Can increase hypoglycemic effects of diabetes medications

NURSING ACTIONS

- Question clients about concurrent use with NSAIDs, heparin, and warfarin.
- Monitor for hypoglycemia if the client takes insulin or other medication for diabetes.

Ginkgo biloba

- Promotes vasodilation: Decreases leg pain caused from occlusive arterial disorders
- Decreases platelet aggregation: Can decrease risk of thrombosis
- Decreases bronchospasm
- Increases blood flow to the brain: Thought to improve memory (dementia, Alzheimer's disease), but studies do not indicate effectiveness

ADVERSE EFFECTS AND PRECAUTIONS

- Mild GI upset, headache, and lightheadedness, which can be decreased by reducing dose
- Use with caution in clients at risk for seizures.

INTERACTIONS

- Can interact with medications that lower the seizure threshold (antihistamines, antidepressants, antipsychotics)
- Can interfere with coagulation

NURSING ACTIONS

- Question clients regarding history of antidepressant use (imipramine), which causes a decrease in seizure threshold.
- Question clients about concurrent use with NSAIDs, heparin, and warfarin.

Glucosamine

- Stimulates cells to make cartilage and synovial fluid
- Suppresses inflammation of the joints and cartilage degradation
- Treats osteoarthritis of the knee, hip, and wrist

ADVERSE EFFECTS AND PRECAUTIONS

- Mild GI upset (nausea, heartburn)
- Use with caution with shellfish allergy.

INTERACTIONS: Use caution if taking antiplatelet or anticoagulant medication.

NURSING ACTIONS: Question clients about concurrent use with NSAIDs, heparin, and warfarin.

Kava

! Causes liver injury Qs

- Possibly acts on gamma-aminobutyric acid (GABA) receptors in the CNS
- Promotes sleep
- Decreases anxiety
- Promotes muscle relaxation without affecting concentration

ADVERSE EFFECTS AND PRECAUTIONS

- Chronic use causes dry, flaky skin and jaundice.
- Chronic use and large doses can cause liver damage, including severe liver failure.

INTERACTIONS: Can cause sedation when taken concurrently with CNS depressants

NURSING ACTIONS

- Question clients taking any CNS depressant, including alcohol, about use of kava.
- Ask clients who have any liver condition about concurrent use.

Ma huang

! Can cause hypertension, tachycardia, stroke, myocardial infarction. Qs

- Stimulates the CNS
- Suppresses the appetite
- Used for weight loss
- Constricts arterioles: Increases heart rate and blood pressure
- Bronchodilator: Treats colds, influenza, and allergies
- Products that include more than 10 mg/dose are forbidden to be sold in the U.S.

ADVERSE EFFECTS AND PRECAUTIONS

- Because it contains ephedrine, ma huang can stimulate the cardiovascular system. At high doses, it can cause death from hypertension and dysrhythmias.
- Stimulation of CNS can cause euphoria. In high doses, it can cause psychosis.

INTERACTIONS

- Interacts with CNS stimulants to potentiate their effect
- Can cause severe hypertension when taken with monoamine oxidase inhibitor antidepressants
- Interacts with antihypertensive medications, decreasing effects

NURSING ACTIONS: Question clients carefully about other medications.

St. John's wort

- Affects serotonin, producing antidepressant effects: Used for mild depression
- Used orally as an analgesic to relieve pain and inflammation
- Applied topically for infection

ADVERSE EFFECTS

- Mild adverse effects (dry mouth, lightheadedness, constipation, GI distress)
- Skin rash when exposed to sunlight

INTERACTIONS

- Can cause serotonin syndrome when combined with other antidepressants, amphetamine, and cocaine
- Decreases effectiveness of oral contraceptives, cyclosporine, warfarin, digoxin, calcium-channel blockers, steroids, HIV protease inhibitors, and some anticancer medications

NURSING ACTIONS

- Question clients taking any of the medications with which this substance interacts about concurrent use.
- Encourage clients to avoid prolonged sun exposure and use sunscreen.

Saw palmetto

Can decrease prostate manifestations of hyperplasia

ADVERSE EFFECTS AND PRECAUTIONS: Few adverse effects; can cause mild GI effects

INTERACTIONS

- Possible additive effects with finasteride
- Can interact with antiplatelet and anticoagulant medications
- Pregnancy Risk Category X Qs

NURSING ACTIONS

- Question clients about use before prostate-specific antigen tests.
- Question clients about concurrent use with aspirin, heparin, and warfarin.

Valerian

- Increases GABA to prevent insomnia (similar to benzodiazepines)
- Reduces anxiety-related restlessness
- Drowsiness effect increases over time

ADVERSE EFFECTS AND PRECAUTIONS

- Can cause drowsiness, lightheadedness, depression
- Risk of physical dependence

PRECAUTION

- Clients who have mental health disorders should use with caution.
- Should be avoided by women who are pregnant or lactating.

INTERACTIONS: It is unknown whether valerian potentiates effects of CNS depressants

NURSING ACTIONS: Warn clients taking valerian about the possibility of drowsiness when operating motor vehicles and other equipment.

Application Exercises

1. A nurse is reinforcing teaching with a client who has anemia and a new prescription for a liquid iron supplement. Which of the following information should the nurse reinforce in the teaching? (Select all that apply.)

   A. "Add foods that are high in fiber to your diet."

   B. "Rinse your mouth after taking the medication."

   C. "Expect stools to be green or black."

   D. "Take the medication with a glass of milk."

   E. "Add red meat to your diet."

2. A nurse is caring for a client who has increased liver enzymes and is taking herbal supplements. Which of the following herbal supplements should the nurse report to the provider?

   A. Glucosamine

   B. Saw palmetto

   C. Kava

   D. St. John's wort

3. A nurse is assisting with the evaluation of a group of clients at a health fair to identify the need for folic acid therapy. Which of the following clients require folic acid therapy? (Select all that apply.)

   A. 12-year-old child who has iron deficiency anemia

   B. 24-year-old female client who has no health problems

   C. 44-year-old client who has hypertension

   D. 55-year-old client who has alcohol use disorder

   E. 35-year-old client who has type 2 diabetes mellitus

4. A nurse is caring for a client who requests information on the use of feverfew. Which of the following responses should the nurse make?

   A. "It is used to treat skin infections."

   B. "It can decrease the frequency of migraine headaches."

   C. "It can lessen the nasal congestion in the common cold."

   D. "It can relieve nausea of morning sickness during pregnancy."

5. A nurse is completing a review of a client's current medications. The client also reports taking ginkgo biloba. Which of the following medications is contraindicated for a client taking ginkgo biloba?

   A. Acetaminophen

   B. Warfarin

   C. Digoxin

   D. Lisinopril

PRACTICE Active Learning Scenario

A nurse is reinforcing teaching with a client about a new prescription for cyanocobalamin. What should the nurse reinforce in the teaching? Use the ATI Active Learning Template: Medication to complete this item.

EXPECTED PHARMACOLOGICAL ACTION

CLIENT EDUCATION: Describe four points to reinforce teaching with the client.

EVALUATION OF MEDICATION EFFECTIVENESS: Describe two nursing interventions.

Application Exercises Key

1. A. **CORRECT:** Foods high in fiber can prevent constipation, which can occur when taking iron supplements.

   B. **CORRECT:** Iron supplements can stain teeth when taken in a liquid form. The client should rinse the mouth after taking the medication.

   C. **CORRECT:** Dark green or black stools can occur when taking iron supplements. The client should anticipate this effect.

   D. Dairy products and caffeine can decrease the absorption of iron supplements. Iron supplements are maximally absorbed when taken on an empty stomach or 1 hr before meals.

   E. **CORRECT:** Red meats are high in iron and recommended to improve anemia when taken concurrently with iron supplements.

   Ⓝ *NCLEX® Connection: Pharmacological Therapies, Expected Actions/Outcomes*

2. A. Glucosamine can increase bleeding and should be used cautiously in clients who are taking antiplatelet medications or anticoagulants.

   B. Saw palmetto can cause mild GI effects and should be used cautiously in clients who are taking antiplatelet medications or anticoagulants.

   C. **CORRECT:** Chronic use or high doses of kava can cause liver damage, including severe liver failure.

   D. Garlic can cause GI distress and should be used cautiously in clients who are taking antiplatelet medications or anticoagulants.

   Ⓝ *NCLEX® Connection: Pharmacological Therapies, Adverse Effects/ Contraindications/Side Effects/Interactions*

3. A. The client who has iron deficiency anemia requires treatment with iron supplements.

   B. **CORRECT:** The female client of childbearing age should take folic acid to prevent neural tube defects in the fetus.

   C. The client who has hypertension requires treatment with diet, exercise, and antihypertensive medication.

   D. **CORRECT:** The client who has alcohol use disorder can require folic acid therapy. Excess alcohol consumption leads to poor dietary intake of folic acid and injury to the liver.

   E. The client who has type 2 diabetes mellitus requires treatment with diet, exercise, and hyperglycemic medication.

   Ⓝ *NCLEX® Connection: Pharmacological Therapies, Expected Actions/Outcomes*

4. A. Aloe is used to treat tissue injury.

   B. **CORRECT:** Feverfew is used to decrease the frequency of migraine headaches, but it has not been proven to relieve an existing migraine headache.

   C. Echinacea is used to can relieve manifestations of the common cold.

   D. Ginger root is used to relieve nausea caused from morning sickness during pregnancy.

   Ⓝ *NCLEX® Connection: Pharmacological Therapies, Expected Actions/Outcomes*

5. A. Aspirin should be used with caution in clients taking ginkgo biloba because ginkgo biloba can suppress coagulation.

   B. **CORRECT:** Warfarin is contraindicated for a client taking ginkgo biloba because ginkgo biloba can suppress coagulation and increase the risk of bleeding or hemorrhage.

   C. Decongestants are contraindicated for a client taking ginkgo biloba. Digoxin is not contraindicated for a client taking ginkgo biloba.

   D. Antipsychotic medications are contraindicated for a client taking ginkgo biloba. Lisinopril is not contraindicated for a client taking ginkgo biloba.

   Ⓝ *NCLEX® Connection: Pharmacological Therapies, Adverse Effects/ Contraindications/Side Effects/Interactions*

PRACTICE Answer

Using the ATI Active Learning Template: Medication

EXPECTED PHARMACOLOGICAL ACTION: Cyanocobalamin converts folic acid from an inactive form to an active form. It corrects megaloblastic anemia related to a deficiency of vitamin B_{12}.

CLIENT EDUCATION
- Monitor for manifestations of hypokalemia.
- Use potassium supplements, if prescribed.
- Consume foods high in potassium.
- Consume foods high in vitamin B_{12}.
- Administer intranasal cyanocobalamin 1 hr before or after eating hot foods when nasal secretions are decreased.
- Periodic laboratory testing of Hgb, Hct, RBC, reticulocyte count, and folate levels is advised.

EVALUATION OF MEDICATION EFFECTIVENESS
- Review laboratory values for increased reticulocyte count and macrocytes, and Hgb and Hct levels within the expected reference range.
- Monitor for improvement of neurologic manifestations (numbness, tingling of hands and feet).

Ⓝ *NCLEX® Connection: Pharmacological and Parenteral Therapies, Medication Administration*

NCLEX® Connections

When reviewing the following chapters, keep in mind the relevant topics and tasks of the NCLEX outline, in particular:

Pharmacological Therapies

ADVERSE EFFECTS/CONTRAINDICATIONS/SIDE EFFECTS/INTERACTIONS: Monitor the client for actual and potential adverse effects of medications (prescribed, over-the-counter, herbal supplements).

MEDICATION ADMINISTRATION: Collect required data prior to medication administration.

UNIT 7   MEDICATIONS AFFECTING THE REPRODUCTIVE SYSTEM

CHAPTER 27   *Medications Affecting the Reproductive Tract*

Medications that affect the reproductive system include hormones that stimulate puberty (estrogen and progesterone in females, testosterone in males), replace a hormone deficiency (male or female), or prevent pregnancy (oral contraceptives).

Medications used to treat benign prostatic hyperplasia (BPH) include 5-alpha reductase inhibitors and alpha₁ adrenergic antagonists. Phosphodiesterase type 5 (PDE5) inhibitors are used to treat erectile dysfunction.

Estrogens

SELECT PROTOTYPE MEDICATIONS: Conjugated estrogens

OTHER MEDICATIONS: Estradiol

ROUTE OF ADMINISTRATION
- **Oral, topical, transdermal, intravaginal, IM, and IV:** Topical therapy reduces the incidence of nausea and vomiting. A smaller dose is prescribed, and there is a reduction of fluctuation of blood estrogen levels and risk of complications.
- **IV and IM:** Rare; primarily used for emergency treatment of uterine bleeding.

PURPOSE

EXPECTED PHARMACOLOGICAL ACTION

Estrogens are hormones needed for growth and maturation of the female reproductive tract, and development of secondary sex characteristics. They are active in the follicular phase of the menstrual cycle. Estrogens block bone resorption and reduce low-density lipoprotein (LDL) levels. At high levels, estrogens suppress the release of a follicle-stimulating hormone (FSH) needed for conception. Estrogens also can promote or suppress blood coagulation.

THERAPEUTIC USES

- Contraception
- Acne in females older than 14 years who want contraception
- Relief of moderate to severe postmenopausal manifestations (hot flashes, mood changes)
- Prevention and treatment of postmenopausal osteoporosis
- Treatment of dysfunctional uterine bleeding, hypogonadism, atrophic vaginitis, and inoperable breast cancer
- Palliative treatment of prostate cancer

COMPLICATIONS

Endometrial and ovarian cancers

When estrogen is used alone for postmenopausal therapy

NURSING ACTIONS: Administer progestins along with estrogen.

CLIENT EDUCATION
- Report persistent vaginal bleeding (if client has an intact uterus).
- Have an endometrial biopsy every 2 years and pelvic exam yearly.

Risk for estrogen-dependent breast cancer

More often in postmenopausal clients who use estrogen with progestin

NURSING ACTIONS: Rule out estrogen-dependent breast cancer prior to starting therapy.

CLIENT EDUCATION: Examine breasts regularly. Obtain yearly breast exams by a provider, and periodic mammograms.

Embolic events

- Myocardial infarction (MI), pulmonary embolism, deep-vein thrombosis, stroke
- Females older than 60 years have increased risk of myocardial infarction and coronary heart disease.

NURSING ACTIONS
- Monitor for pain, swelling, warmth, or erythema of lower legs.
- Advise clients how to reduce risk of cardiovascular disease.

CLIENT EDUCATION: Avoid all nicotine products.

CONTRAINDICATIONS/PRECAUTIONS

- Pregnancy Risk Category X
- Contraindicated for clients who have the following Qs
  - Client or family history of heart disease
  - Atypical vaginal bleeding that is undiagnosed
  - Breast or estrogen-dependent cancer
  - History or risk of thromboembolic disease
- Use cautiously during breastfeeding because estrogens decrease quantity and quality of milk and are excreted in breast milk.
- Use cautiously in prepubescent clients. If administered, monitor bone growth and check periodically for early epiphyseal plate closure.

INTERACTIONS

Estrogens can reduce the effectiveness of warfarin.
- Warfarin doses might need to be adjusted.
- NURSING ACTIONS: If used concurrently, monitor international normalized ratio (INR) and prothrombin time (PT).

Concurrent use of phenytoin can decrease the effectiveness of estrogens and increase the risk of breakthrough bleeding.
NURSING ACTIONS
- Monitor for decreased estrogen effects. An alternative form of birth control might be indicated.
- Monitor for increased vaginal bleeding.

Concurrent use of corticosteroids can increase effects of the corticosteroid.
NURSING ACTIONS: Monitor for increased corticosteroid effects.

Smoking increases risk for thrombophlebitis.
CLIENT EDUCATION: Do not smoke. Use alternative treatment if smoking persists.

Concurrent use of anticoagulants, oral hypoglycemics, or thyroid medications can cause a decrease in the action of these medications.
NURSING ACTIONS
- Monitor for decreased effects, and adjust dosages as needed.
- Monitor glucose and thyroid levels.

NURSING ADMINISTRATION

- Instruct clients to take the medication at the same time each day, such as at bedtime.
- Apply estrogen patches to the skin of the trunk. Avoid the breasts.
- Apply transdermal estrogen as directed depending on type of formulation.
- Instruct clients to report menstrual changes (dysmenorrhea, amenorrhea, breakthrough bleeding, breast changes).
- Encourage clients to perform monthly breast self-examinations and schedule annual gynecologic and breast examinations with the provider.
- Advise clients to notify the provider of any swelling or redness in legs, shortness of breath, or chest pain.
- Discontinue prior to knee or hip surgery or any surgical procedures that can cause extensive immobilization.

NURSING EVALUATION OF MEDICATION EFFECTIVENESS

Depending on therapeutic intent, effectiveness is evidenced by the following.
- No evidence of conception
- Control of acne
- Relief of severe postmenopausal manifestations (hot flashes, mood changes)
- Prevention of osteoporosis
- Reduction in dysfunctional uterine bleeding
- Estrogen levels within the expected reference range for clients who have hypogonadism
- Relief of manifestations of atrophic vaginitis
- Decrease in metastasis of prostate or breast cancer

Progestins

SELECT PROTOTYPE MEDICATION: Medroxyprogesterone

OTHER MEDICATIONS
- Norethindrone
- Megestrol acetate

ROUTES OF ADMINISTRATION: Oral, IM, subcutaneous, transdermal, intravaginal

PURPOSE

EXPECTED PHARMACOLOGICAL ACTION

Progestins induce favorable conditions for fetal growth and development and maintain pregnancy. A drop in progesterone levels results in menstruation.

THERAPEUTIC USES

- Alone or with estrogens for contraception
- Counter adverse effects of estrogen in menopausal hormone therapy
- Treat the following
  - Dysfunctional uterine bleeding due to hormonal imbalance
  - Amenorrhea due to hormonal imbalance
  - Endometriosis
  - Advanced cancer of the endometrium
- In clients who are undergoing in vitro fertilization, and in some clients to prevent preterm birth

COMPLICATIONS

Common adverse effects

- Depression
- Tenderness of breast tissue
- Reports of feeling bloated

Breast cancer

In postmenopausal clients in combination with estrogens

CLIENT EDUCATION: Perform regular breast self-examinations and get mammograms.

Thromboembolic events

MI, pulmonary embolism, thrombophlebitis, stroke

NURSING ACTIONS
- Discourage clients from smoking.
- Monitor for pain, swelling, warmth, or erythema of lower legs.

CLIENT EDUCATION: Notify the provider of chest pain or shortness of breath.

Breakthrough bleeding, amenorrhea

CLIENT EDUCATION: Report abnormal vaginal bleeding.

Edema

NURSING ACTIONS: Monitor blood pressure, I&O, and weight gain.

Jaundice

NURSING ACTIONS
- Monitor for indications of jaundice, such as yellowing of the skin and sclera of the eyes.
- Monitor liver enzymes.

Migraine headaches

CLIENT EDUCATION: Notify the provider of severe headache.

Birth defects/spontaneous abortion

CLIENT EDUCATION: Notify the provider if pregnancy is planned or suspected.

CONTRAINDICATIONS/PRECAUTIONS

- Contraindicated in clients who have the following. Qs
  - Undiagnosed vaginal bleeding
  - History of thromboembolic disease, cardiovascular, or cerebrovascular disease
  - History of breast or genital cancers
- Use cautiously in clients who have seizures disorders, asthma, cardiac disorders, and migraine headaches.

INTERACTIONS

Use of carbamazepine, phenobarbital, phenytoin, and rifampin can decrease contraceptive effectiveness.
CLIENT EDUCATION: Additional contraceptive measures can be needed with concurrent use of these medications.

Concurrent use with corticosteroids and anticoagulants can cause decreased bone density.
CLIENT EDUCATION: Increase calcium and vitamin D intake. Avoid concurrent use.

Smoking increases risk for thrombophlebitis, myocardial infarction, and stroke.
- Risk for complications due to smoking is greatest for clients 35 years and older.
- CLIENT EDUCATION: Do not smoke. Use alternative treatment if smoking persists. Qs

NURSING ADMINISTRATION QPcc

- Apply progestin as directed depending on type of formulation. QPcc
- Notify the provider if pregnancy is planned or suspected.

NURSING EVALUATION OF MEDICATION EFFECTIVENESS

Depending on therapeutic intent, effectiveness is evidenced by the following.
- No evidence of conception
- Restoration of hormonal balance with control of uterine bleeding
- Restoration of menses
- Decrease in endometrial hyperplasia in clients who are postmenopausal and receiving concurrent estrogen
- Control of the metastasis of endometrial cancer
- Term pregnancy

Hormonal contraceptives

SELECT PROTOTYPE MEDICATIONS
- Estrogen-progestin combinations contain estrogen and progestin and are referred to as combination oral contraceptives (OCs). OCs that contain progestin only are often referred to as minipills.
- Combination oral contraceptives with estrogen plus a progestin
  - Ethinyl estradiol and norethindrone
  - Combination oral contraceptives are classified as monophasic, biphasic, triphasic, or quadriphasic. With monophasic OCs, the dosage of estrogen to progestin remains the same throughout the cycle. With the other classifications, the estrogen/progestin changes to duplicate a typical menstrual cycle.
- Progestin-only oral contraceptives: Norethindrone

OTHER MEDICATIONS
- Transdermal patch: Ethinyl estradiol and norelgestromin
- Vaginal contraceptive ring: Ethinyl estradiol and etonogestrel
- Parenteral: Depot medroxyprogesterone acetate available for IM use and for subcutaneous use
- Etonogestrel implants

ROUTE OF ADMINISTRATION
- Oral, transdermal, IM, subcutaneous, subdermal
- Combination OCs are given in a cyclic pattern, usually in a 28-day regimen. They can also be given in extended-cycle schedules.

PURPOSE

EXPECTED PHARMACOLOGICAL ACTION: Oral contraceptives stop conception by preventing ovulation. They also thicken the cervical mucus and alter the endometrial lining to reduce the chance of fertilization.

THERAPEUTIC USES: Prevent pregnancy

COMPLICATIONS

Thromboembolic events

MI, pulmonary embolism, thrombophlebitis, stroke

CLIENT EDUCATION
- Do not smoke.
- Report warmth, edema, tenderness, or pain in lower legs.

Hypertension

NURSING ACTIONS: Monitor and take actions to maintain blood pressure.

Breakthrough or irregular uterine bleeding

NURSING ACTIONS: Evaluate for possible pregnancy if two or more menstrual periods are missed.

CLIENT EDUCATION: Record duration and frequency of breakthrough bleeding.

Breast cancer

NURSING ACTIONS: Oral contraceptives can increase growth of a pre-existing breast cancer. Do not give to clients who have breast cancer.

Hyperglycemia

NURSING ACTIONS: Monitor glucose in clients who have diabetes mellitus. Adjust antihyperglycemics as needed.

Hyperkalemia

With combination OC that contains drospirenone

NURSING ACTIONS: Do not use combination OCs with drospirenone in clients at risk for hyperkalemia (impaired kidney function, adrenal insufficiency).

CONTRAINDICATIONS/PRECAUTIONS
- Pregnancy Risk Category X
- Contraindicated for clients who Qs
  - Are smokers and older than age of 35.
  - Have a history of thrombophlebitis and cardiovascular events.
  - Have a family history or risk factors for breast cancer.
  - Are experiencing abnormal vaginal bleeding.
- Use cautiously in clients who have hypertension, diabetes mellitus, gallbladder disease, uterine leiomyoma, seizures, or migraine headaches.

INTERACTIONS

Oral contraceptive effectiveness decreases with use of carbamazepine, phenobarbital, antibiotics (especially penicillins and cephalosporins), phenytoin, and rifampin. Additional contraceptive measures might be needed with concurrent use of these medications.

Oral contraceptives decrease the effects of warfarin and oral diabetic medications.
NURSING ACTIONS: Monitor INR, PT, and glucose levels. Adjust dosages accordingly.

Oral contraceptives can increase the effects of theophylline and imipramine.
NURSING ACTIONS: Monitor for indications of toxicity.

NURSING ADMINISTRATION
- Check for pregnancy prior to start of therapy. Qs
- Instruct clients to take pills at the same time each day.
- Instruct clients to take medication for 21 days followed by 7 days of no medication (or inert pill). For the traditional 28-day cycle OCs, begin the sequence on the first day or first Sunday after the onset of menses.
- If one or more pills are missed in the first week, take one pill as soon as possible and continue with the pack. Use an additional form of contraception for 7 days.

- If one or two pills are missed in the second or third week, take one as soon as possible and continue with the active pills in the pack but skip the placebos and go straight to the new pack once all of the active pills have been taken.
- If three or more pills are missed during the second or third week, follow the same instructions for missing two pills. Use an additional form of contraception for 7 days.
- Extended-cycle OCs are taken for longer than the typical 28-day cycle. Eighty-four days is common, but some preparations are taken continuously.

> For extended-cycle OCs taken for 84 days, the client has withdrawal bleeding four times per year. Some extended-cycle OCs are taken continuously, and the client does not have withdrawal bleeding.

- Encourage clients who smoke to quit.
- Advise clients to report swelling or redness in legs, shortness of breath, or severe headache.

NURSING EVALUATION OF MEDICATION EFFECTIVENESS

Depending on therapeutic intent, effectiveness is confirmed by no evidence of conception.

Androgens

SELECT PROTOTYPE MEDICATION: Testosterone

OTHER MEDICATIONS: Methyltestosterone

ROUTE OF ADMINISTRATION: IM, transdermal, implantable pellets, buccal tablets

PURPOSE

EXPECTED PHARMACOLOGICAL ACTION
The hormone-receptor complex acts on cellular DNA to promote specific mRNA molecules and production of proteins, resulting in the following.
- Development of sex traits in men
- Production and maturation of sperm
- Increase in skeletal muscle
- Increase in synthesis of erythropoietin

THERAPEUTIC USES
- Deficiency of testosterone
- Hypogonadism in males
- Delayed puberty in boys
- Androgen replacement in testicular failure
- Anemia not responsive to traditional therapy
- Postmenopausal breast cancer
- Muscle wasting in male clients who have AIDS

COMPLICATIONS

Androgenic (virilization) effects

- In female clients, these medications can cause irregularity or cessation of menses, hirsutism, weight gain, acne, lowering of voice, growth of clitoris, vaginitis, and baldness.
- In male clients, these medications can cause acne, priapism, increased facial and body hair, and penile enlargement.
- Medication might be discontinued to prevent permanent changes.

NURSING ACTIONS: Advise clients of possible medication effects and to report occurrence of these effects.

Epiphyseal closure

Premature closure of epiphysis in boys can reduce mature height.

NURSING ACTIONS: Monitor epiphysis with serial X-rays.

Cholestatic hepatitis, jaundice

NURSING ACTIONS
- Monitor for indications of jaundice, such as yellowing of the skin and sclera of the eyes.
- Monitor liver enzymes.

Hypercholesterolemia

These medications can decrease high-density lipoproteins (HDL) and increase LDL.

NURSING ACTIONS: Monitor cholesterol levels.

CLIENT EDUCATION: Adjust diet to reduce cholesterol levels.

Increase in growth of prostate cancer

Do not give to clients who have prostate cancer.

NURSING ACTIONS: Monitor for prostate cancer.

Polycythemia

NURSING ACTIONS: Monitor hemoglobin and hematocrit.

Edema from sodium and water retention

Medication might be discontinued.

CLIENT EDUCATION: Monitor for weight gain and swelling of extremities, and report these to the provider.

High potential for misuse

NURSING ACTIONS: Identify high-risk groups, and educate regarding potential for misuse and possible health risks.

CONTRAINDICATIONS/PRECAUTIONS

- Pregnancy Risk Category X
- Avoid use during lactation.
- Contraindicated in older adult clients and males who have prostate cancer, liver disorders, or severe cardiac disease. Ⓖ

INTERACTIONS

Androgens can increase the effects of oral anticoagulants.
NURSING ACTIONS: Monitor PT and INR.

Androgens can increase the effects of insulins and antidiabetic agents.
NURSING ACTIONS
- Monitor for hypoglycemia.
- Monitor glucose level, and adjust dosages.

NURSING ADMINISTRATION

- Instruct clients using gel formulations to wash their hands after every application due to the possibility of skin-to-skin transfer to others. Cover application with clothing after gel has dried and wash off before skin to skin contact with another person.
- Inject IM formulations into a large muscle and rotate injection sites. Qᴘᴄᴄ
- Monitor female clients for acne and manifestations of masculinization (facial hair, baldness, deepened voice).
- Advise clients to use a barrier method of birth control.
- Advise clients to reduce cholesterol in the diet.
- Advise clients about the risk for misuse.
- Obtain daily weights.

NURSING EVALUATION OF MEDICATION EFFECTIVENESS

Depending on therapeutic intent, effectiveness is evidenced by the following.
- Puberty is induced in males.
- Testosterone is increased in males.
- There is a decrease in the progression of breast cancer in females. Medication produces expected results with minimal adverse effects.

5-Alpha-reductase inhibitors

SELECT PROTOTYPE MEDICATIONS: Finasteride

OTHER MEDICATIONS: Dutasteride

ROUTE OF ADMINISTRATION: Oral

PURPOSE

EXPECTED PHARMACOLOGICAL ACTION: Decreases usable testosterone by inhibiting the converting enzyme, causing a reduction of the prostate size and increased hair growth

THERAPEUTIC USES
- Benign prostatic hyperplasia
- Male pattern baldness

COMPLICATIONS

Decreased libido, ejaculate volume

CLIENT EDUCATION: Notify the provider if adverse effects occur.

Gynecomastia

CLIENT EDUCATION: Notify the provider if adverse effects occur.

CONTRAINDICATIONS/PRECAUTIONS

- Pregnancy Risk Category X
- Contraindicated in clients who have medication hypersensitivity.
- Use with caution in clients who have liver disease.

NURSING ADMINISTRATION

- Advise clients that therapeutic effects can take 6 months or longer.
- Pregnant clients should not handle crushed or broken medication. Qₛ
- Advise clients not to donate blood unless medication has been discontinued for at least 1 month.

NURSING EVALUATION OF MEDICATION EFFECTIVENESS

Depending on therapeutic intent, effectiveness is evidenced by the following.
- Prostate size is decreased, and the client is able to urinate effectively.
- Prostate-specific antigen levels have decreased from baseline.
- Client has increased hair growth.

Alpha₁ adrenergic antagonists

SELECT PROTOTYPE MEDICATION
Selective alpha₁ receptor antagonist: Tamsulosin

OTHER MEDICATIONS
- **Selective alpha1 receptor antagonist:** Silodosin
- **Nonselective alpha₁ receptor antagonists**
  - Alfuzosin
  - Terazosin
  - Doxazosin

ROUTE OF ADMINISTRATION: Oral

PURPOSE

EXPECTED PHARMACOLOGICAL ACTION
- Decrease mechanical obstruction of the urethra by relaxing smooth muscles of the bladder neck and prostate.
- Nonselective agents also cause vasodilation and can lower blood pressure. These agents are used for clients who have BPH and hypertension.

THERAPEUTIC USES
- BPH, thus increasing urinary flow
- Off–label use for females for treatment of urinary hesitancy or urinary retention

COMPLICATIONS

Hypotension, dizziness, nasal congestion, sleepiness, faintness

More likely with nonselective antagonists

NURSING ACTIONS: Monitor blood pressure.

CLIENT EDUCATION
- Rise slowly from sitting or lying position.
- Do not drive or operate machinery when starting therapy or with change in dose until response is known.

Problems with ejaculation

Failure, decreased volume with silodosin and tamsulosin

NURSING ACTIONS: Advise clients of possible adverse effects.

CONTRAINDICATIONS/PRECAUTIONS

- Contraindicated in clients who have medication sensitivity. Qs
- Alfuzosin is contraindicated in female clients and in clients who have severe liver failure.
- Silodosin is contraindicated in clients who have kidney failure or liver failure.
- Doxazosin should be used cautiously in clients who have liver impairment.
- Tamsulosin should be used cautiously in clients who have hepatic or kidney impairment.
- Females of childbearing age should not handle crushed or broken tablets due to the risk of absorption and teratogenic effects.

INTERACTIONS

Cimetidine can decrease clearance of tamsulosin.
NURSING ACTIONS: Use concurrently with caution.

NURSING ADMINISTRATION

- Monitor blood pressure, especially at the start of therapy and with changes of dose. Qpcc
- Advise clients to take medication daily as prescribed.
  - Tamsulosin: 30 min after a meal at the same time each day
  - Silodosin: With the same meal each day
  - Alfuzosin: Right after the same meal each day
  - Terazosin: At bedtime
  - Doxazosin: At the same time each day

NURSING EVALUATION OF MEDICATION EFFECTIVENESS

Depending on therapeutic intent, effectiveness is evidenced by improved urinary flow with minimal adverse effects.

Phosphodiesterase type 5 inhibitors

SELECT PROTOTYPE MEDICATIONS: Sildenafil

OTHER MEDICATIONS
- Tadalafil
- Vardenafil

PURPOSE

EXPECTED PHARMACOLOGICAL ACTION: Augments the effects of nitric oxide released during sexual stimulation, resulting in enhanced blood flow to the corpus cavernosum and penile erection

THERAPEUTIC USES: Erectile dysfunction

COMPLICATIONS

Common adverse reactions

- Headache
- Flushing
- Nasal drainage and congestion
- Nausea

Priapism

CLIENT EDUCATION: Notify the provider if erection lasts more than 4 hr.

Sudden hearing loss

CLIENT EDUCATION: Discontinue medication if hearing is affected.

CONTRAINDICATIONS/PRECAUTIONS

- Contraindicated in clients taking medications in the nitrate family, such as nitroglycerin, due to the risk of severe hypotension. Avoid use of nitrates within 24 hr of taking a phosphodiesterase type 5 (PDE5) inhibitor.
- Use cautiously with antihypertensive medications due to the risk of hypotension.
- Advise clients that grapefruit juice can increase plasma concentrations and possible adverse effects of medication.

INTERACTIONS

Organic nitrates (nitroglycerin, isosorbide) can lead to fatal hypotension.
NURSING ACTIONS: Do not use with organic nitrates.

Ketoconazole, erythromycin, cimetidine, ritonavir, and grapefruit juice inhibit metabolism of sildenafil, thereby increasing plasma levels of medication.
NURSING ACTIONS: Use these medications cautiously in clients taking PDE5 inhibitors.

NURSING ADMINISTRATION

- Administer orally before sexual activity. The time required prior to sexual activity depends on the specific medication prescribed. Qpcc
- Instruct clients that tadalafil is approved to be taken daily or prior to sexual activity.

NURSING EVALUATION OF MEDICATION EFFECTIVENESS

Depending on therapeutic intent, effectiveness is evidenced by erection sufficient for sexual intercourse.

Application Exercises

1. A nurse is reviewing the health care record of a client who is asking about conjugated estrogens. This medication is contraindicated in which of the following conditions?

   A. Atrophic vaginitis

   B. Dysfunctional uterine bleeding

   C. Osteoporosis

   D. Thrombophlebitis

2. A nurse is reinforcing teaching with a female client who is taking testosterone to treat advanced breast cancer. Which of the following are adverse effects of this medication? (Select all that apply.)

   A. Deepening voice

   B. Weight gain

   C. Decreased LDL

   D. Dry mucous membranes

   E. Facial hair

3. A nurse is explaining the mechanism of action of combination oral contraceptives to a group of clients. Which of the following actions occur with the use of combination oral contraceptives? (Select all that apply.)

   A. Thickening cervical mucus

   B. Inducing maturation of ovarian follicle

   C. Increasing development of the corpus luteum

   D. Altering endometrial lining

   E. Inhibiting ovulation

4. A nurse is reinforcing teaching with a client who will start alfuzosin for treatment of benign prostatic hyperplasia. Which of the following is an adverse effect of this medication?

   A. Bradycardia

   B. Edema

   C. Hypotension

   D. Tremor

5. A nurse is caring for a client who has angina and asks about obtaining a prescription for sildenafil to treat erectile dysfunction. Which of the following medications is contraindicated with sildenafil?

   A. Aspirin

   B. Isosorbide

   C. Clopidogrel

   D. Atorvastatin

PRACTICE Active Learning Scenario

A nurse in a provider's office is discussing with a client the use of traditional 28-day cycle oral contraceptives for the prevention of pregnancy. The client asks, "What should I do if I forget to take a pill?" Use the ATI Active Learning Template: Medication to complete this item.

CLIENT EDUCATION: Identify information the nurse should provide the client about administration and steps the client should take if a dose is missed.

Application Exercises Key

1. A. Atrophic vaginitis occurs when there is estrogen deficiency. This medication is used to treated atrophic vaginitis.

   B. Dysfunctional uterine bleeding can occur when there is estrogen deficiency. This medication is used to treat dysfunctional uterine bleeding.

   C. Clients are at risk for osteoporosis after the onset of menopause. Estrogen is used to prevent and slow the progression of osteoporosis.

   D. **CORRECT:** Estrogen increases the risk of thrombolytic events. Estrogen use is contraindicated for a client who has a history of thrombophlebitis.

   Ⓝ *NCLEX® Connection: Pharmacological Therapies, Adverse Effects/ Contraindications/Side Effects/Interactions*

2. A. **CORRECT:** Virilization, the development of adult male characteristics in a female, is an adverse effect of testosterone. The nurse should tell the client that a deepening voice is an adverse effect of testosterone.

   B. **CORRECT:** Edema and weight gain are adverse effects of testosterone.

   C. Decreased HDL and increased LDL are adverse effects of testosterone.

   D. Dry mucous membranes are an indication of dehydration. Edema and fluid retention are adverse effects of testosterone.

   E. **CORRECT:** Virilization is an adverse effect of testosterone. The nurse should tell the client that the development of facial hair is an adverse effect of testosterone.

   Ⓝ *NCLEX® Connection: Pharmacological Therapies, Adverse Effects/ Contraindications/Side Effects/Interactions*

3. A. **CORRECT:** Oral contraceptives cause thickening of the cervical mucus, which slows sperm passage.

   B. Inducing maturation of ovarian follicle is not an action of oral contraceptives.

   C. Increasing the development of the corpus luteum is not an action of oral contraceptives.

   D. **CORRECT:** Oral contraceptives alter the lining of the endometrium, which inhibits implantation of the fertilized egg.

   E. **CORRECT:** Oral contraceptives prevent pregnancy by inhibiting ovulation.

   Ⓝ *NCLEX® Connection: Pharmacological Therapies, Expected Actions/Outcomes*

4. A. Bradycardia is not an adverse effect of alfuzosin.

   B. Edema is not an adverse effect of alfuzosin.

   C. **CORRECT:** Alfuzosin relaxes muscle tone in veins and cardiac output decreases, which leads to hypotension. Clients taking this medication should rise slowly from a sitting or lying position.

   D. Tremor is not an adverse effect of alfuzosin.

   Ⓝ *NCLEX® Connection: Pharmacological Therapies, Adverse Effects/ Contraindications/Side Effects/Interactions*

5. A. Aspirin is contraindicated in clients who have a bleeding disorder, but there are no contradictions for concurrent use of sildenafil.

   B. **CORRECT:** Isosorbide is an organic nitrate that manages pain from angina. Concurrent use is contraindicated because fatal hypotension can occur. The client should avoid taking a nitrate medication for 24 hr after taking sildenafil.

   C. Clopidogrel is contraindicated in clients who are actively bleeding, but there is no contradiction for concurrent use of clopidogrel and sildenafil.

   D. Atorvastatin is contraindicated in clients who have hepatic disease, but there is no contradiction for concurrent use of atorvastatin and sildenafil.

   Ⓝ *NCLEX® Connection: Pharmacological Therapies, Adverse Effects/ Contraindications/Side Effects/Interactions*

PRACTICE Answer

Using the ATI Active Learning Template: Medication

CLIENT EDUCATION
- Take pills at the same time each day.
- Take medication for 21 days followed by 7 days of no medication (or inert pill). For the traditional 28-day cycle OCs, begin the sequence on the first day or first Sunday after the onset of menses.
- If one or more pills are missed in the first week, take one pill as soon as possible and continue with the pack. Use an additional form of contraception for 7 days.
- If one or two pills are missed in the second or third week, take one as soon as possible and continue with the active pills in the pack but skip the placebos and go straight to the new pack once all of the active pills have been taken.
- If three or more pills are missed during the second or third week, follow the same instructions for missing two pills. Use an additional form of contraception for 7 days.

Ⓝ *NCLEX® Connection: Pharmacological and Parenteral Therapies, Medication Administration*

Ⓝ NCLEX® Connections

When reviewing the following chapters, keep in mind the relevant topics and tasks of the NCLEX outline, in particular:

Pharmacological Therapies

ADVERSE EFFECTS/CONTRAINDICATIONS/SIDE EFFECTS/ INTERACTIONS: Monitor for anticipated interactions among the client's prescribed medications and fluids (oral, IV, subcutaneous, IM, topical).

EXPECTED ACTIONS/OUTCOMES: Monitor the client's use of medications over time (prescription, over-the-counter, home remedies).

MEDICATION ADMINISTRATION: Reconcile and maintain a medication list or medication administration record (prescribed medications, herbal supplements, over-the-counter medications).

CHAPTER 28

CHAPTER 28 *Connective Tissue Disorders*

Rheumatoid arthritis (RA) is a chronic disorder with autoimmune and inflammatory components. Pharmacological management provides manifestation relief and some delay in progression of the disorder without resulting in cure. Categories of medications in this section include disease-modifying antirheumatic drugs (DMARDs), glucocorticoids, immunosuppressants, and nonsteroidal anti-inflammatory drugs (NSAIDs), which can be used individually or in combination to manage RA.

Systemic lupus erythematous (SLE) is an autoimmune condition that can cause damage to joints, skin, blood vessels, and organs. Medications for treating lupus include anti-inflammatory medications, NSAIDs, corticosteroids, antimalarials, immunomodulators, and monoclonal antibodies. Topical cortisone can reduce inflammation of the typical skin rash of SLE.

Fibromyalgia is a syndrome characterized by muscle pain and fatigue. There are three FDA-approved medications for treating this syndrome: pregabalin, duloxetine, and milnacipran. Other medications used to treat fibromyalgia syndrome (but not FDA-approved for this use) include amitriptyline, cyclobenzaprine, tramadol, NSAIDs, and opioids. In addition, medications that facilitate sleep (such as zolpidem) and treat restless leg syndrome (such as gabapentin) are sometimes prescribed for manifestations of this condition.

Gout (gouty arthritis) is a painful type of arthritis that is caused by elevated levels of uric acid, which can accumulate and cause localized inflammation in synovial areas. Antigout medications act either by reducing inflammation or decreasing serum uric acid levels. Antigout medications include anti-inflammatory agents, NSAIDs, glucocorticoids, and agents for hyperuricemia.

Disease-modifying antirheumatic drugs

DMARDS I: Major nonbiologic DMARDs
- Immunomodulator medications: methotrexate, leflunomide
- Antimalarial agent: hydroxychloroquine
- Anti–inflammatory medication: sulfasalazine
- Tetracycline antibiotic: minocycline

DMARDS II: Major biologic DMARDs
- Tumor necrosis factor antagonists
  - Etanercept
  - Infliximab
  - Adalimumab
  - Certolizumab
  - Golimumab
- B–lymphocyte–depleting agent: Rituximab
- Interleukin-1 receptor antagonist: Abatacept

DMARDS III: Minor nonbiologic and nonbiologic DMARDs
- Gold salts: Auranofin
- Penicillamine
- Immunosuppressant medications
  - Azathioprine
  - Cyclosporine

GLUCOCORTICOIDS
- Prednisone
- Prednisolone

NSAIDS
- Aspirin
- Ibuprofen
- Diclofenac
- Indomethacin
- Meloxicam
- Naproxen
- Celecoxib

PURPOSE

EXPECTED PHARMACOLOGICAL ACTION

- DMARDs slow the joint degeneration and progression of rheumatoid arthritis.
- Glucocorticoids provide manifestation relief of inflammation and pain.
- NSAIDs provide rapid manifestation relief of inflammation and pain.

THERAPEUTIC USES

- Analgesia for pain, swelling, and joint stiffness
- Maintenance of joint function
- Slow/delay the worsening of the disease (DMARDs, glucocorticoids)
- Short-term therapy (with NSAIDs, glucocorticoids) until long-acting DMARDs take effect
- Prevention of organ rejection in clients who have transplants such as kidney, liver, and heart (glucocorticoids, immunosuppressants)
- Management of inflammatory bowel disease (glucocorticoids, immunosuppressants, DMARDs)

COMPLICATIONS

Cytotoxic agent/immunomodulator (methotrexate)

Increased risk of infection
CLIENT EDUCATION: Notify the provider immediately for manifestations of infection (fever, sore throat).

Hepatic fibrosis and toxicity
- NURSING ACTIONS: Monitor liver function tests.
- CLIENT EDUCATION: Observe for anorexia, abdominal fullness, and jaundice. Notify the provider if manifestations occur.

Bone marrow suppression
NURSING ACTIONS: Obtain baseline CBC, including platelet counts. Repeat every 3 to 6 months.

Ulcerative stomatitis/other GI ulcerations
- Early finding with toxicity
- NURSING ACTIONS
  - Inspect mouth, gums, and throat daily for ulcerations, bleeding, or color changes.
  - Stop the medication if manifestations occur.
- CLIENT EDUCATION: Take the medication with food or 8 oz water.

Fetal death/congenital abnormalities
- NURSING ACTIONS: Avoid use during pregnancy.
- Client education: Use adequate contraception if taking this medication.

Gold salts (auranofin)

Toxicity (severe pruritus, rashes, stomatitis)
NURSING ACTIONS: Notify the provider if these manifestations occur.

Renal toxicity, such as proteinuria
NURSING ACTIONS: Monitor I&O, BUN, creatinine, and UA.

Hematologic disorders
- Thrombocytopenia, leukopenia, agranulocytosis, aplastic anemia
- NURSING ACTIONS: Monitor CBC, WBC, and platelet counts periodically.
- CLIENT EDUCATION: Observe for bruising and gum bleeding, and notify the provider if these occur.

Hepatitis
NURSING ACTIONS: Monitor liver function tests.

GI discomfort (nausea, vomiting, abdominal pain)
NURSING ACTIONS: Observe for manifestations, and notify the provider if they occur.

Sulfasalazine

GI discomfort
- Nausea, vomiting, diarrhea, abdominal pain
- NURSING ACTIONS: Use an enteric-coated preparation, and divide dosage daily.

Hepatic dysfunction (rare)
NURSING ACTIONS: Monitor liver function tests.

Bone marrow suppression (rare)
NURSING ACTIONS: Monitor CBC, including platelet counts.

ANTIMALARIAL AGENT (HYDROXYCHLOROQUINE)

Retinal damage (blindness)
- Rare but most serious toxicity
- CLIENT EDUCATION
  - Have baseline eye examination and follow-up eye exams every 6 months with an ophthalmologist. Qs
  - Stop the medication and notify the provider if blurred vision occurs.

Tumor necrosis factor antagonists (etanercept, infliximab)

Subcutaneous injection-site irritation
- Redness, swelling, pain, itching
- NURSING ACTIONS: Monitor the injection site, and stop the medication if manifestations of irritation occur.

IV infusion reactions (infliximab)
- Flu-like findings, hypotension, possible anaphylaxis
- NURSING ACTIONS
  - Ensure the infusion is stopped and notify provider immediately for severe reaction.
  - Continue to monitor for reaction 2 hr after IV infusion.

Risk of infection
- Especially TB and reactivation of hepatitis B
- NURSING ACTIONS: Test for hepatitis B and TB.
- Client education: Monitor for infection (fever, sore throat, inflammation), and notify the provider if manifestations occur. Medication should be discontinued.

Severe skin reactions
- Including Stevens-Johnson syndrome
- CLIENT EDUCATION: Monitor for adverse skin reactions, and notify the provider if manifestations occur. Medication should be discontinued.

Heart failure
NURSING ACTIONS: Monitor for development or worsening of heart failure (distended neck veins, crackles in lungs, dyspnea). Medication should be discontinued.

Hematologic disorders
NURSING ACTIONS: Monitor for manifestations of bleeding, bruising, or fever. Medication should be discontinued.

Penicillamine

Bone marrow suppression
NURSING ACTIONS: Obtain baseline CBC including platelet counts, and repeat every 3 to 6 months.

Toxicity (severe pruritus, rashes)
NURSING ACTIONS
- Stop the medication.
- Notify the provider if manifestations occur.

Cyclosporine

Risk of infection
- Flu-like manifestations, painful urination
- CLIENT EDUCATION: Notify the provider immediately if manifestations occur.

Hepatotoxicity (jaundice)
NURSING ACTIONS: Monitor liver function, and adjust dosage.

Nephrotoxicity
NURSING ACTIONS
- Monitor BUN and creatinine throughout treatment.
- Monitor I&O.

Hirsutism
This effect is reversible with discontinuation of the medication.

Gingival hyperplasia
NURSING ACTIONS: Advise clients on importance of good dental hygiene and regular dental check-ups.

Glucocorticoids (prednisone)

Risk of infection (fever, sore throat)
CLIENT EDUCATION: Notify the provider immediately if manifestations occur.

Osteoporosis
CLIENT EDUCATION: Take calcium supplements, vitamin D, and/or bisphosphonate (etidronate).

Adrenal suppression
- Nausea, vomiting, hypotension, and confusion can occur if glucocorticoids are stopped abruptly.
- NURSING ACTIONS
  - Monitor administration of IV fluids (0.9% sodium chloride, hydrocortisone).
  - Increase in glucocorticoid dosage can be needed during times of stress (surgery, acute illness). Qᴛᴄ
- CLIENT EDUCATION
  - Do not discontinue the medication suddenly.
  - Observe for manifestations, and notify the provider if manifestations occur.

Fluid retention
NURSING ACTIONS: Monitor for manifestations of fluid excess (crackles, weight gain, edema).

GI discomfort/gastric ulceration
- H_2-receptor antagonists can be used prophylactically.
- CLIENT EDUCATION
  - Observe for manifestations, and notify the provider if manifestations occur.
  - Report manifestations of GI bleeding (coffee-ground emesis; black, tarry stools).

Hyperglycemia
NURSING ACTIONS: Monitor blood glucose level. Clients who have diabetes mellitus might need to adjust hypoglycemic agent.

Hypokalemia
- NURSING ACTIONS
  - Monitor serum potassium levels.
  - Administer potassium supplements.
- CLIENT EDUCATION: Eat potassium-rich foods.

CONTRAINDICATIONS/PRECAUTIONS

Methotrexate
- This medication is Pregnancy Risk Category X. Qs
- Methotrexate is contraindicated in clients who have liver failure, alcohol use disorder, or hematologic disorders.
- Use with caution in clients who have liver or kidney dysfunction, cancer and suppressed bone marrow function, peptic ulcer disease, ulcerative colitis, impaired nutritional status, or infections.
- Use cautiously with children, or clients who are breastfeeding.

Etanercept is contraindicated in clients who have malignancies, active infection, hematologic disorder, or during lactation. Use caution in clients who have heart failure, central nervous system (CNS) demyelinating disorders such as multiple sclerosis, or hematologic disorders.

Cyclosporine is contraindicated in pregnancy, recent vaccination with live virus vaccines, and recent contact with or active infection of chickenpox or herpes zoster.

Glucocorticoids
- Glucocorticoids are contraindicated in systemic fungal infections and live virus vaccines.
- Warn clients against abrupt discontinuation of glucocorticoids. Dosage of glucocorticoids is always adjusted and withdrawn gradually.

INTERACTIONS

Methotrexate

Salicylates, other NSAIDs, sulfonamides, penicillin, and tetracyclines can cause methotrexate toxicity.
NURSING ACTIONS: Monitor for toxic effects.

Folic acid changes the body's response to methotrexate, decreasing its effect.
NURSING ACTIONS: Avoid folic acid supplements or vitamins containing folic acid (even though folic acid can reduce GI toxicity).

Etanercept

Concurrent use of etanercept with a live vaccine increases the risk of getting or transmitting infection.
NURSING ACTIONS: Avoid live vaccines.

Concurrent use with immunosuppressants increases the chance of serious infection.
NURSING ACTIONS: Use precautions against illness if taking immunosuppressants.

Cyclosporine

Concurrent use of phenytoin, phenobarbital, rifampin, carbamazepine, and trimethoprim-sulfamethoxazole decreases cyclosporine level, which can lead to organ rejection.
NURSING ACTIONS: Monitor cyclosporine levels, and adjust dosage accordingly.

Concurrent use of ketoconazole, erythromycin, and amphotericin B can increase cyclosporine levels, leading to toxicity.
NURSING ACTIONS: Monitor cyclosporine dosage, and adjust accordingly to prevent toxicity.

Amphotericin B, aminoglycoside, and NSAIDs are nephrotoxic. Concurrent use with cyclosporine increases the risk for kidney dysfunction.
NURSING ACTIONS: Monitor BUN, creatinine, and I&O.

Consumption of grapefruit juice increases cyclosporine levels by 50%, which poses an increased risk of toxicity.
CLIENT EDUCATION: Avoid drinking grapefruit juice.

Glucocorticoids

Loop diuretics that promote potassium loss increase the risk of hypokalemia.
NURSING ACTIONS: Monitor potassium level, and administer supplements as needed.

Because of the risk for hypokalemia, concurrent use of glucocorticoids with digoxin increases the risk of digoxin-induced dysrhythmias.
NURSING ACTIONS
- Monitor for digoxin-induced dysrhythmias.
- Monitor potassium levels.

NSAIDs increase the risk of GI ulceration.
CLIENT EDUCATION
- Avoid use of NSAIDs.
- If GI distress occurs, notify the provider.

Glucocorticoids promote hyperglycemia, thereby counteracting the effects of insulin and oral diabetic medications.
The dose of diabetic medications might need to be increased.

NURSING ADMINISTRATION

- Advise clients that effects of DMARDs are delayed and can take 3 to 6 weeks, with full therapeutic effect taking several months. Qpcc
- Administer adalimumab by subcutaneous injection every 2 weeks.
- Administer etanercept by subcutaneous injection once per week. Ensure solution is clear without particles present.
- Glucocorticoids can be used as oral agents or intra-articular injections. Short-term therapy can be used to control exacerbations of manifestations and can also be used while waiting for the effects of DMARDs to develop.

Cyclosporine

- Ensure administration of the initial IV dose of cyclosporine is over 2 to 6 hr.
- Monitor for hypersensitivity reactions. Stay with clients for 30 min after administration of cyclosporine.
- Mix oral cyclosporine with milk or orange juice right before ingestion to increase palatability.
- Instruct clients regarding the importance of lifelong therapy if used to prevent organ rejection.

NURSING EVALUATION OF MEDICATION EFFECTIVENESS

Depending on the therapeutic intent, effectiveness can be evidenced by the following.
- Improvement of manifestations of rheumatoid arthritis (reduced swelling of joints, absence of joint stiffness, ability to maintain joint function, absence of pain)
- Decrease in systemic complications (weight loss, fatigue)

Medication for systemic lupus erythematosus

MONOCLONAL ANTIBODY MEDICATION: Belimumab

PURPOSE

EXPECTED PHARMACOLOGICAL ACTION: Disrupts activation of B-lymphocytes through interference with B-lymphocyte stimulator, a protein needed for B-cell activation

THERAPEUTIC USES: SLE

COMPLICATIONS

GI effects (nausea, vomiting, diarrhea)

CLIENT EDUCATION: Natural GI remedies include ginger tea and hard candy. If severe GI distress occurs, notify the provider.

Headache, depressed mood

CLIENT EDUCATION: If suicidal thoughts are present, notify the provider.

Insomnia

CLIENT EDUCATION: Strategies to promote adequate sleep include making sure the bedroom is quiet, dark, and relaxing, and avoiding large meals before bedtime.

Infusion reaction

Erythema, edema, pruritus around IV site
- Anaphylaxis can occur.
- Premedication might be prescribed to minimize hypersensitivity reactions.

NURSING ACTIONS: Ensure the medication is infused slowly over an hour. If anaphylaxis occurs, discontinue infusion and begin emergency treatment.

Increased risk of infection

CLIENT EDUCATION
- Avoid being around individuals who are ill.
- Do not receive live virus vaccines within 30 days of medication.
- Notify provider of fever, painful urination, or bloody diarrhea.

CONTRAINDICATIONS/PRECAUTIONS

- Pregnancy Risk Category C. Avoid breastfeeding.
- Not for use in clients who have severe kidney impairment or SLE affecting CNS.
- Use caution in older adult clients, as well as clients who have depression, cardiac disorders, or infections. Ⓒ

INTERACTIONS

Cyclophosphamide or immune suppressants increase risk for infection.
CLIENT EDUCATION
- Avoid being around others who are ill.
- Do not receive live virus vaccines within 30 days of medication.
- Notify the provider of fever, painful urination, or bloody diarrhea.

NURSING ADMINISTRATION

- Ensure IV infusion administration follows these guidelines.
  - Reconstitute with sterile water, and dilute only with 0.9% saline solution. Ⓠ EBP
  - Refrigerate solution no longer than 8 hr after reconstitution. Allow solution to stand at room temperature for 10 to 15 min before using.
  - When administered by IV infusion, ensure the medication is given slowly, over about 1 hr. Monitor closely for infusion reactions and hypersensitivity.
  - Discard unused solution.
- Administer the oral form of the medication with food.

NURSING EVALUATION OF MEDICATION EFFECTIVENESS

Depending on the therapeutic intent, effectiveness can be evidenced by a decrease in manifestations of SLE.

Medications for fibromyalgia

SEROTONIN-NOREPINEPHRINE REUPTAKE INHIBITORS
- Duloxetine
- Milnacipran

GAMMA-AMINOBUTYRIC ACID ANALOGUE (GABA): Pregabalin

PURPOSE

Serotonin-norepinephrine reuptake inhibitors

EXPECTED PHARMACOLOGICAL ACTION: Restores balance of neurotransmitters, serotonin and norepinephrine

THERAPEUTIC USES
- Fibromyalgia (duloxetine, milnacipran)
- Depression (duloxetine)
- Diabetic peripheral neuropathy (duloxetine)

GABA

EXPECTED PHARMACOLOGICAL ACTION: It is thought that pregabalin binds to alpha-2-delta in CNS tissue.

THERAPEUTIC USES: Fibromyalgia, seizures, neuropathic pain

COMPLICATIONS

Serotonin-norepinephrine reuptake inhibitors

Drowsiness, dizziness, blurred vision
CLIENT EDUCATION
- Do not drive or operate heavy machinery while taking this medication.
- Change positions slowly.
- Employ fall prevention strategies (sensible shoes, removing home hazards).

Nausea, anorexia, weight loss
NURSING ACTIONS: Monitor weight and food intake.

Headache, insomnia, anxiety
NURSING ACTIONS: Monitor for these findings.

Hypertension, tachycardia
NURSING ACTIONS: Monitor vital signs and report changes.

Withdrawal syndrome
- Results in headache, nausea, visual disturbances, anxiety, dizziness, and tremors
- CLIENT EDUCATION: Withdraw from medication gradually.

Sexual dysfunction
- Inability to have an orgasm, decreased libido, impotence, menstrual changes
- CLIENT EDUCATION: Report sexual dysfunction to the provider.

GABA

Drowsiness, fatigue, dizziness, blurred vision, lightheadedness
CLIENT EDUCATION
- Do not drive or operate heavy machinery while taking this medication.
- Change positions slowly.
- Use fall prevention strategies (sensible shoes, removing home hazards).

Increased appetite, weight gain, constipation, abdominal pain
CLIENT EDUCATION
- Prevent weight gain. (Eat a balanced diet. Eliminate high-fat, high-sugar foods from the diet.)
- Develop an exercise plan.

Hypersensitivity reactions (angioedema)
CLIENT EDUCATION: Stop taking the medication and notify the provider or call 911 immediately for rash, hives, dyspnea, or swelling of the face or tongue.

Rhabdomyolysis
- Acute onset of severe muscle weakness and tenderness with elevation of serum creatinine kinase
- Client education: Notify the provider of manifestations. Medication will need to be discontinued if rhabdomyolysis occurs.

Erectile dysfunction and anorgasmia
CLIENT EDUCATION: Report manifestations of sexual dysfunction.

CONTRAINDICATIONS/PRECAUTIONS

Serotonin-norepinephrine reuptake inhibitors

- Pregnancy Risk Category C
- Contraindicated in clients who have hepatic or kidney impairment or those taking MAOIs within 14 days.
- Use with caution in clients who have cardiac problems, hypertension, diabetes, gastrointestinal disorders, and glaucoma.

GABA

- Pregnancy Risk Category C
- Dose might need to be adjusted in older adult clients and clients who have kidney impairment. Ⓖ
- Use with caution in clients who have cardiac problems, hypertension, diabetes, kidney impairment, mental illness, angioedema, and thrombocytopenia.

INTERACTIONS

Serotonin-norepinephrine reuptake inhibitors

SSRIs increase risk for serotonin syndrome.
CLIENT EDUCATION: Notify the provider of suicidal thoughts.

Anticoagulants, warfarin, and NSAIDs, which increase the risk of bleeding (GI bleed)
NURSING ACTIONS: Notify provider for manifestations of internal bleeding (blood in stools).

Diuretics increase risk of low serum sodium levels.
NURSING ACTIONS: Monitor serum sodium levels.

GABA

ACE inhibitors increase risk of angioedema.
CLIENT EDUCATION: Use cool compresses and notify the provider.

Benzodiazepines increase drowsiness.
CLIENT EDUCATION: Do not drive or operate heavy machinery.

Thiazolidinedione (antidiabetic agent) increases risk of weight gain and peripheral edema.
CLIENT EDUCATION
- Follow a healthy, well-balanced diet and get regular activity to help counteract weight gain.
- Elevate extremities for peripheral edema.

Alcohol increases drowsiness and dizziness.
CLIENT EDUCATION: Do not consume alcohol while taking this medication.

NURSING ADMINISTRATION

Serotonin-norepinephrine reuptake inhibitors

- Administered orally without regard to food.
- Swallow capsule whole, do not crush or open capsule.
- Taper withdrawal gradually over 2 weeks.

GABA

- Administered orally with or without food.
- Notify provider if suicidal thoughts are present. Qs
- Taper withdrawal gradually over at least 1 week.

NURSING EVALUATION OF MEDICATION EFFECTIVENESS

Depending on the therapeutic intent, effectiveness can be evidenced by a decrease in manifestations of fibromyalgia.

Antigout medication

ANTI-INFLAMMATORY AGENTS

SELECT PROTOTYPE MEDICATION: Colchicine
- Once considered the medication of choice for acute gout, colchicine is now usually reserved for clients who do not respond to or cannot tolerate safer agents.

OTHER MEDICATIONS
- **NSAIDs**
  - Indomethacin
  - Naproxen
  - Diclofenac
- **Glucocorticoids:** Prednisone

PURPOSE

EXPECTED PHARMACOLOGICAL ACTION
- Colchicine is only effective for inflammation caused by gout.
- These medications decrease inflammation.

THERAPEUTIC USES
- Abort an acute gout attack in response to precursor manifestations
- Treatment of acute attacks
- Decrease incidence of acute attacks for clients who have chronic gout
- Prednisone is used for clients who have acute gout who are unable to take or unresponsive to NSAIDs. This medication is not for use in clients who have hyperglycemia.

ROUTE OF ADMINISTRATION: Colchicine (oral)

AGENTS FOR HYPERURICEMIA

For clients who have chronic gout or frequent gout attacks

SELECT PROTOTYPE MEDICATION: Allopurinol

OTHER MEDICATIONS: Febuxostat, probenecid

PURPOSE

EXPECTED PHARMACOLOGICAL ACTION: Allopurinol and febuxostat inhibit uric acid production. Probenecid inhibits uric acid reabsorption by renal tubules

THERAPEUTIC USES: Hyperuricemia due to chronic gout or secondary to cancer chemotherapy.

ROUTE OF ADMINISTRATION
- Allopurinol (oral, IV)
- Colchicine (oral)

COMPLICATIONS

Colchicine

Mild GI distress, which can progress to GI toxicity
- Abdominal pain, diarrhea, nausea, vomiting
- NURSING ACTIONS: Provide antidiarrheal agents.
  - Client education
  - Take oral medications with food.
  - If severe GI distress occurs, stop colchicine and notify the provider.

Thrombocytopenia, bone marrow suppression
CLIENT EDUCATION: Notify the provider of bleeding, bruising, or sore throat.

Sudden onset of muscle pain, tenderness
- Rhabdomyolysis
- CLIENT EDUCATION: Notify the provider for new onset of these findings.

Probenecid

Renal calculi and kidney injury
- Occur with higher excretion of uric acid
- CLIENT EDUCATION: Drink 2.5 to 3 L fluid daily to decrease risk.

Gastrointestinal effects
CLIENT EDUCATION: Take medication with food to decrease GI effects.

Hypersensitivity reactions (rash)
CLIENT EDUCATION: Report any rash to the provider.

Acute exacerbation of gout
Treatment should be delayed until the acute attack has been controlled.

Allopurinol

Hypersensitivity reaction, fever, rash, kidney and liver damage
NURSING ACTIONS: If administering IV, ensure the infusion is stopped. Severe reaction can require hemodialysis or glucocorticoids.

Kidney injury
NURSING ACTIONS
- Alkalinize the urine and encourage intake of 2 to 3 L of fluids/day.
- Monitor I&O, BUN, and creatinine.

Hepatitis
NURSING ACTIONS: Monitor liver enzymes.

GI distress (nausea, vomiting)
NURSING ACTIONS: Administer with food.

Increase in gout attacks
- During the first months of treatment
- CLIENT EDUCATION: Report increased gout attacks to the provider. Colchicine or an NSAID can be prescribed with allopurinol to prevent this.

CONTRAINDICATIONS/PRECAUTIONS

Colchicine

- Pregnancy Risk Category C
- Contraindicated for clients who have severe kidney, cardiac, hepatic, or gastrointestinal dysfunction
- Use cautiously in older adults and clients who are debilitated or have blood disorders or mild to moderate hepatic dysfunction. ⓒ

Probenecid

- Pregnancy Risk Category C
- Can precipitate acute gout. Do not give within 2 to 3 weeks of an acute attack.

Allopurinol

- Pregnancy Risk Category C
- Contraindicated in clients who have medication hypersensitivity or idiopathic hemochromatosis
- Rhabdomyolysis is most likely with long-term use. Risk is higher in clients taking statins for high cholesterol and those who have impaired kidneys or liver.

INTERACTIONS

Colchicine

Grapefruit or grapefruit juice can increase adverse effects.
CLIENT EDUCATION: Avoid eating grapefruit or drinking grapefruit juice when taking colchicine.

Probenecid

Salicylates can lessen the effectiveness of probenecid and can precipitate gout.
CLIENT EDUCATION: Do not use salicylates during colchicine/probenecid therapy.

Probenecid inhibits renal excretion of some medications (indomethacin, sulfonamides).
Dosage of medications might need to be reduced.

Allopurinol

Allopurinol slows the metabolism of warfarin within the liver, which places clients at risk for bleeding.
- Allopurinol should not be combined with theophylline.
- NURSING ACTIONS: Monitor prothrombin time and INR levels, and adjust warfarin dosages accordingly.
- CLIENT EDUCATION: Observe for manifestations of bleeding (bruising, petechiae, hematuria).

NURSING ADMINISTRATION

- Monitor uric acid levels, CBC, urinalysis, and liver and kidney function tests.
- Ensure allopurinol IV is well diluted and administered as an infusion over 30 to 60 min.
- Advise clients to take oral gout medication with food or after meals to minimize GI distress.
- **Allopurinol and probenecid:** If a rash develops, advise clients to stop the medication and report the occurrence to the provider.
- Instruct clients to concurrently take preventive measures, such as avoiding alcohol and foods high in purine (red meat, scallops). Assist clients in determining what foods precipitate their gout attacks and in avoiding these foods. Clients should ensure an adequate intake of water, exercise regularly, and maintain an appropriate body weight. Qᴘᴄᴄ

NURSING EVALUATION OF MEDICATION EFFECTIVENESS

Depending on the therapeutic intent, effectiveness can be evidenced by the following.
- Improvement of pain caused by a gout attack (decrease in joint swelling, redness, uric acid levels)
- Decrease in number of gout attacks
- Decrease in uric acid levels

Application Exercises

1. A nurse is reinforcing teaching with a client who has gout and a new prescription for allopurinol. For which of the following adverse effects should the client monitor? (Select all that apply.)

   A. Stomatitis

   B. Insomnia

   C. Nausea

   D. Rash

   E. Increased gout pain

2. A nurse is caring for a client who has a new prescription for adalimumab for rheumatoid arthritis. Based on the route of administration of adalimumab, which of the following should the nurse plan to monitor?

   A. The vein for thrombophlebitis during IV administration

   B. The subcutaneous site for redness following injection

   C. The oral mucosa for ulceration after oral administration

   D. The skin for irritation following removal of transdermal patch

3. A nurse is caring for a client who has a new diagnosis of fibromyalgia. Which of the following medications should the nurse anticipate being prescribed for this client?

   A. Colchicine

   B. Hydroxychloroquine

   C. Auranofin

   D. Duloxetine

4. A nurse is reinforcing teaching with a client who has rheumatoid arthritis and a new prescription for methotrexate. Which of the following client statements indicates understanding?

   A. "I will be sure to return to the clinic yearly to have my blood drawn while I'm taking methotrexate."

   B. "I will take this medication on an empty stomach."

   C. "I'll let the doctor know if I develop sores in my mouth while taking this medication.

   D. "I should stop taking oral contraceptives while I'm taking methotrexate."

5. A nurse is caring for a client who has a prescription for cyclosporine to treat rheumatoid arthritis. Which of the following medications increases the risk of toxicity when taken concurrently with cyclosporine?

   A. Phenytoin

   B. Rifampin

   C. Carbamazepine

   D. Erythromycin

PRACTICE Active Learning Scenario

A nurse is reinforcing teaching with a client who has rheumatoid arthritis (RA) and a new prescription for etanercept. What should the nurse reinforce with the client about this medication? Use the ATI Active Learning Template: Medication to complete this item.

THERAPEUTIC USES: Describe the therapeutic use for etanercept in this client.

COMPLICATIONS: Describe at least three adverse effects the client should monitor for.

NURSING INTERVENTIONS: Describe one for each of the adverse effects above.

MEDICATION ADMINISTRATION: Describe at least three important factors.

Application Exercises Key

1. A. Stomatitis occurs with medications that increase the risk of infection, such as many of the DMARDs used to treat rheumatoid arthritis. Allopurinol does not increase a client's risk for infection.

   B. Insomnia is not an adverse effect of allopurinol.

   C. **CORRECT:** Nausea and vomiting can be caused by allopurinol.

   D. **CORRECT:** Rash and other hypersensitivity reactions can be caused by allopurinol. The client should contact the provider for manifestations of hypersensitivity so that the medication can be discontinued.

   E. **CORRECT:** An increase in gout attacks can occur during the first few months of taking allopurinol.

   Ⓝ *NCLEX® Connection: Pharmacological Therapies, Adverse Effects/ Contraindications/Side Effects/Interactions*

2. A. Adalimumab is not administered IV. Monitoring for thrombophlebitis during administration is not necessary.

   B. **CORRECT:** Adalimumab is administered subcutaneously, and injection-site redness and swelling are common. The nurse should monitor the site for redness following injection.

   C. Adalimumab is not administered orally. Monitoring oral mucosa for ulceration following administration is not necessary.

   D. Adalimumab is not administered transdermally. Inspecting the skin for irritation is not necessary.

   Ⓝ *NCLEX® Connection: Pharmacological Therapies, Medication Administration*

3. A. Colchicine is an anti-inflammatory medication used to treat gout.

   B. Hydroxychloroquine is an anti-malarial medication used as a DMARD along with methotrexate to treat rheumatoid arthritis.

   C. Auranofin is a gold salt used to relief joint pain and stiffness in clients who have rheumatoid arthritis.

   D. **CORRECT:** Duloxetine is a serotonin-norepinephrine reuptake inhibitor used to treat fibromyalgia. Other uses for this medication include treating depression and diabetic peripheral neuropathy.

   Ⓝ *NCLEX® Connection: Pharmacological Therapies, Expected Actions/Outcomes*

4. A. CBC (including platelet count), liver, and kidney function tests are monitored at baseline and frequently during treatment with methotrexate to check for adverse effects.

   B. Methotrexate should be taken with food to decrease gastrointestinal distress.

   C. **CORRECT:** Ulcerations in the mouth, tongue, or throat are often the first findings of methotrexate toxicity and should be reported to the provider immediately.

   D. Methotrexate is a Pregnancy Category X medication and can cause severe fetal damage. The client should have a pregnancy test before starting the medication and should use a reliable form of birth control during methotrexate therapy. Oral contraceptives are not contraindicated with methotrexate therapy.

   Ⓝ *NCLEX® Connection: Pharmacological Therapies, Expected Actions/Outcomes*

5. A. Phenytoin can decrease cyclosporine levels and would not cause cyclosporine toxicity.

   B. Rifampin can decrease cyclosporine levels and would not cause cyclosporine toxicity.

   C. Carbamazepine can decrease cyclosporine levels and would not cause cyclosporine toxicity.

   D. **CORRECT:** Erythromycin increases cyclosporine levels. Cyclosporine toxicity can result when the two medications are taken concurrently.

   Ⓝ *NCLEX® Connection: Pharmacological Therapies, Adverse Effects/ Contraindications/Side Effects/Interactions*

PRACTICE Answer

Using the ATI Active Learning Template: Medication

THERAPEUTIC USES: Etanercept is a biologic DMARD classified as a tumor necrosis factor antagonist. It suppresses manifestations of moderate to severe RA and slows the progression of the disorder.

COMPLICATIONS
- Severe infections (tuberculosis, reactivation of hepatitis B)
- Heart failure
- Severe skin reactions, such as Stevens-Johnson syndrome
- Hematologic disorders

NURSING INTERVENTIONS
- Instruct clients to monitor for infection, and to report sore throat and other manifestations.
- Discuss reasons for TB testing and possible hepatitis B testing.
- Instruct clients to notify the provider for edema, shortness of breath, and other manifestations of heart failure.
- Report skin rash to the provider.
- Report easy bruising, bleeding, or unusual fatigue to the provider.

MEDICATION ADMINISTRATION
- Administer by subcutaneous injection twice weekly.
- Discard solutions that are discolored or contain particulate matter.
- Monitor for injection-site reactions, and report them to the provider.
- Rotate injection sites.
- Avoid skin areas that are bruised or reddened when injecting.

Ⓝ *NCLEX® Connection: Pharmacological and Parenteral Therapies, Medication Administration*

UNIT 8   MEDICATIONS FOR JOINT AND BONE CONDITIONS

CHAPTER 29 *Bone Disorders*

Calcium is necessary for the proper functioning of the heart, bones, nerves, muscles, and blood coagulation. It can be given as a supplement when dietary intake is insufficient. Other medications are also used for prevention and treatment of osteoporosis and prevention of fractures.

Medication classifications include calcium supplements, selective estrogen receptor modulators (also known as estrogen agonist/antagonists), bisphosphonates, and calcitonin.

Calcium supplements

SELECT PROTOTYPE MEDICATION: Calcium citrate

OTHER MEDICATIONS
- Calcium carbonate
- Calcium acetate
- **For IV administration**
  - Calcium chloride
  - Calcium gluconate

PURPOSE

EXPECTED PHARMACOLOGICAL ACTION

- Maintenance of musculoskeletal, neurological, and cardiovascular function
- Maintenance of calcium levels

THERAPEUTIC USES

- Oral calcium supplements are used for clients who have hypocalcemia or deficiencies of parathyroid hormone, vitamin D, or dietary calcium.
- Oral dietary supplements are used for adolescents, older adults, and clients who are postmenopausal, pregnant, or breastfeeding. Ⓖ
- IV medications are used for clients who have critically low levels of calcium.

COMPLICATIONS

Hypercalcemia

Calcium level greater than 10.5 mg/dL
- Initial findings include tachycardia and elevated blood pressure eventually leading to bradycardia and hypotension. Other findings include muscle weakness, hypotonia, constipation, nausea, vomiting, abdominal pain, lethargy, and confusion.
- Medications used to prevent hypercalcemia include bisphosphonates (alendronate, oral inorganic phosphates).

NURSING ACTIONS
- Monitor serum calcium levels to maintain between 9 and 10.5 mg/dL.
- Monitor infusion of 0.9% sodium chloride IV.
- Medications used to reverse hypercalcemia include IV furosemide, and calcium chelators (plicamycin).

CLIENT EDUCATION: Monitor for manifestations and report them to the provider.

CONTRAINDICATIONS/PRECAUTIONS

- Calcium supplements are contraindicated in clients who have hypercalcemia, renal calculi, hypophosphatemia, digoxin toxicity, or ventricular fibrillation. Qs
- Use cautiously in clients who have kidney disease or a decrease in GI function.

INTERACTIONS

Concurrent use of glucocorticoids reduces absorption of calcium.
NURSING ACTIONS: Give at least 1 hr apart.

Concurrent use of calcium decreases absorption of tetracyclines and thyroid hormone.
NURSING ACTIONS: Give at least 1 hr apart.

Concurrent administration of thiazide diuretics increases risk of hypercalcemia.
NURSING ACTIONS
- Monitor for hypercalcemia.
- Avoid concurrent use.

Spinach, rhubarb, beets, bran, and whole grains can decrease calcium absorption.
- NURSING ACTIONS: Do not administer calcium with foods that decrease absorption.
- CLIENT EDUCATION: Avoid consuming these foods at the same time as taking calcium.

IV calcium precipitates with phosphates, carbonates, sulfates, and tartrates.
NURSING ACTIONS: Ensure parenteral calcium is not mixed with compounds that cause precipitation.

Concurrent use of digoxin and parenteral calcium can lead to severe bradycardia.
NURSING ACTIONS: Ensure IV injection of calcium is given slowly with careful monitoring of client cardiac status. Qs

NURSING ADMINISTRATION

- Instruct clients to take a calcium supplement at least 1 hr apart from glucocorticoids, tetracyclines, or thyroid hormone.
- Chewable tablets provide more consistent bioavailability.
- Recommended doses of oral calcium vary depending on the specific calcium preparation. Instruct the client to follow the prescription.
- Advise clients to take oral calcium with 8 oz water.
- Ensure that prior to administration, IV infusions of calcium are body temperature.
- Ensure IV infusions are administered at a rate of 0.5 to 2 mL/min.

NURSING EVALUATION OF MEDICATION EFFECTIVENESS

Depending on therapeutic intent, effectiveness is evidenced by serum calcium level within expected reference range: 9.0 to 10.5 mg/dL.

Selective estrogen receptor modulator (agonist/antagonist)

SELECT PROTOTYPE MEDICATION: Raloxifene

PURPOSE

EXPECTED PHARMACOLOGICAL ACTION

- Works as endogenous estrogen in bone, lipid metabolism, and blood coagulation
- Decreases bone resorption, which slows bone loss and preserves bone mineral density
- Works as an antagonist to estrogen on breast and endometrial tissue
- Can decrease plasma levels of cholesterol

THERAPEUTIC USES

- Prevent and treat postmenopausal osteoporosis to prevent spinal fractures in female clients
- Protect against breast cancer

COMPLICATIONS

Increased risk for pulmonary embolism and deep-vein thrombosis (DVT)

Medication should be stopped prior to scheduled immobilization, such as surgery. Medication can be resumed when the client is fully mobile.

NURSING ACTIONS
- Monitor for manifestations of DVT, such as red, swollen calves.
- Discourage long periods of sitting and inactivity.

Hot flashes

CLIENT EDUCATION: The medication can exacerbate hot flashes.

CONTRAINDICATIONS/PRECAUTIONS

- Raloxifene is Pregnancy Risk Category X.
- This medication is contraindicated in clients who have a history of venous thrombosis.
- The medication should be stopped 3 days before periods in which risk of DVT is high, such as surgical procedures. Qs

INTERACTIONS

Concurrent use with estrogen hormone therapy is discouraged.

NURSING ADMINISTRATION

- For maximum benefit of the medication, encourage clients to consume adequate amounts of calcium (such as from dairy products) and vitamin D (such as from egg yolks). Inadequate amounts of dietary calcium and vitamin D cause release of parathyroid hormone, which stimulates calcium release from the bone.
- Take medication with or without food once per day.
- Monitor bone density. Clients should undergo a bone density scan every 12 to 18 months.
- Monitor serum calcium. Expected reference range is 9 to 10.5 mg/dL.
- Monitor liver function tests. Raloxifene levels can increase in clients who have hepatic impairment.
- Encourage clients to perform weight-bearing exercises (such as walking 30 to 40 min) daily.

NURSING EVALUATION OF MEDICATION EFFECTIVENESS

Depending on therapeutic intent, effectiveness is evidenced by the following.
- Increase in bone density
- No fractures

Bisphosphonates

SELECT PROTOTYPE MEDICATION: Alendronate

OTHER MEDICATIONS
- Ibandronate
- Risedronate
- **For IV infusion:** Zoledronic

PURPOSE

EXPECTED PHARMACOLOGICAL ACTION

Bisphosphonates decrease the number and action of osteoclasts, and inhibit bone resorption.

THERAPEUTIC USES

- Prophylaxis and treatment of postmenopausal osteoporosis
- For male clients who have osteoporosis
- Prophylaxis and treatment of osteoporosis produced by long-term glucocorticoid use
- For clients who have Paget's disease of the bone

COMPLICATIONS

Esophagitis, esophageal ulceration (oral formulations)

CLIENT EDUCATION
- Sit upright or ambulate for 30 min after taking this medication orally. Q_{EBP}
- If taking ibandronate, remain upright and do not ingest food or other medications for 1 hr after taking the medication orally.
- Take tablets with at least 240 mL (8 oz) water and liquid formulation with at least 60 mL (2 oz).
- Discontinue the medication and contact the provider for difficulty swallowing or new heartburn.

GI disturbances (all bisphosphonates)

Abdominal pain, nausea, diarrhea, constipation

NURSING ACTIONS: Notify the provider for GI problems that prevent adequate intake.

Musculoskeletal pain

CLIENT EDUCATION
- Take a mild analgesic.
- Notify the provider if pain persists. Alternate medication can be prescribed.

Visual disturbances

Blurred vision, eye pain

CLIENT EDUCATION: Watch for manifestations and report them to the provider. Medication should be discontinued.

Bisphosphonate-related osteonecrosis of the jaw

With IV infusion

CLIENT EDUCATION
- See a dentist prior to beginning treatment.
- Avoid dental work during administration of medication.

Kidney toxicity with IV infusion

NURSING ACTIONS: Monitor kidney function and hydration status.

CONTRAINDICATIONS/PRECAUTIONS

- Most bisphosphonates are Pregnancy Risk Category C. Zoledronic acid is Pregnancy Risk Category D.
- These medications are contraindicated for clients who have dysphagia, esophageal stricture, esophageal disorders, serious kidney impairment, or hypocalcemia.
- These medications should not be administered to clients who cannot sit upright or stand for at least 30 min after medication administration.
- Use cautiously for clients who are lactating or have upper GI disorders, infection, or liver impairment.
- Older adults are at slight risk for femoral fractures, which can occur without trauma while taking bisphosphonates. Ⓖ

INTERACTIONS

Alendronate absorption decreases when taken with calcium, iron, magnesium supplements, antacids, orange juice, and caffeine.
CLIENT EDUCATION
- Take the medication on an empty stomach with at least 240 mL (8 oz) water.
- Wait 30 min after administration to take antacids or supplements.

NURSING ADMINISTRATION

- Tablets are prescribed once per day or once per week. The liquid form is prescribed once per week.
- Monitor bone density. Clients should have a bone density scan every 12 to 18 months.
- Monitor serum calcium. Expected reference range is 9 to 10.5 mg/dL.

CLIENT EDUCATION Q_{PCC}
- Take the medication first thing in the morning after getting out of bed.
- Take oral medication on an empty stomach, drinking at least 240 mL (8 oz) water with tablets and at least 60 mL (2 oz) water with liquid formulation.
- Sit, stand, or ambulate for 30 min after taking the medication.
- Avoid all foods and liquids or any medications within 30 min of taking alendronate.

- Avoid chewing or sucking on the tablet.
- Perform weight-bearing exercises (such as walking 30 to 40 min) daily.
- Notify the provider of difficulty swallowing, painful swallowing, or new or worsening heartburn.
- If a dose is skipped, wait until the next day 30 min before eating breakfast to take the dose. Do not take two tablets on the same day.
- For maximum benefit of the medication, consume adequate amounts of calcium and vitamin D.

NURSING EVALUATION OF MEDICATION EFFECTIVENESS

Depending on therapeutic intent, effectiveness is evidenced by the following.
- Increase in bone density
- No fractures

Calcitonin

SELECT PROTOTYPE MEDICATION: Calcitonin-salmon

PURPOSE

EXPECTED PHARMACOLOGICAL ACTION
- Decreases bone resorption by inhibiting the activity of osteoclasts in osteoporosis
- Increases renal calcium excretion by inhibiting tubular resorption

THERAPEUTIC USES: Treat (but not prevent) postmenopausal osteoporosis, moderate to severe Paget's disease, hypercalcemia caused by hyperparathyroidism, and cancer

COMPLICATIONS

Nausea

CLIENT EDUCATION: Nausea is usually self-limiting.

Nasal dryness and irritation with intranasal route

CLIENT EDUCATION
- Alternate nostrils daily.
- Inspect nasal mucosa periodically for ulceration.

CONTRAINDICATIONS/PRECAUTIONS

- This medication is Pregnancy Risk Category C.
- The medication is contraindicated in clients who have hypersensitivity to the medication or fish protein. Perform an allergy skin test prior to administration if the client is at risk.
- Use cautiously with children and clients who are lactating or have kidney disease.
- Intranasal spray is only approved for treatment of postmenopausal osteoporosis.

INTERACTIONS

Concurrent use with lithium can decrease serum lithium levels.
NURSING ACTIONS: Monitor lithium levels closely.

NURSING ADMINISTRATION

- Calcitonin-salmon is most commonly given by nasal spray. It can also be given IM or subcutaneously. Rotate injection sites to prevent inflammation. Qpcc
- Keep the container in an upright position.
- Instruct clients to alternate nostrils daily.
- Check for Chvostek's or Trousseau's signs to monitor for hypocalcemia.
- Monitor bone density scans periodically.
- Encourage clients to consume a diet high in calcium and vitamin D.

NURSING EVALUATION OF MEDICATION EFFECTIVENESS

Depending on therapeutic intent, effectiveness is evidenced by the following.
- Increase in bone density
- Serum calcium level within the expected reference range of 9 to 10.5 mg/dL

Application Exercises

1. A nurse is reinforcing teaching with a client who is taking raloxifene to prevent postmenopausal osteoporosis. Which of the following are possible adverse effects of this medication? (Select all that apply.)

   A. Hot flashes

   B. Lump in breast

   C. Swelling or redness in calf

   D. Shortness of breath

   E. Difficulty swallowing

2. A nurse is assisting with the care of a client who has hypocalcemia and is receiving IV calcium gluconate. The nurse should monitor the client for which of the following manifestations as an indication of hypercalcemia? (Select all that apply.)

   A. Nausea

   B. Diarrhea

   C. Muscle weakness

   D. Blurred vision

   E. Abdominal pain

3. A nurse is caring for a client who has a new prescription for calcitonin-salmon for osteoporosis. Which of the following tests should the nurse expect before beginning this medication?

   A. Skin test for allergy to the medication

   B. ECG to rule out cardiac dysrhythmias

   C. Mantoux test to rule out exposure to tuberculosis

   D. Liver function tests to determine risk for medication toxicity

4. A nurse is caring for a young adult client whose serum calcium is 8.8 mg/dL. Which of the following medications should the nurse anticipate administering to this client?

   A. Calcitonin-salmon

   B. Calcium carbonate

   C. Zoledronic acid

   D. Ibandronate

5. A nurse is reinforcing teaching with a client who has a new prescription for calcitonin-salmon for postmenopausal osteoporosis. Which of the following instructions should the nurse provide?

   A. Swallow tablets on an empty stomach with plenty of water.

   B. Watch for skin rash and redness when applying calcitonin-salmon topically.

   C. Mix the liquid medication with juice and take it after meals.

   D. Alternate nostrils each time calcitonin-salmon is inhaled.

PRACTICE Active Learning Scenario

A nurse in a provider's office is reinforcing teaching with a client who is postmenopausal and at high risk for osteoporosis about a new prescription for alendronate. What information should the nurse reinforce with the client about this medication? Use the ATI Active Learning Template: Medication to complete this item.

THERAPEUTIC USES: Identify the therapeutic use for alendronate.

COMPLICATIONS: List two adverse effects of this medication.

DIAGNOSTIC TESTS: Describe two diagnostic tests to monitor.

NURSING INTERVENTIONS: Describe two nursing actions.

Application Exercises Key

1. A. **CORRECT:** Raloxifene can cause hot flashes or increase existing hot flashes.

   B. Raloxifene does not cause breast lumps. It is used therapeutically to protect against breast and endometrial cancer.

   C. **CORRECT:** Raloxifene increases the risk for thrombophlebitis, which can cause swelling or redness in the calf.

   D. **CORRECT:** Raloxifene increases the risk for pulmonary embolism, which can cause shortness of breath.

   E. Difficulty swallowing due to esophagitis is an adverse effect of bisphosphonates (such as alendronate), but is not an adverse effect of raloxifene.

   Ⓝ *NCLEX® Connection: Pharmacological Therapies, Adverse Effects/ Contraindications/Side Effects/Interactions*

2. A. **CORRECT:** Nausea is a manifestation of hypercalcemia.

   B. Constipation, not diarrhea, is a manifestation of hypercalcemia.

   C. **CORRECT:** Muscle weakness is a manifestation of hypercalcemia.

   D. Blurred vision is not a manifestation of hypercalcemia.

   E. **CORRECT:** Abdominal pain is a manifestation of hypercalcemia.

   Ⓝ *NCLEX® Connection: Pharmacological Therapies, Expected Actions/Outcomes*

3. A. **CORRECT:** Anaphylaxis can occur if the client is allergic to calcitonin-salmon. A skin test to determine allergy can be done before starting this medication. The nurse also should ask the client about allergies to fish.

   B. An ECG to rule out cardiac dysrhythmias is not necessary before beginning calcitonin-salmon. This medication does not affect heart rhythm.

   C. A Mantoux test to rule out exposure to tuberculosis is not necessary before beginning calcitonin-salmon. This medication does not affect resistance to TB.

   D. Liver function tests are not necessary before beginning calcitonin-salmon. This medication is metabolized in the kidneys and does not affect the liver.

   Ⓝ *NCLEX® Connection: Pharmacological Therapies, Expected Actions/Outcomes*

4. A. Calcitonin-salmon increases excretion of calcium and should not be given to a client who has a serum calcium of 8.8 mg/dL.

   B. **CORRECT:** The client's serum calcium level is below the expected reference range. Calcium carbonate is an oral form of calcium used to increase serum calcium to the expected reference range.

   C. Zoledronic acid is an IV bisphosphonate used to treat osteoporosis. This medication can decrease serum calcium levels by inhibiting bone resorption of calcium, and should not be given to a client who has a serum calcium of 8.8 mg/dL.

   D. Ibandronate is a bisphosphonate used to treat osteoporosis. This medication can decrease serum calcium levels by inhibiting bone reabsorption of calcium. It should not be given to a client who has a serum calcium of 8.8 mg/dL.

   Ⓝ *NCLEX® Connection: Pharmacological Therapies, Medication Administration*

5. A. Clients should drink at least 240 mL (8 oz) water with alendronate tablets and take it on an empty stomach to promote absorption and prevent esophagitis.

   B. Calcitonin-salmon is not available as a topical preparation.

   C. Clients should drink at least 60 mL (2 oz) water with alendronate liquid solution.

   D. **CORRECT:** Calcitonin-salmon can be administered IM or subcutaneously, but is commonly administered intranasally for postmenopausal osteoporosis. The client should alternate nostrils daily.

   Ⓝ *NCLEX® Connection: Pharmacological Therapies, Expected Actions/Outcomes*

PRACTICE Answer

Using the ATI Active Learning Template: Medication

THERAPEUTIC USES: In the client who is at high risk for osteoporosis, the purpose of alendronate is to prevent osteoporosis from occurring by decreasing resorption of bone. The medication also is used to treat osteoporosis and Paget's disease.

COMPLICATIONS: Alendronate can cause esophagitis, esophageal ulceration, and other GI effects (nausea, diarrhea, constipation); muscle pain; and visual disturbances. Rarely, it can cause atraumatic femoral fracture.

DIAGNOSTIC TESTS: Serum calcium, bone density scans

Ⓝ *NCLEX® Connection: Pharmacological and Parenteral Therapies, Medication Administration*

NURSING INTERVENTIONS
- Check the client's ability to follow administration directions (must be able to sit or stand for at least 30 min after taking alendronate).
- Instruct the client to take this medication first thing in the morning with at least 240 mL (8 oz) water and wait 30 min before eating or drinking anything else or taking any other medications or supplements.
- Reinforce teaching with the client about other ways to help prevent osteoporosis, such as performing weight-bearing exercises daily and obtaining adequate amounts of calcium and vitamin D.

NCLEX® Connections

When reviewing the following chapters, keep in mind the relevant topics and tasks of the NCLEX outline, in particular:

Pharmacological Therapies

MEDICATION ADMINISTRATION: Identify the client's need for PRN medications.

PHARMACOLOGICAL PAIN MANAGEMENT
Monitor and document the client's response to pharmacological interventions (pain rating scale, verbal reports).

Maintain pain control devices (epidural, patient-controlled analgesia, peripheral nerve catheter).

UNIT 9   MEDICATIONS FOR PAIN AND INFLAMMATION

CHAPTER 30 *Nonopioid Analgesics*

Nonopioid analgesics can have anti-inflammatory, antipyretic, and analgesic actions. These medications include nonsteroidal anti-inflammatory drugs (NSAIDs) and acetaminophen.

Nonsteroidal anti-inflammatory drugs

SELECT PROTOTYPE MEDICATIONS

- **First-generation NSAIDs (COX-1 and COX-2 inhibitors)**
  - Aspirin
  - Ibuprofen
  - Naproxen
  - Indomethacin
  - Diclofenac
  - Ketorolac
  - Meloxicam
- **Second-generation NSAIDs (selective COX-2 inhibitor):** Celecoxib

PURPOSE

EXPECTED PHARMACOLOGICAL ACTION

Inhibition of cyclooxygenase: Inhibition of COX-1 can result in decreased platelet aggregation and kidney damage, while inhibition of COX-2 results in decreased inflammation, fever, and pain and does not decrease platelet aggregation.

THERAPEUTIC USES

- Inflammation suppression
- Analgesia for mild to moderate pain, such as with osteoarthritis and rheumatoid arthritis
- Fever reduction
- Dysmenorrhea
- Inhibition of platelet aggregation, which protects against ischemic stroke and myocardial infarction (aspirin)

COMPLICATIONS

Gastrointestinal (GI) effects

Dyspepsia, abdominal pain, heartburn, nausea
- Damage to gastric mucosa can lead to GI bleeding and perforation, especially with long-term use.
- Risks increase for older adults, clients who smoke or have alcohol use disorder, and those who have a history of peptic ulcers or previous inability to tolerate NSAIDs.
- Some providers prescribe prophylactic medications, such as misoprostol.

NURSING ACTIONS
- Observe for indications of GI bleeding (passage of black or dark-colored stools, severe abdominal pain, nausea, vomiting).
- Administer a proton pump inhibitor (such as omeprazole) or an H_2 receptor antagonist (such as ranitidine) to decrease the risk of ulcer formation.

CLIENT EDUCATION
- Take the medication with food or with 240 mL (8 oz) water or milk.
- Avoid alcohol.

Impaired kidney function

Decreased urine output, weight gain from fluid retention, increased BUN, creatinine levels

Older adults and clients who have heart failure are particularly at risk.

NURSING ACTIONS: Monitor I&O and kidney function (BUN, creatinine).

Increased risks of heart attack, stroke

With nonaspirin NSAIDs

NURSING ACTIONS: Suggest the smallest effective dosage for clients who have cardiovascular disease.

Salicylism (aspirin)

Manifestations include tinnitus, sweating, flushing, headache, dizziness, drowsiness, confusion, nausea, vomiting, diarrhea, tachycardia, tachypnea, and respiratory alkalosis.

CLIENT EDUCATION: Notify the provider and stop taking aspirin if these manifestations occur.

Reye syndrome

Giving aspirin to children and adolescents who have a viral illness (chickenpox, influenza) can cause this rare but serious complication.

CLIENT EDUCATION: Avoid giving aspirin to a child or adolescent who has a viral illness. Qs

Aspirin toxicity

Progresses from the mild findings with salicylism to high fever, acidosis, dehydration, electrolyte imbalances, coma, respiratory depression, respiratory failure
- Aspirin toxicity is a medical emergency.
- Activated charcoal can decrease absorption.
- Hemodialysis might be necessary.

NURSING ACTIONS
- Cool the client with tepid water.
- Assist with correcting dehydration and electrolyte imbalance with IV fluids.
- Assist with reversing acidosis and promoting salicylate excretion with bicarbonate.
- Perform gastric lavage.

CONTRAINDICATIONS/PRECAUTIONS

First-generation NSAIDs

- Pregnancy Risk Category D
- Peptic ulcer disease
- Bleeding disorders (hemophilia, vitamin K deficiency)
- Hypersensitivity to aspirin and other NSAIDs
- Children and adolescents who have chickenpox or influenza (aspirin)

NURSING ACTIONS: Use NSAIDs cautiously for the following.
- Older adult clients Ⓖ
- Clients who smoke cigarettes
- Clients who have *Helicobacter pylori* infection, hypovolemia, asthma, chronic urticaria, bleeding disorders, or a history of alcohol use disorder
- Clients taking anticoagulants, glucocorticoids, ACE inhibitors, or ARBs

Advanced kidney disease is a contraindication for receiving ketorolac. Use should be no longer than 5 days because of the risk for kidney damage. Qs

Second-generation NSAIDs

Clients who have cardiovascular disease require caution when taking second-generation NSAIDs.

Celecoxib suppresses inflammation, relieves pain, decreases fever, and protects against colorectal cancer.
- Celecoxib, an NSAID COX-2 inhibitor, is a last-choice medication for chronic pain due to the increased risks of myocardial infarction (MI) and stroke due to secondary suppression of vasodilation.
- An allergy to sulfonamides is a contraindication for receiving celecoxib.

INTERACTIONS

Anticoagulants (heparin, warfarin) increase the risk of bleeding.
- NURSING ACTIONS: Monitor PTT, PT, and INR.
- CLIENT EDUCATION: There is an increased risk of bleeding when taking an NSAID concurrently with an anticoagulant. Report indications of bleeding.

Glucocorticoids increase the risk of gastric bleeding.
CLIENT EDUCATION: Take antiulcer prophylaxis, such as misoprostol, to decrease the risk of gastric ulcer.

Alcohol increases the risk of bleeding.
CLIENT EDUCATION: Avoid consuming alcoholic beverages to decrease the risk of GI bleeding.

Ibuprofen decreases the antiplatelet effects of the low-dose aspirin clients take to prevent MI.
CLIENT EDUCATION: Do not take ibuprofen concurrently with aspirin.

Ketorolac and concurrent use of other NSAIDs increase the risk of known adverse effects.
CLIENT EDUCATION: Do not take ketorolac concurrently with other NSAIDs.

Many of these medications interact when taken concurrently or with other over-the-counter medications (antacids, herbal and natural products).
CLIENT EDUCATION: Tell the provider about any over-the-counter medications, vitamins, or herbal supplements before taking them.

NURSING ADMINISTRATION

- Advise clients to stop aspirin 1 week before elective surgery or expected date of childbirth. Q EBP
- Advise clients to take NSAIDs with food, milk, or 240 mL (8 oz) water to help prevent or minimize gastric discomfort.
- Instruct clients not to chew or crush enteric-coated or sustained-release aspirin tablets.
- Advise clients to notify the provider if manifestations of gastric discomfort or ulceration occur.
- Advise clients to notify the provider if manifestations of salicylism occur. They should stop taking aspirin and resume at a lower dosage after the manifestations resolve.
- Ketorolac is for short-term treatment of moderate to severe pain, such as during postoperative recovery.
  - Concurrent use with opioids allows for lower dosages of opioids and thus minimizes adverse effects (constipation, respiratory depression).
  - Clients receive ketorolac parenterally at first and then PO. Use should not be longer than 5 days because of the risk for kidney damage.

NURSING EVALUATION OF MEDICATION EFFECTIVENESS

Indications of effectiveness include the following.
- Reduction in inflammation
- Reduction of fever
- Relief from mild to moderate pain
- Absence of injury

Acetaminophen

PURPOSE

EXPECTED PHARMACOLOGICAL ACTION: Slows the production of prostaglandins in the CNS

THERAPEUTIC USES
- Analgesic (relief of pain) effects
- Antipyretic (reduction of fever) effects

COMPLICATIONS

Adverse effects are rare at therapeutic dosages.

Acute toxicity

Results in liver damage with early manifestations of nausea, vomiting, diarrhea, sweating, and abdominal discomfort progressing to hepatic failure, coma, and death

NURSING ACTIONS: Administer the antidote, acetylcysteine.

CLIENT EDUCATION
- Take acetaminophen at safe dosages and not to exceed 4 g/day. Carefully follow the provider's advice about administration to children.
- For concurrent malnutrition, limit acetaminophen to 3 g/day.
- If consuming more than three alcoholic drinks per day, limit acetaminophen to 2 g/day.
- Limit over-the-counter dosage of acetaminophen when taking a prescription for combination analgesics that contain acetaminophen.

CONTRAINDICATIONS/PRECAUTIONS

Clients who consume three or more alcoholic drinks per day and those taking warfarin require caution when taking acetaminophen. Qs

INTERACTIONS

Alcohol increases the risk of liver damage.
CLIENT EDUCATION: There is potential risk of liver damage with consumption of alcohol.

Acetaminophen slows the metabolism of warfarin, leading to increased levels of warfarin. This places clients at risk for bleeding.
- NURSING ACTIONS: Monitor prothrombin time and INR levels, and report them to the provider for dosage adjustment of warfarin.
- CLIENT EDUCATION: Observe for indications of bleeding (bruising, petechiae, hematuria).

NURSING ADMINISTRATION

- Acetaminophen is a component of many prescription and over-the-counter medications. Keep an ongoing total of daily acetaminophen intake, and follow prescribed dosages (no more than 4 g/day) to prevent toxicity. QEBP
- Administer acetaminophen with 240 mL (8 oz) water with or without food.
- The FDA recommends that clients take only one product containing acetaminophen at a time. Instruct clients to read medication labels carefully to determine the amount of acetaminophen in each dose.
- In the event of an overdose, clients receive acetylcysteine (the antidote for acetaminophen) IV or PO to prevent liver damage. PO administration through a nasogastric tube prevents emesis and subsequent aspiration.

NURSING EVALUATION OF MEDICATION EFFECTIVENESS

Indications of effectiveness include the following.
- Relief of pain
- Reduction of fever

Application Exercises

1. A nurse is collecting data from a client who has salicylism. Which of the following findings should the nurse expect? (Select all that apply.)

    A. Dizziness

    B. Diarrhea

    C. Jaundice

    D. Tinnitus

    E. Headache

2. A nurse is assisting with the admission of a toddler who has had an acetaminophen overdose. Which of the following medications should the nurse anticipate administering to this client?

    A. Acetylcysteine

    B. Pegfilgrastim

    C. Misoprostol

    D. Naltrexone

3. A nurse is reinforcing teaching with a client about celecoxib. Which of the following information should the nurse include?

    A. Increases the risk of a myocardial infarction

    B. Decreases the risk of stroke

    C. Inhibits COX-1

    D. Increases platelet aggregation

4. A nurse is collecting data from a client who reports taking aspirin about four times daily to relieve the pain of a wrist sprain. Which of the following medications interacts adversely with aspirin?

    A. Digoxin

    B. Levothyroxine

    C. Warfarin

    D. Nitroglycerin

5. A nurse in an urgent care center is collecting data from a client who has severe aspirin toxicity. Which of the following findings should the nurse expect?

    A. Body temperature 35° C (95° F)

    B. Lung crackles

    C. Cool, dry skin

    D. Respiratory depression

PRACTICE Active Learning Scenario

A nurse at a provider's office is reinforcing teaching with a client who has osteoarthritis and is starting long-term therapy with NSAIDs. What information should the nurse include, and what actions should the nurse take? Use the ATI Active Learning Template: Medication to complete this item.

THERAPEUTIC USES

COMPLICATIONS: Describe two adverse effects.

NURSING INTERVENTIONS: Describe three nursing actions, including two laboratory values the nurse should monitor.

Application Exercises Key

1. A. **CORRECT:** Manifestations of salicylism include dizziness, drowsiness, and confusion.

   B. **CORRECT:** Manifestations of salicylism include diarrhea, nausea, and vomiting.

   C. Clients who take aspirin metabolize the medication through the liver. Jaundice is not an expected finding with salicylism.

   D. **CORRECT:** Manifestations of salicylism include tinnitus, sweating, and flushing.

   E. **CORRECT:** Manifestations of salicylism include headache, tachycardia, and tachypnea.

   Ⓝ *NCLEX® Connection: Pharmacological Therapies, Adverse Effects/ Contraindications/Side Effects/Interactions*

2. A. **CORRECT:** The nurse should administer acetylcysteine, which is the antidote for acetaminophen overdose.

   B. To increase the production of neutrophils, the nurse should administer pegfilgrastim.

   C. To prevent the formation of gastric ulcers, the nurse should administer misoprostol, which is a prostaglandin hormone.

   D. To prevent alcohol craving, the nurse should administer naltrexone, which is an opioid antagonist.

   Ⓝ *NCLEX® Connection: Pharmacological Therapies, Adverse Effects/ Contraindications/Side Effects/Interactions*

3. A. **CORRECT:** Celecoxib increases the risks for a myocardial infarction because it suppresses vasodilation.

   B. Celecoxib increases the risk for stroke because it suppresses vasodilation.

   C. Celecoxib inhibits COX-2, which suppresses inflammation, relieves pain, decreases fever, and protects against colorectal cancer.

   D. Celecoxib does not have an effect on platelet aggregation; it can cause GI bleeding.

   Ⓝ *NCLEX® Connection: Pharmacological Therapies, Expected Actions/Outcomes*

4. A. Digoxin does not interact adversely with aspirin. Examples of medications that interact adversely with aspirin include cefotetan and valproic acid.

   B. Levothyroxine does not interact adversely with aspirin. Examples of medications that interact adversely with aspirin include oral hypoglycemic medications and penicillins.

   C. **CORRECT:** Aspirin, which inhibits platelet aggregation, increases the effects of warfarin and other anticoagulants. This client would have an increased risk for bleeding.

   D. Nitroglycerin does not interact adversely with aspirin. Examples of medications that interact adversely with aspirin include phenytoin and methotrexate.

   Ⓝ *NCLEX® Connection: Pharmacological Therapies, Adverse Effects/ Contraindications/Side Effects/Interactions*

5. A. Hyperthermia is an expected manifestation of severe aspirin toxicity.

   B. Dehydration is an expected manifestation of severe aspirin toxicity. Lung crackles are not an expected finding.

   C. Diaphoresis is an expected manifestation of severe aspirin toxicity. Cool, dry skin is not an expected finding.

   D. **CORRECT:** Respiratory depression due to increasing acidosis is an expected manifestation of severe aspirin toxicity.

   Ⓝ *NCLEX® Connection: Pharmacological Therapies, Adverse Effects/ Contraindications/Side Effects/Interactions*

PRACTICE Answer

Using ATI Active Learning Template: Medication

THERAPEUTIC USES: NSAIDs treat mild to moderate joint pain and stiffness and decrease the inflammation osteoarthritis causes.

COMPLICATIONS

- Gastrointestinal effects (anorexia, abdominal pain, nausea, vomiting, heartburn) can occur.
- GI bleeding can occur because NSAIDs affect platelet function.
- Nephrotoxicity can occur.
- NSAIDs can cause CNS effects (dizziness, headache, blurry vision, tinnitus).
- Allergy can occur, including cross allergy with other NSAIDs, such as aspirin.

NURSING INTERVENTIONS

- Monitor Hgb, Hct, and kidney function tests.
- Ask the client about any previous allergic reactions to NSAIDs.
- Collect data about the GI system, and ask about any history of GI bleeding or peptic ulcer disease.
- Advise the client to take the medication with food, milk, or 240 mL (8 oz) water to prevent GI distress.
- Advise the client to tell the provider about any over-the-counter medications, vitamins, or herbal supplements before taking them.

Ⓝ *NCLEX® Connection: Pharmacological and Parenteral Therapies, Medication Administration*

UNIT 9   MEDICATIONS FOR PAIN AND INFLAMMATION

CHAPTER 31 *Opioid Agonists*
and Antagonists

Opioid analgesics treat moderate to severe pain. Most opioid analgesics reduce pain by attaching to a receptor in the CNS, altering the perception and response to pain.

Opioids are agonists, agonist-antagonists, or antagonists. An agonist attaches to a receptor and produces a response. An agonist-antagonist binds to one receptor, causing a response, and binds to another receptor that prevents a response. An antagonist attaches to a receptor site and prevents a response.

The desired outcome is to reduce pain and increase activity with few adverse effects. Opioid agonists are in Schedule II under the Controlled Substances Act.

Opioid agonists

SELECT PROTOTYPE MEDICATION: Morphine

OTHER MEDICATIONS
- Fentanyl
- Meperidine
- Methadone
- Codeine
- Oxycodone
- Hydromorphone

ROUTE OF ADMINISTRATION
- Morphine: Oral, subcutaneous, IM, IV, epidural, intrathecal
- Fentanyl: IV, IM, transmucosal, transdermal
- Meperidine: Oral, subcutaneous, IM, IV
- Codeine: Oral, subcutaneous, IM, IV
- Methadone: Oral, subcutaneous, IM
- Oxycodone: Oral, rectal
- Hydromorphone: Oral, subcutaneous, IM, IV

PURPOSE

EXPECTED PHARMACOLOGICAL ACTION: Opioid agonists and other morphine-like medications (fentanyl), act on the mu receptors, and to a lesser degree on kappa receptors. Activation of mu receptors produces analgesia, respiratory depression, euphoria, and sedation; kappa receptor activation produces analgesia, sedation, and decreased GI motility. Activation of mu receptors can also lead to physical dependence.

THERAPEUTIC USES
- Relief of moderate to severe pain: postoperative, myocardial infarction (MI), postpartum, cancer
- Sedation
- Reduction of bowel motility
- Cough suppression (codeine)
- Relief of anxiety due to dyspnea from pulmonary edema

COMPLICATIONS

Respiratory depression

NURSING ACTIONS
- Monitor vital signs.
- Withhold opioids for a respiratory rate less than 12/min, and notify the provider.
- Have naloxone and resuscitation equipment available.
- Discourage the use of opioids with other CNS depressants (barbiturates, benzodiazepines, alcohol).

Constipation

NURSING ACTIONS
- Administer a stimulant laxative (such as bisacodyl) to counteract decreased bowel motility or a stool softener (such as docusate sodium) to prevent constipation.
- For clients who have end-stage disorders (cancer, AIDS) and are opioid-dependent, administer an opioid antagonist (such as methylnaltrexone) to treat severe constipation.

CLIENT EDUCATION: Increase fluid and fiber intake and physical activity.

Orthostatic hypotension

NURSING ACTIONS: Provide assistance with ambulation as necessary.

CLIENT EDUCATION
- Sit or lie down if feeling lightheaded or dizzy.
- Due to the dilation effect on the peripheral arterioles and veins, avoid sudden changes in position by slowly moving from a lying to a sitting or standing position. Qs

Urinary retention

NURSING ACTIONS
- Monitor I&O.
- Check the bladder for distention by palpating the lower abdomen every 4 to 6 hr, because opioid medication can suppress awareness that the bladder is full.

CLIENT EDUCATION
- Urinate every 4 hr.
- Medications with anticholinergic properties (tricyclic antidepressants, antihistamines) can worsen this manifestation.

Cough suppression

NURSING ACTIONS: Auscultate the lungs for crackles.

CLIENT EDUCATION
- Cough at regular intervals to prevent the accumulation of secretions in the airway.
- Increase intake of fluid to liquefy secretions.

Sedation

CLIENT EDUCATION: Avoid hazardous activities (driving, operating heavy machinery).

Biliary colic

NURSING ACTIONS: Avoid giving morphine to clients who have a history of biliary colic. Meperidine is an alternative.

Nausea, vomiting

NURSING ACTIONS: Administer an antiemetic.

Opioid overdose triad

Coma, respiratory depression, pinpoint pupils

NURSING ACTIONS
- Monitor vital signs.
- Assist with providing mechanical ventilation.
- Administer naloxone, an opioid antagonist that reverses respiratory depression and other overdose manifestations.

CONTRAINDICATIONS/PRECAUTIONS

- Biliary tract surgery is a contraindication for receiving morphine. Qs
- Prematurity is a contraindication for receiving morphine during and after delivery because of its respiratory depressant effects.
- Kidney failure is a contraindication for receiving meperidine because of the accumulation of normeperidine, which can result in seizures and neurotoxicity.

- The following clients require caution when receiving these medications.
  - Clients who have asthma, emphysema, or head injuries; infants; older adult clients (risk of respiratory depression) Ⓖ
  - Clients who are pregnant (risk of physical dependence of the fetus)
  - Clients in labor (risk of respiratory depression in the newborn and inhibition of labor by decreasing uterine contractions)
  - Clients who have inflammatory bowel disease (risks of megacolon, paralytic ileus)
  - Clients who have an enlarged prostate (risk of acute urinary retention)
  - Clients who have hepatic or kidney disease

INTERACTIONS

CNS depressants (barbiturates, phenobarbital, benzodiazepines, alcohol) have additive CNS depression action.
- NURSING ACTIONS: Warn clients about taking these medications concurrently with opioid agonists.
- CLIENT EDUCATION: Avoid drinking alcohol.

Anticholinergic agents (atropine, scopolamine), antihistamines (diphenhydramine), and tricyclic antidepressants (amitriptyline) have additive anticholinergic effects (constipation, urinary retention).
CLIENT EDUCATION: Increase intake of fluids and dietary fiber to prevent constipation.

Meperidine can interact with monoamine oxidase inhibitors (MAOIs) and cause hyperpyrexic coma (excitation, seizures, respiratory depression).
NURSING ACTIONS: Discourage the use of meperidine with MAOIs to prevent this syndrome.

Antihypertensives have additive hypotensive effects.
CLIENT EDUCATION: Refrain from taking opioids with antihypertensive agents.

Additional medications (amphetamines, clonidine, dextromethorphan) can increase opioid-induced analgesia.
CLIENT EDUCATION: Avoid taking other medications that have a CNS effect with opioid medication.

NURSING ADMINISTRATION

- Determine pain levels on a regular basis. Document client responses.
- Measure baseline vital signs. If the respiratory rate is less than 12/min, notify the provider and withhold the medication.
- Follow controlled-substance procedures.
- Double-check opioid doses with another nurse prior to administration.
- Have naloxone and resuscitation equipment available.
- Warn clients not to increase dosages without consulting the provider.

- For clients who have cancer, administer opioids on a fixed schedule around the clock. Administer supplemental doses PRN. Q_EBP
- Advise clients who have a physical dependence not to stop taking opioids abruptly. They should withdraw them slowing, tapering the dosage over 3 days.
- Closely monitor patient-controlled analgesia (PCA) pump settings (dose, lockout interval, 4-hr limit). Reassure clients about safety measures that protect against self-administration of excessive doses. Encourage clients to use PCA prophylactically prior to painful activities. Q_PCC
- When clients switch from PCA to oral doses of opioids, make sure they receive adequate PCA dosing until the onset of oral medication takes place.
- The first administration of a transdermal fentanyl patch will take several hours to achieve the desired therapeutic effect. Administer short-acting opioids prior to the onset of therapeutic effects and for breakthrough pain.

NURSING EVALUATION OF MEDICATION EFFECTIVENESS

Indications of effectiveness include the following.
- Relief of moderate to severe pain (postoperative pain, cancer pain, myocardial pain)
- Cough suppression
- Resolution of diarrhea

Opioid agonist-antagonists

SELECT PROTOTYPE MEDICATION: Butorphanol

OTHER MEDICATION
- Nalbuphine
- Buprenorphine
- Pentazocine

ROUTE OF ADMINISTRATION
- Butorphanol: IV, IM, intranasal
- Nalbuphine: IV, IM, subcutaneous
- Buprenorphine: IV, sublingual, transdermal
- Pentazocine: IV, IM, subcutaneous

PURPOSE

EXPECTED PHARMACOLOGICAL ACTION

- These medications act as antagonists on mu receptors and agonists on kappa receptors (except for buprenorphine, which has agonist/antagonist activity on opposite receptors).
- Agonist-antagonists have the following difference compared with pure opioid agonists.
  - Low potential for abuse, causing little euphoria (high doses can even cause adverse effects: anxiety, restlessness, confusion)
  - Less respiratory depression
  - Less analgesia

THERAPEUTIC USES

- Relief of moderate to severe pain
- Treatment of opioid dependence (buprenorphine)
- Adjunct to balanced anesthesia
- Relief of labor pain

COMPLICATIONS

Abstinence syndrome

- Cramping, hypertension, vomiting, fever, anxiety
- This syndrome can result when clients who are physically dependent on opioid agonists receive these medications.

NURSING ACTIONS: Avoid giving these medications to clients when suspecting opioid use.

CLIENT EDUCATION: Stop taking opioid agonists, such as morphine, before taking agonist-antagonist medications.

Sedation, respiratory depression

NURSING ACTIONS
- Have naloxone and resuscitation equipment available.
- Monitor for respiratory depression.

Dizziness

CLIENT EDUCATION: Use caution when standing up and avoid driving and using heavy machinery.

Headache

NURSING ACTIONS
- Monitor for headache.
- Check level of consciousness.

CONTRAINDICATIONS/PRECAUTIONS

Clients who have a history of MI, kidney or liver disease, respiratory depression, or head injury, and clients who are physically dependent on opioids, require caution when receiving these medications. Q_S

INTERACTIONS

CNS depressants and alcohol can cause additive effects.
NURSING ACTIONS
- Use caution with concurrent use.
- Monitor respirations.

Opioid agonists can antagonize and reduce the analgesic effects.
NURSING ACTIONS: Do not administer these medications concurrently.

NURSING ADMINISTRATION

- Measure baseline vital signs. If the respiratory rate is less than 12/min, withhold the medication and notify the provider. Q$_{EBP}$
- Have naloxone and resuscitation equipment available.
- Screen clients for opioid dependence prior to administration. Agonist-antagonists can trigger withdrawal manifestations.
- Warn clients not to increase dosages without consulting the provider.
- Advise clients to use caution when getting out of bed or standing. Clients should not operate heavy machinery or drive until they know if the CNS effects will make these activities unsafe.

NURSING EVALUATION OF MEDICATION EFFECTIVENESS

Indications of effectiveness include improvement of manifestations, such as relief of pain.

Opioid antagonists

SELECT PROTOTYPE MEDICATION: Naloxone

OTHER MEDICATIONS
- Naltrexone
- Methylnaltrexone
- Alvimopan

ROUTE OF ADMINISTRATION
- Naloxone: IV, IM, subcutaneous, intranasal
- Naltrexone: Oral, IM
- Methylnaltrexone: Subcutaneous
- Alvimopan: Oral

PURPOSE

EXPECTED PHARMACOLOGICAL ACTION

Opioid antagonists interfere with the action of opioids by competing for opioid receptors. Opioid antagonists have no effect in the absence of opioids.

THERAPEUTIC USES

- Treatment of opioid use disorder by preventing euphoria (naltrexone)
- Reversal of the effects of opioids, such as respiratory depression (naloxone)
- Reversal of respiratory depression in newborns (naloxone)
- Reversal of severe opioid-induced constipation in clients who have late-stage cancer or other disorders (methylnaltrexone, alvimopan)

COMPLICATIONS

Tachycardia, tachypnea

NURSING ACTIONS
- Monitor heart rhythm (risk of ventricular tachycardia) and respiratory function.
- Have resuscitative equipment, including oxygen, available during administration.

Abstinence syndrome

- Cramping, hypertension, vomiting, reversal of analgesia
- These manifestations can occur when clients who are physically dependent on opioid agonists receive these medications.

CONTRAINDICATIONS/PRECAUTIONS

- Opioid antagonists are Pregnancy Risk Category B. Q$_S$
- Due to the risk of withdrawal manifestations, clients should be free of opioids prior to the administration of naltrexone.
- Acute hepatitis and liver failure are contraindications for receiving naltrexone.

NURSING ADMINISTRATION

- Naloxone has rapid first-pass inactivation, so IV, IM, subcutaneous, or intranasal administration is necessary.
- Observe for withdrawal manifestations or the abrupt onset of pain. Be prepared to address the need for analgesia if clients receive it to reverse postoperative opioid-induced respiratory depression. Q$_{EBP}$
- Rapid infusion of naloxone can cause hypertension, tachycardia, nausea, and vomiting.
- The half-life of opioid analgesia can exceed the half-life of naloxone (60 to 90 min). Monitor respirations for up to 2 hr after use to identify the recurrence of respiratory depression and the need for repeat dosing of naloxone.
- Methylnaltrexone and alvimopan reverse the constipation opioids cause but without reversing their analgesic or respiratory effects.
- Alvimopan administration for longer than 7 days increases the risk for MI.

NURSING EVALUATION OF MEDICATION EFFECTIVENESS

Indications of effectiveness include the following.
- Reversal of respiratory depression
  - Regular respirations
  - No shortness of breath
  - Respiratory rate within the expected reference range
- Reduced euphoria and craving for alcohol for clients who have alcohol use disorder
- Relief of severe opioid-induced constipation (methylnaltrexone, alvimopan)

Application Exercises

1. A nurse is preparing to administer an opioid agonist to a client who has acute pain. The nurse should monitor for which of the following complications?

    A. Urinary retention

    B. Tachypnea

    C. Tinnitus

    D. Joint pain

2. A nurse is caring for a client who has end-stage cancer and is receiving morphine. The client's daughter asks why the provider prescribed methylnaltrexone. Which of the following responses should the nurse make?

    A. "The medication will increase your mother's respiratory rate."

    B. "The medication will prevent dependence on morphine."

    C. "The medication will relieve your mother's constipation."

    D. "The medication works with morphine to increase pain relief."

3. A nurse is preparing to administer butorphanol to a client who has a history of substance use disorder. The nurse should be aware of which of the following information about butorphanol?

    A. Butorphanol has a greater risk for misuse than morphine.

    B. Butorphanol causes a higher incidence of respiratory depression than morphine.

    C. Opioid antagonists cannot reverse the effects of butorphanol.

    D. Butorphanol can cause abstinence syndrome in clients who have opioid dependency.

4. A nurse is caring for a client who is receiving morphine postoperatively. Which of the following actions should the nurse take?

    A. Have alvimopan available to reverse excessive sedation.

    B. Protect the client's skin from the severe diarrhea that morphine causes.

    C. Withhold this medication for respiratory rate less than 16/min.

    D. Encourage the client to cough at regular intervals.

5. A nurse is reviewing the medication administration record of a client who is receiving transdermal fentanyl for the relief of severe pain. Which of the following medications should the nurse expect to cause an adverse effect if the client receives it concurrently with fentanyl?

    A. Ampicillin

    B. Diazepam

    C. Furosemide

    D. Prednisone

PRACTICE Active Learning Scenario

A nurse is reinforcing discharge teaching with a client who is postoperative and has a new prescription for an opioid medication for incisional pain. What information should the nurse include and what actions should the nurse take? Use the ATI Active Learning Template: Medication to complete this item.

THERAPEUTIC USES: Describe for oxycodone.

COMPLICATIONS: List three adverse effects for oxycodone.

CLIENT EDUCATION: List three teaching points to reinforce.

Application Exercises Key

1. A. **CORRECT:** The nurse should monitor for urinary retention by palpating the client's abdomen regularly because morphine can suppress awareness that the bladder is full.

   B. The nurse should monitor for bradypnea, not tachypnea, because the activation of mu receptors can cause respiratory depression.

   C. Opioid medications do not typically cause tinnitus, but they can cause diplopia, miosis, and blurry vision.

   D. Opioid medications do not typically cause joint pain, but they can cause headaches.

   Ⓝ *NCLEX® Connection: Pharmacological Therapies, Pharmacological Pain Management*

2. A. Methylnaltrexone does not reverse analgesia or respiratory depression.

   B. Methylnaltrexone does not prevent dependence on opioids, such as morphine.

   C. **CORRECT:** Methylnaltrexone is an opioid antagonist that treats severe constipation that has not responded to laxatives in clients who have opioid dependency. The medication blocks the mu opioid receptors in the GI tract.

   D. Methylnaltrexone is not an adjunct to opioids for pain relief.

   Ⓝ *NCLEX® Connection: Pharmacological Therapies, Expected Actions/Outcomes*

3. A. Butorphanol has less risk for misuse than morphine does.

   B. Butorphanol is less likely to cause respiratory depression than morphine is.

   C. An opioid antagonist can reverse the manifestations of a butorphanol overdose.

   D. **CORRECT:** Opioid agonist/antagonist medications, such as butorphanol, can cause abstinence syndrome in clients who have opioid dependency. Manifestations include hypertension, vomiting, fever, and anxiety.

   Ⓝ *NCLEX® Connection: Pharmacological Therapies, Expected Actions/Outcomes*

4. A. Alvimopan only counteracts the constipating effects of opioids.

   B. The nurse should plan to monitor for constipation because morphine affects the mu opioid receptors in the GI tract.

   C. The nurse should withhold opioids if the respiratory rate is 12/min or less, and notify the charge nurse and provider.

   D. **CORRECT:** The nurse should remind the client to cough at regular intervals to prevent the accumulation of secretions in the airway, because opioid medications can cause cough suppression.

   Ⓝ *NCLEX® Connection: Pharmacological Therapies, Expected Actions/Outcomes*

5. A. Ampicillin, an antibiotic, does not interact with fentanyl. Examples of antibiotics that interact with fentanyl are erythromycin and clarithromycin.

   B. **CORRECT:** Diazepam, a benzodiazepine, is a CNS depressant, which can interact by causing excessive sedation when the client receives it concurrently with an opioid agonist or agonist/antagonist.

   C. Furosemide, a loop diuretic, does not interact with fentanyl. Examples of medications that interact with fentanyl are diltiazem and verapamil.

   D. Prednisone, a glucocorticoid, does not interact with fentanyl. Examples of medications that interact with fentanyl are ketoconazole and ritonavir.

   Ⓝ *NCLEX® Connection: Pharmacological Therapies, Medication Administration*

PRACTICE Answer

Using the ATI Active Learning Template: Medication

THERAPEUTIC USES:
Opioid medication relieves moderate to severe pain.

COMPLICATIONS
- Sedation
- Nausea
- Vomiting
- Constipation
- Orthostatic hypotension
- Urinary retention

NURSING INTERVENTIONS
- Do not drive or perform other hazardous activities while taking this medication.
- Notify the provider for severe nausea or vomiting.
- Prevent constipation by increasing intake of liquids and foods with fiber and taking a stool softener or laxatives if necessary.
- Move slowly from lying or sitting to standing to minimize the effects of orthostatic hypotension.
- Urinate every 4 hr, and contact the provider for manifestations of dysuria.

Ⓝ *NCLEX® Connection: Pharmacological and Parenteral Therapies, Medication Administration*

CHAPTER 32 *Adjuvant Medications for Pain*

Adjuvant medications work with a primary pain medication, usually an opioid agonist, to increase pain relief while reducing the dosage of the opioid agonist. Lower dosages of the opioid reduce adverse reactions (respiratory depression, sedation, constipation). Targeting pain stimuli with different types of medications often improves pain relief.

Categories of medications include tricyclic antidepressants, anticonvulsants, CNS stimulants, antihistamines, glucocorticoids, bisphosphonates, and NSAIDs. Pain relief is an off-label use of many of these medications.

SELECT PROTOTYPE MEDICATIONS
- **Tricyclic antidepressants:** Amitriptyline (oral)
- **Anticonvulsants:** Carbamazepine, gabapentin, pregabalin (oral)
- **CNS stimulants:** Methylphenidate (oral, transdermal)
- **Antihistamines:** Hydroxyzine (oral, IM)
- **Glucocorticoids:** Dexamethasone (oral, IV, IM)
- **Bisphosphonates:** Etidronate (oral)
- **NSAIDs:** Ibuprofen (oral, IV)

OTHER MEDICATIONS
- **Tricyclic antidepressants:** Imipramine (oral)
- **Anticonvulsants:** Phenytoin (oral, IV)
- **CNS stimulants:** Dextroamphetamine (oral)
- **Glucocorticoids:** Prednisone (oral)
- **Bisphosphonates:** Pamidronate (IV)
- **NSAIDs:** Ketorolac (oral, IM, IV, intranasal)

PURPOSE

EXPECTED PHARMACOLOGICAL ACTION

Adjuvant medications for pain enhance the therapeutic effects of opioids. Q EBP

THERAPEUTIC USES

These medications work in combination with opioids; they are not a substitute for opioids.
- **Tricyclic antidepressants** treat depression, fibromyalgia syndrome, and neuropathic pain (aching, burning, darting, sharp stabbing).
- **Anticonvulsants** relieve neuropathic pain and neuralgia.
- **CNS stimulants** augment analgesia and decrease sedation.
- **Antihistamines** decrease anxiety, prevent insomnia, and relieve nausea and vomiting.
- **Glucocorticoids** improve appetite and decrease pain from intracranial pressure, spinal cord compression, and rheumatoid arthritis.
- **Bisphosphonates** manage hypercalcemia and bone pain.
- **NSAIDs** treat inflammation and fever, and relieve mild to moderate pain and dysmenorrhea.

COMPLICATIONS

Tricyclic antidepressants (amitriptyline)

Orthostatic hypotension
- NURSING ACTIONS
  - Provide assistance with ambulation if necessary.
  - Monitor orthostatic blood pressures.
  - Withhold the medication and notify the provider for hypotension or tachycardia.
- CLIENT EDUCATION: Sit or lie down if feeling lightheaded or dizzy, and change positions slowly.

Sedation
CLIENT EDUCATION: Avoid hazardous activities (driving, operating heavy machinery).

Anticholinergic effects
- Dry mouth, urinary retention, constipation, blurry vision
- NURSING ACTIONS: Monitor I&O. Check the bladder for distention by palpating the lower abdomen every 4 to 6 hr.
- CLIENT EDUCATION
  - Increase fluid intake. Sip fluids throughout the day. Chew gum or suck on hard candy. Use an alcohol-free mouthwash.
  - Increase daily fiber intake.
  - Increase physical activity by engaging in a regular exercise routine.
  - Take a stimulant laxative, such as bisacodyl, to counteract decreased bowel motility.
  - Take a stool softener, such as docusate sodium, to prevent constipation.
  - Urinate just prior to taking the medication and then every 4 hr. Report urinary retention to the provider.
  - If blurry vision is present, avoid hazardous activities, wear dark glasses for intolerance to light, and report blurry vision to the provider.

Anticonvulsants (carbamazepine, gabapentin, pregabalin)

Bone marrow suppression
- NURSING ACTIONS: Periodically monitor CBC, including platelets.
- CLIENT EDUCATION: Observe for indications of bone marrow suppression (easy bruising and bleeding, fever, sore throat) and notify the provider if they occur.

Gastrointestinal (GI) distress
- Nausea, vomiting, diarrhea, constipation
- CLIENT EDUCATION
  - Take the medication with food.
  - If constipation occurs, increase physical activity and daily fluid and fiber intake. Take a stimulant laxative (such as bisacodyl) and a stool softener (such as docusate sodium).

Drowsiness
CLIENT EDUCATION: Avoid activities that require alertness.

Rash
CLIENT EDUCATION: Stop taking the medication and notify the provider.

CNS stimulants (methylphenidate)

Weight loss
NURSING ACTIONS
- Monitor the client's weight.
- Encourage good nutrition.

Insomnia
CLIENT EDUCATION
- Take the last dose of the day no later than 1600.
- Decrease caffeine consumption.

Antihistamines (hydroxyzine)

Sedation
- Older adult clients require lower dosages. ©
- CLIENT EDUCATION: Avoid hazardous activities (driving, operating heavy machinery).

Dry mouth
CLIENT EDUCATION: Increase fluid intake. Sip fluids throughout the day. Chew gum or suck on hard candy.

Glucocorticoids (dexamethasone)

Adrenal insufficiency
- Hypotension, dehydration, infection, weakness, lethargy, vomiting, diarrhea (with prolonged use)
- CLIENT EDUCATION: Observe for these manifestations and notify the provider if they occur.

Osteoporosis
CLIENT EDUCATION: Take calcium supplements, vitamin D, and/or a bisphosphonate.

Fluid and electrolyte disturbances
- Hypokalemia
- Sodium and water retention
- NURSING ACTIONS: Monitor potassium levels. Suggest potassium supplements if necessary.
- CLIENT EDUCATION
  - Eat potassium-rich foods (potatoes, bananas, citrus fruits).
  - Restrict sodium intake.
  - Report fluid retention and edema to the provider.

Glucose intolerance
NURSING ACTIONS: Monitor blood glucose levels.

Peptic ulcer disease
- NURSING ACTIONS: Regularly check stools for occult blood.
- CLIENT EDUCATION
  - Take the medication with meals.
  - Report black, tarry stools.
  - Use an antiulcer medication.

Bisphosphonates (etidronate, pamidronate)

Transient flu-like manifestations (pamidronate)
- NURSING ACTIONS: Monitor for fever.
- Client education: Notify the provider if manifestations occur.

Abdominal cramps, nausea, diarrhea, esophagitis (etidronate)
CLIENT EDUCATION
- Take this medication with 240 mL (8 oz) water and sit or stand upright for 30 to 60 min after taking it. Qs
- For maximum absorption, wait 2 hr before ingesting food, antacids, or vitamins.

Venous irritation at the injection site (pamidronate)
NURSING ACTIONS: Monitor the injection site. Make sure clients receive sufficient IV fluids.

Hypocalcemia
- NURSING ACTIONS: Monitor calcium, magnesium, potassium, and phosphate levels.
- CLIENT EDUCATION
  - Report numbness or tingling around the mouth, spasms, and seizures to the provider.
  - Take supplemental calcium and vitamin D.

NSAIDs (ibuprofen)

Bone marrow suppression
- NURSING ACTIONS: Periodically monitor CBC, including platelets.
- CLIENT EDUCATION: Observe for indications of easy bruising and bleeding, fever, and sore throat. Notify the provider if they occur.

Gastrointestinal (GI) distress
- Abdominal pain, ulceration, nausea, vomiting, diarrhea, constipation
- NURSING ACTIONS: Monitor for GI bleeding (coffee-ground emesis; bloody or black tarry stools; abdominal pain).
- CLIENT EDUCATION: Take the medication with food, milk, or an antacid.

Myocardial infarction (MI) or stroke
NURSING ACTIONS: Monitor cardiac and neurological status, especially in older adult clients and those who have a history of cardiac disease or risk factors for MI or stroke.

CONTRAINDICATIONS/PRECAUTIONS

Tricyclic antidepressants (amitriptyline)

- Recovery from an MI and having taken an MAOI within 14 days are contraindications for taking tricyclic antidepressants.
- Clients who have a seizure disorder, urinary retention, prostatic hyperplasia, angle-closure glaucoma, hyperthyroidism, or liver or kidney disease require caution when taking tricyclic antidepressants.

Anticonvulsants (carbamazepine, gabapentin)

- Carbamazepine is Pregnancy Risk Category D. Gabapentin and pregabalin are Pregnancy Risk Category C.
- Bone marrow suppression and having taken an MAOI within 14 days are contraindications for taking these anticonvulsants.

CNS stimulants (methylphenidate)

- Clients should not take methylphenidate within 14 days of taking a MAOI.
- Clients who have hypertension require caution. Methylphenidate can result in hypertensive crisis.
- Clients who have agitation, tics, or history of substance use disorder require caution.

Antihistamines (hydroxyzine)

- Clients who have acute asthma should not take hydroxyzine.
- Clients who are in the first trimester of pregnancy or breastfeeding should not take hydroxyzine.
- Older adults and those in the second or third trimester of pregnancy require caution when taking hydroxyzine (Pregnancy Risk Category C).

Glucocorticoids (dexamethasone)

- Fungal infections, seizure disorders, ulcerative colitis, and coagulopathy are contraindications for taking glucocorticoids.
- Clients who have hypertension, hypothyroidism, diabetes mellitus, osteoporosis, or liver disease require caution when taking glucocorticoids.

Bisphosphonate (etidronate, pamidronate)

- Achalasia, esophageal structure, and osteomalacia are contraindications for receiving bisphosphonates.
- Clients who have kidney disease require caution when taking bisphosphonates.

NSAIDs (ibuprofen)

- A history of bronchospasm with aspirin or other NSAIDs and severe kidney or hepatic disease are contraindications for taking NSAIDs.
- Clients who have GI bleeding or cardiac disorders require caution when taking NSAIDs.
- Older adult clients require caution when taking NSAIDs.

INTERACTIONS

Tricyclic antidepressants (amitriptyline)

Barbiturates, CNS depressants, antihistamines, over-the-counter (OTC) sleep aids, and alcohol can cause additive CNS depression.
CLIENT EDUCATION: Do not take these medications concurrently.

Anticonvulsants (carbamazepine, gabapentin)

Carbamazepine decreases the effects of oral contraceptives and warfarin.
- NURSING ACTIONS: Monitor for therapeutic effects of warfarin with PT and INR. Providers might adjust dosages.
- CLIENT EDUCATION: Discuss possible contraceptive changes with the provider.

Carbamazepine can result in CNS toxicity with lithium, and a fatal reaction with MAOIs.
CLIENT EDUCATION: Do not take these medications concurrently.

Grapefruit juice inhibits metabolism, and thus increases carbamazepine levels.
CLIENT EDUCATION: Do not drink grapefruit juice.

Phenytoin and phenobarbital decrease the effects of carbamazepine.
CLIENT EDUCATION: Do not take these medications concurrently.

CNS depression occurs with gabapentin and all other CNS depressants (alcohol, sedatives, antihistamines).
CLIENT EDUCATION: Do not take these medications concurrently.

CNS stimulants (methylphenidate)

Alkalizing medications can increase reabsorption.
NURSING ACTIONS: Monitor for increases in amphetamine effects.

Acidifying medications can increase the excretion of amphetamine.
NURSING ACTIONS: Monitor for decreases in amphetamine effects.

Insulin and oral antidiabetes medications can decrease glucose levels.
NURSING ACTIONS: Monitor glucose levels.

Methylphenidate decreases the effect of antihypertensives.
NURSING ACTIONS: Monitor blood pressure. Check it more often for clients who have cardiac disease.

MAOIs can cause severe hypertension.
CLIENT EDUCATION: Do not take these medications concurrently.

Caffeine can increase stimulant effects.
CLIENT EDUCATION: Avoid caffeine.

OTC medications with sympathomimetic actions can increase CNS stimulation.
CLIENT EDUCATION: Check with the provider before taking OTC medications.

Antihistamines (hydroxyzine)

Barbiturates, CNS depressants, and alcohol can cause additive CNS depression.
CLIENT EDUCATION: Do not take these medications concurrently.

Glucocorticoids (dexamethasone)

Glucocorticoids promote hyperglycemia, thereby counteracting the effects of insulin and oral hypoglycemics.
The provider might increase the dosage of hypoglycemic medications.

Concurrent use of salicylates and NSAIDs can increase the risk for GI bleeding.
NURSING ACTIONS
- Monitor for GI bleeding.
- Use caution in clients who take these medications concurrently.

Because of the risk for hypokalemia, there is an increased risk of dysrhythmias resulting from digoxin.
- NURSING ACTIONS
  - Monitor potassium levels and cardiac rhythm.
  - Suggest potassium supplements if necessary.
- CLIENT EDUCATION: Eat potassium-rich foods.

Diuretics that promote potassium loss increase the risk for hypokalemia.
- NURSING ACTIONS
  - Monitor potassium levels.
  - Suggest potassium supplements if necessary.
- CLIENT EDUCATION: Eat potassium-rich foods.

Glucocorticoids decrease the antibody response to vaccines and increase the risk of infection from live virus vaccines.
CLIENT EDUCATION: Do not receive immunizations during glucocorticoid therapy.

Bisphosphonates (etidronate, pamidronate)

Calcium and iron supplements and high-calcium foods decrease the absorption of these medications.
CLIENT EDUCATION: Take etidronate on an empty stomach 2 hr before meals, with 240 mL (8 oz) water.

NSAIDs (ibuprofen)

NSAIDs can reduce the effectiveness of antihypertensives, furosemide, thiazide diuretics, and oral antidiabetes medications.
NURSING ACTIONS: Monitor for medication effectiveness.

Aspirin, corticosteroids, alcohol, and tobacco can increase GI effects.
CLIENT EDUCATION: Do not take these medications concurrently.

NSAIDs can increase levels of oral anticoagulants and lithium.
NURSING ACTIONS: Monitor medication levels.

There is an increased risk of bleeding with the use of other NSAIDs, thrombolytics, antiplatelets, anticoagulants, and salicylates.
NURSING ACTIONS
- Use caution in clients who take these medications together.
- Monitor for bleeding.

NURSING ADMINISTRATION

- The client's self-report is the key element in evaluating pain. Qpcc
- Clients should receive a pain management plan.
- Encourage clients who have cancer to voice their fears and concerns about cancer, cancer pain, and pain management.
- Advise clients to take pain medications on a fixed schedule around the clock, and not just when they need them. QEBP
- Inform clients that physical dependence is not addiction.
- Older adult clients need careful monitoring because they are at risk for increased adverse effects and adverse medication interactions with pain medications.
- Because pain relief is an off-label use for some adjuvant medications, it is important to explain to clients that they are taking these medications to reduce pain, and not for their original purpose.

NURSING EVALUATION OF MEDICATION EFFECTIVENESS

Indications of effectiveness include the following.

- Relief of depression, seizures, dysrhythmias, and other manifestations that increase the client's pain level
- Decreased opioid adverse effects
- Relief of neuropathic pain
- Decreased cancer bone pain
- Relief of neuralgia

PRACTICE Active Learning Scenario

A nurse in an acute care facility is reinforcing teaching with a client who has metastatic cancer and is receiving morphine and carbamazepine for pain relief. What information should the nurse provide about these medications? Use the ATI Active Learning Template: Medication to complete this item.

THERAPEUTIC USES: Describe the therapeutic use for carbamazepine in this client.

COMPLICATIONS: Describe two adverse effects the client should monitor for.

INTERACTIONS: Describe two interactions with carbamazepine.

CLIENT EDUCATION: Describe two teaching points to reinforce.

Application Exercises

1. A nurse is caring for a client who has cancer and is taking morphine and carbamazepine for pain relief. Which of the following effects should the nurse monitor for? (Select all that apply.)
   - A. The need for a lower dosage of the opioid
   - B. Reduced adverse effects of the opioid
   - C. Increased analgesic effects
   - D. Enhanced CNS stimulation
   - E. Increased opioid tolerance

2. A nurse is assisting with the plan of care for a client who has brain cancer and reports headaches. Which of the following adjuvant medications should the nurse expect the provider to prescribe?
   - A. Dexamethasone
   - B. Methylphenidate
   - C. Hydroxyzine
   - D. Amitriptyline

3. A nurse is reinforcing teaching with a client who has a new prescription for etidronate to help relieve bone pain. Which of the following instructions should the nurse include?
   - A. Wait 30 min after taking the medication before eating any food.
   - B. Take the medication with 30 mL (1 oz) water.
   - C. Sit upright or stand for 30 min after taking the medication.
   - D. Increase fluid and fiber intake to prevent the constipation the medication causes.

4. A nurse is assisting with the plan of care for a client who has cancer and is taking a glucocorticoid as an adjuvant medication for pain control. Which of the following interventions should the nurse include? (Select all that apply.)
   - A. Monitor for urinary retention.
   - B. Monitor glucose level.
   - C. Monitor potassium level.
   - D. Monitor for gastric bleeding.
   - E. Monitor for respiratory depression.

5. A nurse is administering amitriptyline to a client who has cancer pain. For which of the following manifestations should the nurse monitor as an adverse effect of this medication?
   - A. Decreased appetite
   - B. Severe diarrhea
   - C. Decreased heart rate
   - D. Orthostatic hypotension

Application Exercises Key

1. A. **CORRECT:** The provider can reduce the dosage of the opioid when adding adjuvant medications for pain.

   B. **CORRECT:** Adjuvant medications can reduce the adverse effects of the opioid.

   C. **CORRECT:** Adjuvant medications increase the analgesic effects of the opioid.

   D. Concurrent administration of morphine and carbamazepine do not increase CNS stimulation.

   E. An adjuvant medication can help reduce opioid tolerance.

   (N) *NCLEX® Connection: Pharmacological Therapies, Adverse Effects/ Contraindications/Side Effects/Interactions*

2. A. **CORRECT:** Dexamethasone, a glucocorticoid, decreases inflammation and swelling. It can reduce cerebral edema and relieve intracranial pressure from the tumor.

   B. The use of methylphenidate as an adjuvant is for elevating mood and increasing pain relief.

   C. The use of hydroxyzine as an adjuvant is for decreasing anxiety and helping the client sleep.

   D. The use of amitriptyline as an adjuvant is for relieving neuropathic pain and elevating mood.

   (N) *NCLEX® Connection: Pharmacological Therapies, Expected Actions/Outcomes*

3. A. For maximum absorption, clients should wait 2 hr before ingesting food, antacids, or vitamins.

   B. The nurse should instruct the client to take this medication with 240 mL (8 oz) water to minimize the risk of esophagitis.

   C. **CORRECT:** The nurse should instruct the client to sit or stand upright for 30 to 60 min after taking it to minimize the risk of esophagitis.

   D. Adverse effects of etidronate include abdominal cramps, nausea, and diarrhea, not constipation.

   (N) *NCLEX® Connection: Pharmacological Therapies, Expected Actions/Outcomes*

4. A. Monitoring for urinary retention is not necessary because glucocorticoids do not cause this effect.

   B. **CORRECT:** Monitoring serum glucose is important because glucocorticoids raise the glucose level, especially in clients who have diabetes mellitus.

   C. **CORRECT:** Monitoring serum potassium level is important because glucocorticoids can cause hypokalemia.

   D. **CORRECT:** Monitoring for gastric bleeding is important because glucocorticoids irritate the gastric mucosa and put the client at risk for a peptic ulcer.

   E. Monitoring for respiratory depression is not necessary because glucocorticoids do not depress respirations.

   (N) *NCLEX® Connection: Pharmacological Therapies, Expected Actions/Outcomes*

5. A. Amitriptyline can cause increased appetite and weight gain.

   B. Amitriptyline can cause constipation.

   C. Amitriptyline can increase the heart rate.

   D. **CORRECT:** Amitriptyline can cause orthostatic hypotension. The nurse should monitor for this effect and instruct the client to move slowly from lying down or sitting after taking this medication.

   (N) *NCLEX® Connection: Pharmacological Therapies, Adverse Effects/ Contraindications/Side Effects/Interactions*

PRACTICE Answer

Using the ATI Active Learning Template: Medication

THERAPEUTIC USES:
Carbamazepine relieves neuropathic (nerve) pain, which is often sharp, burning, or aching.

COMPLICATIONS: Adverse effects of carbamazepine include GI manifestations (abdominal pain, nausea, vomiting). It also can cause bone marrow suppression, affecting all blood cell types.

INTERACTIONS
- The medication can cause hypertensive crisis if the client takes it within 14 days of taking an MAOI antidepressant.
- Toxicity can result if the client drinks grapefruit juice while taking carbamazepine.

CLIENT EDUCATION
- It is necessary to monitor CBC, including platelet counts.
- Report abnormal bleeding, bruising, or indications of infection.
- Watch for GI manifestations, and take the medication with food if they occur.

(N) *NCLEX® Connection: Pharmacological and Parenteral Therapies, Medication Administration*

UNIT 9   MEDICATIONS FOR PAIN AND INFLAMMATION

CHAPTER 33 *Miscellaneous Pain Medications*

Pain is subjective and can indicate current or impending tissue injury. Pain can result from the release of chemical mediators, inflammation, or pressure.

Migraine headaches can result from the inflammation and vasodilation of cerebral blood vessels. Medications for migraine headaches can stop a migraine (abortive) or prevent one from occurring (prophylactic). First-line treatment for migraine headaches includes nonspecific analgesics (such as aspirin-like medications) and migraine-specific medications (such as serotonin receptor agonists [triptans]). Ergot alkaloids are second-line treatment for migraines, and prophylactic medications include beta blockers, anticonvulsants, tricyclic antidepressants, and estrogens.

Local anesthetics block motor and sensory neurons to a specific area. Administration can be topical; via injection directly into an area; or regional, epidural, or into the subarachnoid (spinal) space.

Migraine medications

SELECT PROTOTYPE MEDICATIONS
- **Aspirin-like medications:** Acetaminophen, NSAIDs (aspirin, naproxen)
- **Serotonin receptor agonists (triptans):** Sumatriptan (oral, subcutaneous, inhalation, transdermal)
- **Ergot alkaloids**
  - Ergotamine (oral, sublingual, rectal)
  - Dihydroergotamine (IV, IM, subcutaneous, intranasal)
- **Beta blockers:** Propranolol (oral)
- **Anticonvulsants:** Divalproex (oral), topiramate
- **Tricyclic antidepressants:** Amitriptyline (oral)
- **Estrogens:** Estrogen (gel, patches)

OTHER MEDICATIONS
- **Triptans:** Almotriptan, frovatriptan, naratriptan, zolmitriptan
- **Ergot alkaloids:** Ergotamine/caffeine
- **Combination OTC analgesics:** Acetaminophen/aspirin/caffeine
- **Other combinations:** Isometheptene/dichloralphenazone/acetaminophen
  - Isometheptene relieves headaches through vasoconstriction of arterioles.
  - Dichloralphenazone has sedative properties.
  - Acetaminophen is a mild analgesic.

PURPOSE

EXPECTED PHARMACOLOGICAL ACTION: Migraine medications prevent inflammation and dilation of the intracranial blood vessels, thereby relieving migraine pain.

THERAPEUTIC USES
- Some medications provide abortive therapy to stop a migraine after it begins or after prodromal manifestations start. These include NSAIDs and combination anti-inflammatory medications, triptans, and ergot alkaloids.
- Other medications provide prophylactic therapy to help prevent a migraine headache. Preventive agents include beta blockers, anticonvulsants, amitriptyline, and estrogens.

COMPLICATIONS

Aspirin-like medications (NSAIDs, acetaminophen combination)

Bone marrow suppression
- NURSING ACTIONS: Periodically monitor CBC, including platelets.
- CLIENT EDUCATION: Observe for indications of easy bruising and bleeding, fever, or sore throat. Notify the provider if they occur.

Gastrointestinal (GI) distress
- Abdominal pain, ulceration, nausea, vomiting, diarrhea, constipation
- NURSING ACTIONS: Monitor for GI bleeding (coffee-ground emesis; bloody or black tarry stools; abdominal pain).
- CLIENT EDUCATION: Take the medication with food, milk, or an antacid.

Myocardial infarction (MI) or stroke
NURSING ACTIONS: Monitor cardiac status, especially for older adult clients and clients who have a history of cardiac disease. Ⓒ

Serotonin receptor antagonists (sumatriptan)

Chest pressure (heavy arms, chest tightness)
CLIENT EDUCATION
- Adverse effects are self-limiting and not dangerous.
- Notify the provider for continuous or severe chest pain.

Coronary artery vasospasm, angina
Clients who have or are at risk for coronary artery disease (CAD) should not take triptans.

Dizziness or vertigo
CLIENT EDUCATION: Avoid driving and operating machinery until the medication's effects are known.

Teratogenesis
Clients who are pregnant, trying to become pregnant, or are not using adequate contraception should not take triptans.

Ergot alkaloids (ergotamine, dihydroergotamine)

GI discomfort (nausea, vomiting)
NURSING ACTIONS: Administer an antiemetic, such as metoclopramide.

Acute or chronic overdose (ergotism)
- Muscle pain, paresthesias in fingers and toes; peripheral ischemia
- NURSING ACTIONS: Withhold the medication, and immediately notify the provider if these manifestations occur.

Physical dependence
CLIENT EDUCATION
- Do not to exceed the prescribed dosage.
- Do not take these medications daily on a long-term basis.
- Manifestations of withdrawal include headache, nausea, vomiting, and restlessness. Notify the provider if these manifestations occur.

Fetal harm or abortion
CLIENT EDUCATION
- Do not take these medications during pregnancy.
- Use multiple forms of contraception while taking these medications.

Beta blockers (propranolol)

Extreme tiredness, fatigue, depression, asthma exacerbation
CLIENT EDUCATION: Observe for manifestations and notify the provider if they occur.

Bradycardia, hypotension
- NURSING ACTIONS: Monitor heart rate and blood pressure.
- CLIENT EDUCATION
  - Check heart rate prior to taking the medication.
  - Notify the provider of any significant change.

Anticonvulsants (divalproex)

GI distress
- Nausea, vomiting, diarrhea, dyspepsia, indigestion
- NURSING ACTIONS: Report manifestations to the provider.

Fetal neural tube defects
CLIENT EDUCATION
- Do not take these medications during pregnancy.
- Use additional contraception when taking this medication.

Hepatitis
NURSING ACTIONS
- Monitor liver enzymes.
- Notify the provider of lethargy or fever.

Pancreatitis
CLIENT EDUCATION: Report abdominal pain, nausea, vomiting, and anorexia. If these occur, the provider should discontinue the medication.

Tricyclic antidepressants (amitriptyline)

Anticholinergic effects
- Dry mouth, constipation, urinary retention, tachycardia, blurry vision
- CLIENT EDUCATION
  - Increase fluid intake. Sip fluids throughout the day. Chew gum or suck on hard candy. Use an alcohol-free mouthwash.
  - Increase daily fiber intake.
  - Increase physical activity by engaging in regular exercise.
  - Stimulant laxatives (such as bisacodyl) counteract reduced bowel motility. Stool softeners (such as docusate sodium) prevent constipation.
  - Urinate just before taking the medication and then every 4 hr. Report urinary retention to the provider.
  - Report blurry vision.

Drowsiness or dizziness
CLIENT EDUCATION: Avoid driving or operating machinery until the medication's effects are known.

CONTRAINDICATIONS/PRECAUTIONS

Ergotamine
- Kidney and liver dysfunction, sepsis, hypertension, pregnancy, CAD, and history of MI are contraindications.
- Pregnancy Risk Category X

Triptans
- Liver failure, ischemic heart disease, history of MI, uncontrolled hypertension, and other heart diseases are contraindications.
- Pregnancy Risk Category C

Propranolol
- Heart block, bradycardia, bronchial asthma, cardiogenic shock, and heart failure are contraindications.
- Clients taking other antihypertensives or who have liver or kidney impairment, diabetes mellitus, or Wolff-Parkinson-White syndrome require caution when taking these medications.
- Pregnancy Risk Category C

Divalproex
- Liver disease is a contraindication.
- Pregnancy Risk Category D; Category X for migraine headaches

Amitriptyline
- Recent MI and having taken an MAOI within 14 days are contraindications.
- Clients who have a seizure history, urinary retention, prostatic hyperplasia, angle-closure glaucoma, hyperthyroidism, or liver or kidney disease require caution when taking these medications.
- Pregnancy Risk Category C

Aspirin-like medications
- Severe kidney impairment and hepatic disease are contraindications.
- Older adults and clients who have GI bleeding or cardiac disorders require caution when taking these medications.

Acetaminophen

Acetaminophen should be an adjunct to other medications; alone, it is ineffective for treating migraines.

INTERACTIONS

Aspirin-like medications (NSAIDs, acetaminophen combination)

NSAIDs can reduce the effectiveness of antihypertensives, furosemide, thiazide diuretics, and oral antidiabetes medications.
NURSING ACTIONS: Monitor for medication effectiveness.

Corticosteroids, alcohol, and tobacco can increase GI effects.
CLIENT EDUCATION: Do not take these together.

NSAIDs can increase levels of oral anticoagulants and lithium.
NURSING ACTIONS: Monitor medication levels.

There is an increased risk of bleeding with the use of other NSAIDs, thrombolytics, antiplatelets, anticoagulants, and salicylates.
- NURSING ACTIONS: Monitor for bleeding.
- CLIENT EDUCATION: Use caution if taking these medications together.

Serotonin receptor antagonists (sumatriptan)

Concurrent use of MAOIs can lead to MAO toxicity.
CLIENT EDUCATION: Do not take triptans within 2 weeks of stopping MAOIs.

Concurrent use with ergotamine or another triptan can cause a vasospastic reaction.
NURSING ACTIONS: Discourage concurrent use of these medications.

Taking selective serotonin reuptake inhibitors (SSRIs) with triptans can cause serotonin syndrome (confusion, agitation, hyperthermia, diaphoresis, possible death).
CLIENT EDUCATION: Do not take these medications concurrently.

Ergotamine and dihydroergotamine

Concurrent use with triptans can cause a vasospastic reaction.
CLIENT EDUCATION: Take triptans at least 24 hr apart from taking an ergotamine medication.

Some HIV protease inhibitors, antifungal medications, macrolide antibiotics, and grapefruit juice can increase ergotamine levels, increasing vasospasm.
CLIENT EDUCATION: Do not take these medications concurrently.

Beta blockers (propranolol)

Verapamil and diltiazem have additive cardiosuppression effects.
NURSING ACTIONS: If clients must take these medications concurrently, monitor the ECG, heart rate, and blood pressure.

Diuretics and antihypertensive medications have additive hypotensive effects.
NURSING ACTIONS: Monitor blood pressure. Withhold and notify the provider if the systolic blood pressure is less than 90 mm Hg.

Propranolol can mask the hypoglycemic effect of insulin and prevent the breakdown of fat in response to hypoglycemia.
NURSING ACTIONS
- Administer with caution.
- Monitor blood glucose levels.

Anticonvulsants (divalproex)

NSAIDs, erythromycin, and salicylates can cause divalproex toxicity.
NURSING ACTIONS: Monitor medication levels.

Benzodiazepines, opioids, antihistamines, and alcohol can cause central nervous system (CNS) depression.
CLIENT EDUCATION: Do not take these medications concurrently.

Divalproex can increase levels of phenobarbital and phenytoin.
NURSING ACTIONS: Monitor medication levels.

These medications increase the effects of warfarin.
NURSING ACTIONS
- Monitor for therapeutic effects of warfarin with PT and INR. Providers might make dosage adjustments.
- Monitor for bleeding.

Tricyclic antidepressants (amitriptyline)

Barbiturates, CNS depressants, antihistamines, over-the-counter sleep aids, and alcohol can cause additive CNS depression.
CLIENT EDUCATION: Do not take these medications concurrently.

Cimetidine can increase amitriptyline levels.
NURSING ACTIONS: Monitor medication effects.

MAOIs can increase CNS excitation or cause seizures.
CLIENT EDUCATION: Do not take amitriptyline within 2 weeks of taking MAOIs.

NURSING ADMINISTRATION

- Advise clients not to use abortive medications more often than 2 days a week.
- Advise clients who have migraines to avoid trigger factors that cause stress and fatigue, such as consumption of alcohol and tyramine-containing foods (wine, aged cheese).
- Advise clients that lying down in a dark, quiet place can help ease manifestations. Q_{EBP}
- Antiemetics, preferably metoclopramide, are useful as adjunct medications for migraine treatment.
- Advise clients to check their heart rate before taking propranolol.
- Clients can take some medications with food to reduce GI distress (divalproex) and to increase absorption (propranolol).
- Advise clients to protect their skin and eyes from the sun (amitriptyline) and avoid driving or operating machinery until they know how the medication will affect them.
- Advise caution due to orthostatic hypotension (amitriptyline, propranolol). Qs

NURSING EVALUATION OF MEDICATION EFFECTIVENESS

Indications of effectiveness include the following.
- Reduction in the intensity and frequency of migraine attacks
- Prophylaxis against migraine attacks
- Termination of migraine headaches
- Reduction in the size and frequency of medication dosages

Local anesthetics

SELECT PROTOTYPE MEDICATIONS
- **Amide type:** Lidocaine

OTHER MEDICATIONS
- **Ester type:** Tetracaine, procaine
- **Amide type:** Eutectic mixture of 2.5% lidocaine/2.5% prilocaine (EMLA)

PURPOSE

EXPECTED PHARMACOLOGICAL ACTION

These medications decrease pain by blocking the conduction of pain impulses in a specific area. Loss of consciousness does not occur.

THERAPEUTIC USES

PARENTERAL ADMINISTRATION
- Pain management for dental procedures, minor surgical procedures, labor and delivery, diagnostic procedures
- Regional anesthesia (spinal, epidural)

TOPICAL ADMINISTRATION
- Skin and mucous membrane disorders
- Control laryngeal and esophageal reflexes prior to endoscopic procedures
- Minor procedures, such as IV insertion, injection (pediatric), and wart removal

COMPLICATIONS

CNS excitation

Seizures, followed by respiratory depression, leading to unconsciousness

NURSING ACTIONS
- Monitor for indications of seizure activity, sedation, and changes in mental status (decreases in level of consciousness).
- Monitor vital signs and respiratory status.
- Have equipment ready for resuscitation.
- Administer benzodiazepines (midazolam, diazepam) to treat seizures.

Hypotension, cardiosuppression

Bradycardia, heart block, cardiac arrest (common with spinal anesthesia due to sympathetic blockade)

NURSING ACTIONS
- Monitor vital signs and the ECG.
- If manifestations occur, follow prescriptions for treatment.

Allergic reactions

More likely with ester-type agents, such as procaine
- Clients who are allergic to one ester-type agent are likely allergic to all other ester-type agents.
- Amide-type anesthetic agents are less likely to cause allergic reactions, and therefore are better for injection.

NURSING ACTIONS
- Observe for manifestations of an allergy to anesthetics (allergic dermatitis, anaphylaxis).
- Treat with antihistamines.

Prolonged labor, fetal effects

- A decrease in uterine contractility can prolong labor.
- Local anesthetics can cross the placenta and result in fetal bradycardia and CNS depression.
- Clients who are in labor require caution when receiving local anesthetics.

NURSING ACTIONS
- Monitor uterine activity for effectiveness.
- Monitor fetal heart rate for bradycardia and decreased variability.

Spinal headache

NURSING ACTIONS: Monitor for indications of severe headache.

CLIENT EDUCATION: Remain flat in bed for 12 hr postprocedure.

Urinary retention

Can occur with spinal anesthesia

NURSING ACTIONS
- Monitor urinary output.
- Notify the provider if clients have not urinated within 8 hr.

CONTRAINDICATIONS/PRECAUTIONS

- Local anesthetics are Pregnancy Risk Category B.
- Supraventricular dysrhythmias and heart block are contraindications.
- Clients who have liver and kidney dysfunction, heart failure, or myasthenia gravis require caution with the use of local anesthetics.
- Locations on the fingers, nose, and other body parts with end arteries are contraindications for adding epinephrine to local anesthetics. Gangrene can result due to vasoconstriction.
- Advise clients to use caution to prevent self-inflicted injury until the anesthetic effect wears off.

INTERACTIONS

Antihypertensive medications have additive hypotensive effects with parenteral administration of local anesthetics.
NURSING ACTIONS: Monitor heart rate and blood pressure.

NURSING ADMINISTRATION

- Advise clients to avoid hazardous activities when recovering from anesthesia.
- Keep clients in a comfortable position during recovery.

Injection of local anesthetics
- Vasoconstrictors, such as epinephrine, help prevent the spread of the local anesthetic.
  - Containing the anesthetic prolongs the anesthesia and decreases the risk of systemic toxicity.
  - Do not add epinephrine to a local anesthetic for injection into the fingers, nose, or other body parts with end arteries because gangrene can result due to vasoconstriction.
- Prepare the injection site for the local anesthetic by cleansing and shaving it if necessary.
- Monitor vital signs and level of consciousness.
- Maintain IV access for the possible need for administration of emergency medications.
- Have equipment ready for resuscitation.
- For a regional block, protect the area of numbness from injury.

Spinal or epidural nerve blocks
- Monitor clients during insertion for hypotension, anaphylaxis, seizure, and dura puncture. Q_{EBP}
- Monitor for respiratory depression and sedation.
- Monitor the insertion site for hematoma and indications of an infection.
- Determine the level of sensory block. Evaluate leg strength prior to ambulating.
- Prepare IV fluids to administer to compensate for the sympathetic blocking effects of regional anesthetics.
- Have clients lie supine for 12 hr following spinal anesthesia to minimize headache.
- Notify the provider if clients are unable to urinate after 8 hr.

Topical cream (EMLA)
- Apply the cream to intact skin 1 hr before routine procedures or a superficial puncture and 2 hr before more extensive procedures or deep puncture.
- Apply it to the smallest surface area necessary for minimizing systemic absorption. Avoid wrapping or heating the area.
- Prior to the procedure, remove the dressing and clean the skin with an antiseptic solution.
- Keep clients NPO following oral administration until normal pharyngeal sensation returns (approximately 1 hr). Monitor first oral intake.
- Clients can apply EMLA at home prior to visiting a health care facility for a procedure.

CLIENT EDUCATION
- Notify the provider for indications of infection (fever, swelling, redness), increases in pain, severe headache, sudden weakness of the lower extremities, or decreases in bowel or bladder control. Q_S
- Notify the provider for indications of systemic infusion (metallic taste, tinnitus, perioral numbness, seizures).
- Sanitize hands before and after self-administration of a topical anesthetic.

NURSING EVALUATION OF MEDICATION EFFECTIVENESS

Indications of effectiveness include the following.
- No procedural pain
- Pain relief

Application Exercises

1. A nurse is reinforcing teaching with a client who has migraine headaches. Which of the following instructions should the nurse provide? (Select all that apply.)

   A. Take ergotamine to prevent migraine headaches.

   B. Identify and avoid factors that trigger migraine headaches.

   C. Lie down in a dark quiet room at the onset of a migraine headache.

   D. Avoid foods that contain tyramine.

   E. Avoid exercise that can increase heart rate.

2. A nurse is contributing to the plan of care for a client who is to receive tetracaine prior to a bronchoscopy. Which of the following actions should the nurse suggest for the plan of care?

   A. Keep the client NPO until pharyngeal sensation returns.

   B. Monitor the insertion site for a hematoma.

   C. Palpate the bladder to detect urinary retention.

   D. Keep the client in bed for 12 hr after the procedure.

3. A nurse is caring for a client who receives an injection of lidocaine during the repair of a skin laceration. The nurse should monitor for which of the following adverse reactions?

   A. Seizures

   B. Tachycardia

   C. Hypertension

   D. Fever

4. A nurse is reviewing the health history of a client who has migraine headaches and is to begin prophylaxis with propranolol. Which of the following findings should the nurse report to the provider?

   A. The client had a prior MI.

   B. The client takes warfarin for atrial fibrillation.

   C. The client takes an SSRI for depression.

   D. An ECG indicates a first-degree heart block.

5. A nurse is reinforcing teaching with a client who has migraine headaches and a new prescription for ergotamine. The client should stop taking the medication and notify the provider for which of the following adverse effects? (Select all that apply.)

   A. Nausea

   B. Visual disturbances

   C. Positive home pregnancy test

   D. Numbness and tingling in fingers

   E. Muscle pain

PRACTICE Active Learning Scenario

A nurse is reinforcing teaching with a client who has frequent migraine headaches about a new prescription for sumatriptan. What should the nurse remind the client about this medication? Use the ATI Active Learning Template: Medication to complete this item.

THERAPEUTIC USES: Describe the therapeutic use for sumatriptan in this client.

COMPLICATIONS: Describe two adverse effects the client should monitor for.

INTERACTIONS: Describe two interactions the nurse should inform the client about.

NURSING INTERVENTIONS: Describe two for this client.

Application Exercises Key

1. A. Taking ergotamine at the onset of a migraine aborts headache manifestations. Regular use can cause physical dependence and toxicity.

   B. **CORRECT:** Identifying and avoiding trigger factors is an important action that can help prevent some migraine headaches.

   C. **CORRECT:** Lying down in a dark, quiet room at the onset of a migraine headache can prevent the onset of more severe manifestations.

   D. **CORRECT:** Foods that contain tyramine can be a trigger for some migraine headaches. The client should avoid foods that contain tyramine (smoked meats, most cheeses, wine).

   E. Clients should exercise between migraine headaches because it can relieve stress, which can trigger headaches.

   Ⓝ *NCLEX® Connection: Pharmacological Therapies, Expected Actions/Outcomes*

2. A. **CORRECT:** The nurse should keep the client NPO following the procedure until normal pharyngeal sensation returns (approximately 1 hr) and should then monitor the client's first oral intake to make sure aspiration does not occur.

   B. The nurse should monitor the insertion site for a hematoma for clients who receive spinal anesthesia.

   C. The nurse should palpate the bladder to detect urinary retention for clients who receive spinal anesthesia.

   D. Clients who receive spinal anesthesia should rest in bed for 12 hr after the procedure.

   Ⓝ *NCLEX® Connection: Pharmacological Therapies, Expected Actions/Outcomes*

3. A. **CORRECT:** Seizure activity is an adverse effect that can occur as a result of local anesthetic injection.

   B. Bradycardia can occur as a result of local anesthetic injection.

   C. Hypotension can occur as a result of local anesthetic injection.

   D. Fever is not an adverse effect of local anesthetic injection.

   Ⓝ *NCLEX® Connection: Pharmacological Therapies, Adverse Effects/ Contraindications/Side Effects/Interactions*

4. A. A prior MI is not a contraindication for taking propranolol.

   B. Warfarin does not interact adversely with propranolol.

   C. Concurrent use of an SSRI is not a contraindication for taking propranolol. Clients should not take sumatriptan with SSRIs because it can lead to serotonin syndrome

   D. **CORRECT:** First-degree heart block is a contraindication for taking propranolol. The nurse should report this finding to the provider.

   Ⓝ *NCLEX® Connection: Pharmacological Therapies, Expected Actions/Outcomes*

5. A. Nausea commonly occurs with a migraine headache and does not warrant withholding the medication and notifying the provider. Nausea and vomiting also are common adverse effects of ergotamine. If they occur, the provider might prescribe an antiemetic.

   B. Visual disturbances, such as flashing lights, are common findings with migraine headaches and do not warrant withholding the medication and notifying the provider.

   C. **CORRECT:** A client who has a positive home pregnancy test should stop taking ergotamine and notify the provider. Ergotamine is in Pregnancy Risk Category X and can cause abortion.

   D. **CORRECT:** Numbness and tingling in fingers or toes is a finding with ergotamine overdose. The client should stop taking the medication and notify the provider.

   E. **CORRECT:** Unexplained muscle pain is a finding with ergotamine overdose. The client should stop taking the medication and notify the provider.

   Ⓝ *NCLEX® Connection: Pharmacological Therapies, Adverse Effects/ Contraindications/Side Effects/Interactions*

PRACTICE Answer

Using the ATI Active Learning Template: Medication

THERAPEUTIC USES: Sumatriptan aborts a migraine headache and its other manifestations (nausea, vomiting) after the headache begins by causing cranial artery vasoconstriction.

COMPLICATIONS: This medication can cause dizziness, vertigo, chest and arm heaviness and pressure, and anginal pain due to coronary vasospasm.

INTERACTIONS: Toxicity can result if the client takes sumatriptan concurrently or within 2 weeks of taking an MAOI antidepressant. The client should not take sumatriptan concurrently with other triptan medications or within 24 hr of taking ergotamine or dihydroergotamine.

NURSING INTERVENTIONS
- Instruct the client to take sumatriptan at the first sign of migraine manifestations.
- Show the client how to administer sumatriptan if the route is intranasal or subcutaneous.
- Advise the client to notify the provider immediately at the onset of angina pain. Tell the client how to distinguish transient chest or arm heaviness due to sumatriptan from angina pain.

Ⓝ *NCLEX® Connection: Pharmacological and Parenteral Therapies, Medication Administration*

ⓝ NCLEX® Connections

When reviewing the following chapters, keep in mind the relevant topics and tasks of the NCLEX outline, in particular:

Pharmacological Therapies

ADVERSE EFFECTS/CONTRAINDICATIONS/SIDE EFFECTS/INTERACTIONS: Identify potential and actual incompatibilities of the client's medications.

DOSAGE CALCULATIONS: Use clinical decision making when calculating dosages.

MEDICATION ADMINISTRATION

Mix medications from two vials as necessary (insulin).

Reinforce client teaching on self-administration of medications (insulin, subcutaneous insulin pump).

UNIT 10   MEDICATIONS AFFECTING THE
ENDOCRINE SYSTEM

CHAPTER 34 *Diabetes Mellitus*

Diabetes mellitus is a chronic illness that results from an absolute or relative deficiency of insulin, often combined with a cellular resistance to insulin's actions. Various insulins are available to manage diabetes. These medications differ in their onset, peak, and duration.

Oral antidiabetic medications work in various ways to increase available insulin or modify carbohydrate metabolism. Newer injectable medications are used to supplement insulin or oral agents to manage glucose control.

Insulin

SELECT PROTOTYPE MEDICATIONS
- **Rapid-acting:** Lispro insulin
  - ONSET: 15 to 30 min
  - PEAK: 0.5 to 2.5 hr
  - DURATION: 3 to 6 hr
- **Short-acting:** Regular insulin
  - ONSET: 0.5 to 1 hr
  - PEAK: 1 to 5 hr
  - DURATION: 6 to 10 hr
- **Intermediate-acting:** NPH insulin
  - ONSET: 1 to 2 hr
  - PEAK: 6 to 14 hr
  - DURATION: 16 to 24 hr
- **Long-acting:** Insulin glargine
  - ONSET: 70 min
  - PEAK: None
  - DURATION: 18 to 24 hr

OTHER MEDICATIONS
- **Rapid-acting**
  - Insulin aspart
  - Insulin glulisine
- **Short-acting:** Regular insulin
- **Long-acting:** Insulin detemir is dose-dependent. The greater units/kg the client receives, the longer the duration of the insulin. In some cases, the client can receive up to 0.4 units/kg, resulting in a duration of 20 to 24 hr, making it a long-acting insulin.

PREMIXED INSULINS
- **70% NPH and 30% regular:** Mixture of intermediate- and short-acting insulin
- **50% NPH and 50% regular:** Mixture of intermediate- and short-acting insulin
- **70% insulin lispro protamine and 30% insulin lispro:** Mixture of intermediate- and rapid-acting insulin
- **75% insulin lispro protamine and 25% insulin lispro:** Mixture of intermediate- and rapid-acting insulin
- **50% insulin lispro protamine and 50% insulin lispro:** Mixture of intermediate- and rapid-acting insulin

PURPOSE

EXPECTED PHARMACOLOGICAL ACTION

- Promotes cellular uptake of glucose (decreases glucose levels)
- Converts glucose into glycogen
- Moves potassium into cells (along with glucose)

THERAPEUTIC USES

- Insulin is used for glycemic control of diabetes mellitus (type 1, type 2, gestational) to prevent complications.
- Clients who have type 2 diabetes mellitus can require insulin when:
  - Oral antidiabetic medications, diet, and exercise are unable to control blood glucose levels.
  - Severe kidney or liver disease is present.
  - Painful neuropathy is present.
  - Undergoing surgery or diagnostic tests.
  - Experiencing severe stress (infection, trauma).
  - Undergoing emergency treatment of diabetes ketoacidosis (DKA) and hyperosmolar hyperglycemic nonketotic syndrome.
  - Requiring treatment of hyperkalemia.

COMPLICATIONS

Hypoglycemia

- Hypoglycemia occurs when blood glucose is less than 70 mg/dL.
- Hypoglycemia can result from the following.
  - Overdose of insulin
  - Too little food
  - Vomiting and diarrhea
  - Alcohol intake
  - Strenuous exercise
  - Childbirth

NURSING ACTIONS

- Monitor for hypoglycemia. If abrupt onset, client will experience sympathetic nervous system (SNS) effects (tachycardia, palpitations, diaphoresis, shakiness). If gradual onset, client will experience parasympathetic (PNS) manifestations (headache, tremors, weakness, lethargy, disorientation).
- Administer glucose. For conscious clients, administer a snack of 15 g carbohydrate (4 oz orange juice, 2 oz grape juice, 8 oz milk, glucose tablets per manufacturer's suggestion to equal 15 g).
- If the client is not fully conscious, do not risk aspiration. Administer glucose parenterally, such as subcutaneous/IM glucagon, or ask the charge nurse to administer IV glucose.
- Encourage clients to wear a medical alert bracelet and to always have a snack with glucose handy.

Lipohypertrophy

CLIENT EDUCATION: Systematically rotate injection sites and allow 1 inch between injection sites.

INTERACTIONS

Sulfonylureas, meglitinides, beta blockers, and alcohol have additive hypoglycemic effects with concurrent use.
NURSING ACTIONS: Monitor serum glucose levels for hypoglycemia (less than 70 mg/dL) and adjust insulin or oral antidiabetic dosages accordingly.

Concurrent use of thiazide diuretics and glucocorticoids can raise blood glucose levels and thereby counteract the effects of insulin.
NURSING ACTIONS: Monitor serum glucose levels for hyperglycemia, and adjust insulin doses accordingly. Higher insulin doses can be indicated.

Beta blockers can mask SNS response to hypoglycemia (tachycardia, tremors), making it difficult for clients to identify hypoglycemia
CLIENT EDUCATION
- Monitor glucose levels and do not rely on SNS manifestations as an alert to developing hypoglycemia.
- Maintain a regular eating schedule to ensure adequate glucose during times of hypoglycemic action.

NURSING ADMINISTRATION

- Adjust the insulin dosage to meet insulin needs.
  - The dosage might need to be increased in response to increase in caloric intake, infection, stress, growth spurts, and in the second and third trimesters of pregnancy. Q PCC
  - The dosage might need to be decreased in response to level of exercise or first trimester of pregnancy.
- Ensure adequate glucose is available at the time of onset of insulin and during all peak times.
- When mixing short-acting insulin with longer-acting insulin, draw the short-acting insulin up into the syringe first. This prevents the possibility of accidentally injecting some of the longer-acting insulin into the shorter-acting insulin vial. (This can pose a risk for unexpected insulin effects with subsequent uses of the vial.)

- For insulin suspensions, gently rotate the vial between the palms to disperse the particles throughout the vial prior to withdrawing insulin.
- NPH and premixed insulins should appear cloudy. Do not administer other insulins if they are cloudy. Do not administer any insulins that are discolored or if a precipitate is present.
- Insulin glargine and insulin detemir are both clear in color, not administered IV, and should not be mixed in a syringe with any other insulin.
- Administer lispro, aspart, glulisine, and regular insulin by subcutaneous injection. Monitor a client receiving continuous subcutaneous infusion and IV route.
- Administer NPH insulin via the subcutaneous route.
- Instruct clients to administer subcutaneous insulin in one general area to have consistent rates of absorption. Absorption rates from subcutaneous tissue increase from thigh to upper arm to abdomen.
- Use only insulin-specific syringes that correspond to the concentration of insulin being administered. Administer U-100 insulin with a U-100 syringe; administer U-500 insulin with a U-500 syringe.
- Select an appropriate needle length to ensure insulin is injected into subcutaneous tissue vs. intradermal (too short) or intramuscular (too long).
- Encourage clients to enhance diabetes medication therapy with a proper diet and consistent activity.
- Ensure proper storage of insulin.
  - Unopened vials of a single type of insulin can be stored in the refrigerator until their expiration date. Q EBP
  - Vials of premixed insulins can be stored for up to 3 months under refrigeration.
  - Insulins premixed in syringes can be kept for 1 to 2 weeks under refrigeration. Keep the syringes in a vertical position, with the needles pointing up. Prior to administration, the insulin should be resuspended by gently moving the syringe.
  - Store the vial that is in use at room temperature, avoiding proximity to sunlight and intense heat. Discard after 1 month.

Oral antidiabetics

Sulfonylureas

SELECT PROTOTYPE MEDICATIONS
- **1st generation:** Chlorpropamide
- **2nd generation:** Glipizide

OTHER MEDICATIONS
- **1st generation:** Tolazamide
- **2nd generation:** Glyburide, glimepiride

Meglitinides (glinides)

SELECT PROTOTYPE MEDICATION: Repaglinide

OTHER MEDICATION: Nateglinide

Biguanides

SELECT PROTOTYPE MEDICATION: Metformin

Thiazolidinediones (glitazones)

SELECT PROTOTYPE MEDICATION: Pioglitazone

Alpha-glucosidase inhibitors

SELECT PROTOTYPE MEDICATION: Acarbose

OTHER MEDICATIONS: Miglitol

DPP-4 inhibitors (gliptins)

SELECT PROTOTYPE MEDICATION: Sitagliptin

OTHER MEDICATIONS: Saxagliptin, alogliptin, linagliptin

Sodium-glucose co-transporter 2 (SGLT-2) inhibitors

SELECT PROTOTYPE MEDICATION: Canagliflozin

OTHER MEDICATIONS: Dapagliflozin

PURPOSE

EXPECTED PHARMACOLOGICAL ACTION

Sulfonylureas: Insulin release from the pancreas

Meglitinides (glinides): Insulin release from the pancreas

Biguanides
- Reduces the production of glucose within the liver through suppression of gluconeogenesis
- Increases muscles' glucose uptake and use
- First-choice medication for most clients who have type 2 diabetes

Thiazolidinediones (glitazones)
- Increases cellular response to insulin by decreasing insulin resistance
- Increases glucose uptake and decreased glucose production

Alpha-glucosidase inhibitors: Slows carbohydrate absorption and digestion

DPP-4 inhibitors (gliptins)
- Augments naturally occurring incretin hormones, which promote release of insulin and decrease secretion of glucagon
- Lowers fasting and postprandial blood glucose levels

SGLT-2 inhibitors
- Used in combination with insulin for type 1 diabetes
- Limits the rise of glucose postprandial
- Excretes glucose through the urine
- Promotes weight loss

THERAPEUTIC USES

- Antidiabetic agents control blood glucose levels in clients who have type 2 diabetes mellitus and are used in conjunction with diet and exercise lifestyle changes.
- Metformin is also used to treat polycystic ovary syndrome (PCOS) (off-label use).

COMPLICATIONS

Glipizide and repaglinide

Hypoglycemia
- NURSING ACTIONS: Monitor for manifestations of hypoglycemia. If abrupt onset, the client will experience SNS manifestations (tachycardia, palpitations, diaphoresis, shakiness). If gradual onset, the client will experience PNS manifestations (headache, tremors, weakness).
- CLIENT EDUCATION
  ○ Self-administer a snack of 15 g carbohydrate (4 oz orange juice, 2 oz grape juice, 8 oz milk, glucose tablets per manufacturer's suggestion to equal 15 g).
  ○ Notify the provider if there is a recurrent problem.
  ○ If severe hypoglycemia occurs, IV glucose might be needed.
  ○ Wear a medical alert bracelet.

Weight gain
CLIENT EDUCATION: Adhere to a proper diet and increase physical activity.

Metformin

Gastrointestinal effects: Anorexia, nausea, and diarrhea, which frequently result in weight loss of 3 to 4 kg (6.6 to 8.8 lb)
- Effects usually subside with use.
- Dose should be titrated to target dose to minimize severity of GI effects
- NURSING ACTIONS
  ○ Monitor for severity of these effects.
  ○ Discontinue the medication if necessary.

Vitamin B$_{12}$ and folic acid deficiency caused by altered absorption

Lactic acidosis: Hyperventilation, myalgia, sluggishness, somnolence (50% mortality rate)
- CLIENT EDUCATION
  ○ Withhold medication if these manifestations occur, and inform the provider immediately.
  ○ Severe lactic acidosis can be treated with hemodialysis.

Pioglitazone

Fluid retention
NURSING ACTIONS: Monitor for edema, weight gain, and indications of heart failure.

Elevations in low-density lipoproteins (LDL) cholesterol
NURSING ACTIONS: Monitor cholesterol levels.

Bladder cancer
CLIENT EDUCATION: Manifestations of bladder cancer include hematuria, urgency, and dysuria. Inform the provider immediately if these manifestations occur.

Ovulation in anovulatory premenopausal females
NURSING ACTIONS: Instruct client regarding potential for ovulation and contraceptive options.

Fractures in female clients
CLIENT EDUCATION: Measures to maintain bone health include exercise and adequate intake of calcium and vitamin D.

Hepatotoxicity
- NURSING ACTIONS: Perform baseline and periodic liver function tests.
- CLIENT EDUCATION: Report any hepatotoxicity manifestations (jaundice, dark urine).

Acarbose

Gastrointestinal effects: abdominal distention and cramping, hyperactive bowel sounds, diarrhea, excessive gas
- NURSING ACTIONS
  - Monitor impact of these effects on the client.
  - Discontinue the medication if necessary.

Anemia due to the decrease of iron absorption
NURSING ACTIONS
- Monitor hemoglobin and iron levels.
- Discontinue the medication if necessary.

Hepatotoxicity with long-term use
- Liver function will return to normal after the medication is discontinued.
- NURSING ACTIONS
  - Check baseline liver function and perform periodic liver function tests.
  - Discontinue the medication if elevations occur.

Sitagliptin

Generally well tolerated

Pancreatitis
CLIENT EDUCATION
- Manifestations of pancreatitis include severe, persistent abdominal pain with or without vomiting.
- Stop medication immediately and the contact provider if manifestations occur.

Canagliflozin

Cystitis, candidiasis, and polyuria in female clients
NURSING ACTIONS: Monitor for manifestations of infection.

Dizziness and risk for hypotension in older adults with concurrent use of diuretics
CLIENT EDUCATION
- Rise slowly from a seated position, and report episodes of dizziness to the provider.
- Use caution if medications are given together.

CONTRAINDICATIONS/PRECAUTIONS

- PREGNANCY RISK CATEGORY C: Glipizide, repaglinide, pioglitazone, canagliflozin Qs
- PREGNANCY RISK CATEGORY B: Metformin, acarbose, sitagliptin. These oral agents are generally avoided in pregnancy and lactation, but the provider may prescribe them.
- Use cautiously in clients who have kidney failure, hepatic dysfunction, or heart failure due to the risk of medication accumulation and resulting hypoglycemia. Severity of disease can indicate contraindication.
- All oral diabetic medications are contraindicated in the treatment of DKA.
- **Metformin** is contraindicated for clients who have severe infection, shock, and any hypoxic condition. The medication should not be used by clients who have alcohol use disorder.
- **Acarbose** is contraindicated for clients who have gastrointestinal disorders (inflammatory disease, ulceration, obstruction).
- **Pioglitazone** is contraindicated for clients who have severe heart failure, history of bladder cancer, and active hepatic disease. Use cautiously in clients who have mild heart failure and in older adults. ⓖ
- **Canagliflozin** is contraindicated for clients who have kidney failure and are undergoing dialysis.

INTERACTIONS

Glipizide

Use of alcohol can result in disulfiram-like reaction (intense nausea and vomiting, flushing, palpitations).
NURSING ACTIONS: Inform clients about the risk, and encourage them to avoid alcohol.

NSAIDs, sulfonamide antibiotics, ranitidine, and cimetidine have additive hypoglycemic effect.
CLIENT EDUCATION
- Closely monitor glucose levels when these other agents are used concurrently.
- Dosage adjustment of the oral antidiabetic medication might be needed.

Beta blockers can mask SNS response to hypoglycemia (tachycardia, tremors, palpitations, diaphoresis), making it difficult for clients to identify hypoglycemia.
CLIENT EDUCATION
- Monitoring glucose levels and do not rely on SNS manifestations as an alert to developing hypoglycemia.
- Maintain a regular eating schedule to ensure adequate glucose during times of hypoglycemic action.

Beta blockers decrease effectiveness by inhibiting insulin release.
CLIENT EDUCATION: Closely monitor glucose levels.

Repaglinide

Concurrent use of gemfibrozil results in inhibition of repaglinide metabolism, leading to an increased risk for hypoglycemia.
NURSING ACTIONS
- Avoid concurrent use of repaglinide or pioglitazone and gemfibrozil.
- Closely monitor for manifestations of hypoglycemia.

Pioglitazone

Use with insulin can lead to fluid retention.
NURSING ACTIONS: Avoid concurrent use.

Increased levels with atorvastatin and ketoconazole.
NURSING ACTIONS: Monitor glucose levels. Dosage of pioglitazone might need to be reduced.

Decreased levels with rifampin and cimetidine.
NURSING ACTIONS: Monitor glucose levels. Dosage of pioglitazone might need to be increased.

Metformin

Alcohol increases the risk of lactic acidosis with concurrent use.
NURSING ACTIONS: Inform clients of the risks, and encourage clients to avoid consuming alcohol.

Concurrent use of iodine-containing contrast media can result in acute kidney failure.
NURSING ACTIONS: Clients taking metformin should discontinue medication 24 to 48 hr prior to procedure. They can resume medication 48 hr after test if lab results indicate normal kidney function.

Acarbose

Concurrent use of acarbose with sulfonylureas or insulin increases the risk for hypoglycemia.
- If hypoglycemia develops, treatment requires the use of glucose instead of sucrose because the hydrolysis of sucrose to glucose and fructose is inhibited by acarbose.
- NURSING ACTIONS: Monitor carefully for hypoglycemia.

Concurrent use of metformin causes additive gastrointestinal effects and risk for hypoglycemia.
NURSING ACTIONS: Monitor carefully for gastrointestinal effects and hypoglycemia.

Sitagliptin

No significant interactions

Canagliflozin

Decreased effect if used concurrently with rifampin, phenytoin, or phenobarbital
NURSING ACTIONS: Monitor glucose levels, as dosage might need to be increased.

Increases the effect of thiazide and loop diuretics
NURSING ACTIONS: Monitor for dehydration and hypotension. Use caution if medications are used together.

CLIENT EDUCATION

- Exercise consistently and to follow appropriate dietary guidelines.
- Maintain a log of glucose levels and to note patterns that affect glucose levels (increased dietary intake, infection).
- Consider working with a registered dietitian or diabetic nurse educator. Qᴛᴄ
- Administer medications orally and at appropriate times.
  - **Glipizide:** Best taken with breakfast.
  - **Repaglinide:** Eat within 30 min of taking a dose of the medication, three times per day.
  - **Metformin:** Take immediate release tablets two times per day with breakfast and evening meal and to take sustained-release tablets once daily with evening meal.
  - **Pioglitazone:** Take once a day, with or without food.
  - **Acarbose:** Take with the first bite of food, three times per day.
  - **Sitagliptin:** Take once a day with or without food.
  - **Canagliflozin:** Take once a day, before the first meal of the day.
- Formulations can combine two medications.
- If also taking insulin, monitor for manifestations of hypoglycemia.

Amylin mimetics

SELECT PROTOTYPE MEDICATION: Pramlintide

PURPOSE

EXPECTED PHARMACOLOGICAL ACTION

Pramlintide mimics the actions of the naturally occurring peptide hormone amylin, resulting in reduction of postprandial glucose levels from decreased gastric emptying time and inhibition of secretion of glucagon. There is also an increase in the sensation of satiety, which helps decrease caloric intake.

THERAPEUTIC USES

- Supplemental glucose control for clients who have type 1 or type 2 diabetes mellitus
- Can be used in conjunction with insulin or an oral antidiabetic medication, usually metformin and/or a sulfonylurea

COMPLICATIONS

Nausea

CLIENT EDUCATION: Report manifestations to the provider. Dose can be decreased.

Reaction at injection sites

Generally self-limiting

CONTRAINDICATIONS/PRECAUTIONS

- Pregnancy Risk Category C. Qs
- This medication is contraindicated for clients who have kidney failure or are receiving dialysis.
- Use cautiously in clients who have thyroid disease, osteoporosis, or alcohol use disorder.

INTERACTIONS

Insulin increases the risk for hypoglycemia.
NURSING ACTIONS: Concurrent use can require a decrease in insulin dose, usually 50% of rapid- or short-acting insulin. Avoid use in clients unable to self-monitor blood glucose levels.

Concurrent use of pramlintide with medications that slow gastric emptying (such as opioids) or medications that delay food absorption (such as acarbose) can further slow gastric emptying time.
NURSING ACTIONS: Avoid concurrent use.

Oral medication absorption is delayed.
NURSING ACTIONS: Administer oral medications 1 hr before or 2 hr after injection of pramlintide.

NURSING ADMINISTRATION

- Administer subcutaneously prior to meals, using the thigh or abdomen. QEBP
- Instruct clients to keep unopened vials in the refrigerator and not to freeze. Opened vials can be kept cool or at room temperature but should be discarded after 28 days. Keep vials out of direct sunlight.
- Instruct clients not to mix medication with insulin in the same syringe.

Incretin mimetics

SELECT PROTOTYPE MEDICATION: Exenatide

OTHER MEDICATIONS
- Liraglutide
- Albiglutide

PURPOSE

EXPECTED PHARMACOLOGICAL ACTION

Mimics the effects of naturally occurring glucagon-like peptide-1, and thereby promotes release of insulin, decreases secretion of glucagon, and slows gastric emptying. Fasting and postprandial blood glucose levels are lowered. Incretin mimetics decrease appetite, which can lead to weight loss.

THERAPEUTIC USES

- Supplemental glucose control for clients who have type 2 diabetes
- Can be used in conjunction with an oral antidiabetic medication, usually metformin or a sulfonylurea

COMPLICATIONS

GI effects (nausea, vomiting, diarrhea)

CLIENT EDUCATION: Notify the provider if manifestations are intolerable.

Pancreatitis (severe and intolerable abdominal pain)

CLIENT EDUCATION: Withhold medication and notify the provider.

CONTRAINDICATIONS/PRECAUTIONS

- Pregnancy Risk Category C Qs
- Contraindicated for clients who have severe kidney impairment, severe gastrointestinal disease, or a history of pancreatitis.
- Use cautiously in older adult clients and clients who have kidney impairment or thyroid disease. ⓒ

INTERACTIONS

Oral medication absorption is delayed, especially oral contraceptives, antibiotics, and acetaminophen.
NURSING ACTIONS: Administer oral medications 1 hr before injection of exenatide.

Concurrent use of sulfonylurea increases risk of hypoglycemia.
- Clients can require a lower dose of sulfonylurea.
- CLIENT EDUCATION: Monitor blood glucose levels.

NURSING ADMINISTRATION

- This medication is supplied in prefilled injector pens.
- Administer subcutaneously in the thigh, abdomen, or upper arm. QEBP
- Give exenatide injection within 60 min before the morning and evening meal. Never administer after a meal. Exenatide is also available in a longer-acting formula that can be administered once weekly. Liraglutide is administered once a day without regard to meals. Albiglutide is administered once weekly.
- Instruct clients to keep the injection pen in the refrigerator and to discard after 30 days.

NURSING EVALUATION OF MEDICATION EFFECTIVENESS

Depending on therapeutic intent, effectiveness can be evidenced by the following.
- Preprandial glucose levels 90 to 130 mg/dL and postprandial levels less than 180 mg/dL
- HbA1c less than 7%

Hyperglycemic agent

SELECT PROTOTYPE MEDICATION: Glucagon

PURPOSE

EXPECTED PHARMACOLOGICAL ACTION

Increases blood glucose levels by increasing the breakdown of glycogen into glucose; decreasing glycogen synthesis enhances the synthesis of glucose

THERAPEUTIC USES

- Emergency management of hypoglycemic reactions, such as insulin overdose, in clients who are unable to take oral glucose
- Decrease in gastrointestinal motility in clients undergoing radiological procedures of the stomach and intestines

COMPLICATIONS

GI distress (nausea, vomiting)
NURSING ACTIONS: Turn clients onto the left side following administration to reduce the risk of aspiration if emesis occurs.

CONTRAINDICATIONS/PRECAUTIONS

- Glucagon is ineffective for hypoglycemia resulting from inadequate glycogen stores (starvation).
- Pregnancy Risk Category B Qs
- Use cautiously in clients who have cardiovascular disease.

NURSING ADMINISTRATION

- Administer glucagon subcutaneously or IM, or ensure IV administration immediately following reconstitution parameters. QEBP
- Provide food as soon as the client regains full consciousness and is able to swallow.
- Instruct clients to maintain access to a source of glucose and glucagon kit at all times.

NURSING EVALUATION OF MEDICATION EFFECTIVENESS

Depending on therapeutic intent, effectiveness can be evidenced by elevation in blood glucose level to greater than 70 mg/dL.

Application Exercises

1. A nurse is reinforcing teaching with clients in an outpatient facility about the use of insulin to treat type 1 diabetes mellitus. For which of the following types of insulin should clients to expect a peak effect 1 to 5 hr after administration?

   A. Insulin glargine

   B. NPH insulin

   C. Regular insulin

   D. Insulin lispro

2. A nurse is caring for a client in an outpatient facility who has been taking acarbose for type 2 diabetes mellitus. Which of the following laboratory tests should the nurse monitor?

   A. WBC

   B. Serum potassium

   C. Platelet count

   D. Liver function tests

3. A nurse is reinforcing teaching with a client who has type 2 diabetes mellitus and is starting repaglinide. Which of the following statements by the client indicates understanding?

   A. "I'll take this medication once a day."

   B. "I'll take this medicine within 30 minutes before eating."

   C. "I'll take this medicine just before I go to bed."

   D. "I'll take this medication at least 1 hour before I eat."

4. A nurse is reinforcing teaching with a client who has a new prescription for metformin. The nurse should instruct the client to report which of the following manifestations as an adverse effect of metformin?

   A. Somnolence

   B. Constipation

   C. Fluid retention

   D. Weight gain

5. A nurse is reinforcing teaching with a client who has a prescription for pramlintide for type 1 diabetes mellitus. Which of the following instructions should the nurse include? (Select all that apply.)

   A. "Take oral medications 1 hr before injection."

   B. "Use upper arms as preferred injection sites."

   C. "Mix pramlintide with the breakfast dose of insulin."

   D. "Inject pramlintide just before a meal."

   E. "Discard open vials after 28 days."

Application Exercises Key

1. A. Insulin glargine, a long-acting insulin, does not have a peak effect time, but is stable in effect for 24 hr following administration.

    B. NPH insulin has a peak effect of 6 to 14 hr following administration.

    C. **CORRECT:** Regular insulin has a peak effect of 1 to 5 hr following administration.

    D. Insulin lispro has a peak effect of 30 min to 2.5 hr following administration.

    (N) *NCLEX® Connection: Pharmacological Therapies, Medication Administration*

2. A. Infection is not an adverse effect of acarbose. It is not necessary to monitor WBC while the client is taking this medication.

    B. Acarbose does not affect potassium levels. It is not necessary to monitor serum potassium while the client is taking this medication.

    C. Acarbose does not affect platelet levels. It is not necessary to monitor the platelet count while the client is taking this medication.

    D. **CORRECT:** Acarbose can cause liver toxicity when taken long-term. Liver function tests should be monitored periodically while the client takes this medication.

    (N) *NCLEX® Connection: Pharmacological Therapies, Expected Actions/Outcomes*

3. A. The client should take this medication before each meal, rather than once each day to control glucose levels.

    B. **CORRECT:** Repaglinide causes a rapid, short-lived release of insulin. The client should take this medication within 30 min before each meal so that insulin is available when food is digested.

    C. Repaglinide should not be taken just before bedtime.

    D. Repaglinide has a rapid onset and should be taken 30 min prior to a meal.

    (N) *NCLEX® Connection: Pharmacological Therapies, Medication Administration*

4. A. **CORRECT:** Somnolence can indicate lactic acidosis, which is manifested by extreme drowsiness, hyperventilation, and muscle pain. It is a rare but very serious adverse effect caused by metformin and should be reported to the provider.

    B. Diarrhea is an adverse effect of metformin.

    C. Fluid retention is not an adverse effect caused by metformin.

    D. Anorexia and weight loss are adverse effects of metformin.

    (N) *NCLEX® Connection: Pharmacological Therapies, Adverse Effects/ Contraindications/Side Effects/Interactions*

5. A. **CORRECT:** Pramlintide delays oral medication absorption, so oral medications should be taken 1 hr before or 2 hr after pramlintide injection.

    B. The thigh or abdomen, rather than the upper arms, are preferred sites for pramlintide injection.

    C. Pramlintide should not be mixed in a syringe with any type of insulin.

    D. **CORRECT:** Pramlintide can cause hypoglycemia, especially when the client also takes insulin, so it is important to eat a meal after injecting this medication.

    E. **CORRECT:** Unused medication in the open pramlintide vial should be discarded after 28 days.

    (N) *NCLEX® Connection: Pharmacological Therapies, Expected Actions/Outcomes*

A nurse in an acute care facility is reinforcing teaching with a client who has type 2 diabetes mellitus and is taking exenatide and an oral antidiabetic agent. What should the nurse reinforce with the client about this medication? Use the ATI Active Learning Template: Medication to complete this item.

THERAPEUTIC USES: Identify the therapeutic use for exenatide in this client.

COMPLICATIONS: Identify two adverse effects the client should watch for.

NURSING INTERVENTIONS: Describe two laboratory tests the nurse should monitor.

CLIENT EDUCATION: Describe instruction points to give a client taking exenatide.

Using the ATI Active Learning Template: Medication

THERAPEUTIC USES: Exenatide is prescribed along with an oral antidiabetic medication, such as metformin or a sulfonylurea medication, for clients who have type 2 diabetes mellitus to improve diabetes control. Exenatide improves insulin secretion by the pancreas, decreases secretion of glucagon, and slows gastric emptying.

COMPLICATIONS
*   GI effects (nausea, vomiting)
*   Pancreatitis manifested by acute abdominal pain and possibly severe vomiting
*   Hypoglycemia, especially when taken concurrently with a sulfonylurea medication, such as glipizide

NURSING INTERVENTIONS: Monitor daily blood glucose testing by the client, periodic HbA1c tests, and periodic kidney function testing. Use exenatide cautiously in clients who have any kidney impairment.

CLIENT EDUCATION
*   Inject exenatide subcutaneously.
*   Take exenatide within 60 min before the morning and evening meal but not following the meal.
*   Withhold exenatide and notify the provider for severe abdominal pain.
*   How to recognize and treat hypoglycemia.
*   Exenatide should not be given within 1 hr of oral antibiotics, acetaminophen, or an oral contraceptive due to its ability to slow gastric emptying.

(N) *NCLEX® Connection: Pharmacological and Parenteral Therapies, Medication Administration*

CHAPTER 35

UNIT 10   MEDICATIONS AFFECTING THE
           ENDOCRINE SYSTEM

CHAPTER 35 *Endocrine Disorders*

The endocrine system is made up of glands that secrete hormones, which act on specific receptor sites. Hormones target receptor sites to regulate response to stress, growth, metabolism, and homeostasis.

An endocrine disorder usually involves oversecretion or undersecretion of hormones, or an altered response by the target area or receptor.

Medications can be used to treat disorders of the thyroid, anterior and posterior pituitary, and adrenal glands.

Thyroid hormone

SELECT PROTOTYPE MEDICATION: Levothyroxine

OTHER MEDICATIONS
- Liothyronine
- Liotrix
- Thyroid USP

PURPOSE

EXPECTED PHARMACOLOGICAL ACTION: Thyroid hormones are a synthetic form of thyroxine (T_4), a form of liothyronine (T_3), or a combination of T_3 and T_4. They increase metabolic rate, protein synthesis, cardiac output, renal perfusion, oxygen use, body temperature, blood volume, and growth processes.

THERAPEUTIC USES
- Thyroid hormone replacement is used for treatment of hypothyroidism (all ages, all forms).
- Thyroid hormones are used for the emergency treatment of myxedema coma (IV route), a severe deficiency of thyroid hormone.

ROUTE OF ADMINISTRATION: Oral, IV (myxedema coma)

COMPLICATIONS

Overmedication

Overmedication can result in indications of hyperthyroidism (anxiety, tachycardia, palpitations, altered appetite, abdominal cramping, heat intolerance, fever, diaphoresis, weight loss, menstrual irregularities).

CLIENT EDUCATION: Report indications of overmedication to the provider.

Chronic overtreatment

Chronic overtreatment can cause atrial fibrillation and an increased risk of fractures from bone loss, especially in older adults.

NURSING ACTIONS: TSH levels should be monitored at least once a year.

CONTRAINDICATIONS/PRECAUTIONS

- Pregnancy Risk Category A
- Use is contraindicated for clients who have thyrotoxicosis and adrenal insufficiency.
- Due to cardiac stimulant effects, use is contraindicated following a MI.
- Use cautiously in clients who have cardiovascular problems (hypertension, angina pectoris, ischemic heart disease) because of cardiac stimulant effects.
- Use cautiously in older adults. Ⓒ
- Use cautiously in clients who have diabetes.
- Thyroid hormone replacement is not for use in the treatment of obesity.

INTERACTIONS

Binding agents, antiulcer medications, calcium and iron supplements, and food reduce levothyroxine absorption with concurrent use.
- Binding agents include cholestyramine and colestipol. Antiulcer medications include sucralfate, cimetidine, lansoprazole, and antacids.
- NURSING ACTIONS: Allow at least 4 hr between medication administration.

Many antiseizure and antidepressant medications (carbamazepine, phenytoin, phenobarbital, sertraline) and the antibiotic rifampin can increase levothyroxine metabolism.
NURSING ACTIONS: Monitor for therapeutic effects of levothyroxine. Dosages of levothyroxine might need to be increased.

Levothyroxine can increase the anticoagulant effects of warfarin by breaking down vitamin K.
- NURSING ACTIONS
  - Monitor prothrombin time (PT) and international normalized ratio (INR).
  - Decreased dosages of warfarin can be needed.
  - Levothyroxine can alter blood glucose levels requiring increased dosages for insulin.
  - Levothyroxine can alter digoxin levels.
- CLIENT EDUCATION: Report signs of bleeding (bruising, petechiae).

NURSING ADMINISTRATION

- Obtain baseline vital signs, weight, and height, and monitor periodically throughout treatment.
- Monitor and report signs of cardiac excitability (angina, chest pain, palpitations, dysrhythmias).
- Daily therapy begins with a low dose that increases gradually over several weeks. Full effect of medication can take 6 to 8 weeks.
- Monitor T_4 and TSH levels.
- Instruct clients to take the medication daily on an empty stomach 30 to 60 min before breakfast.
- Reinforce client education regarding the importance of lifelong replacement (even after improvement of symptoms). Advise clients not to discontinue the medication without checking with the provider.
- Instruct clients to check with the provider before switching to another brand of levothyroxine because some concerns regarding interchangeability of brands have been raised, and dosage adjustments can be necessary. Qᴛᴄ

NURSING EVALUATION OF MEDICATION EFFECTIVENESS

Depending on therapeutic intent, evidence of effectiveness can include the following.
- Decreased TSH levels
- T_4 levels within expected reference range
- Absence of hypothyroidism manifestations (depression, weight gain, bradycardia, anorexia, cold intolerance, dry skin, menorrhagia)

Thionamides

SELECT PROTOTYPE MEDICATION: Methimazole

OTHER MEDICATION: Propylthiouracil (PTU)

PURPOSE

EXPECTED PHARMACOLOGICAL ACTION

- Blocks the synthesis of thyroid hormones
- Prevents the oxidation of iodide
- Blocks conversion of T_4 into T_3

THERAPEUTIC USES

- Treatment of Graves' disease
- Produces a euthyroid state prior to thyroid removal surgery
- As an adjunct to irradiation of the thyroid gland
- In the emergency treatment of thyrotoxicosis
- Methimazole is considered first-line therapy
- Treatment for thyroid storm (PTU preferred)

ROUTE OF ADMINISTRATION: Oral

COMPLICATIONS

Hypothyroidism

Overmedication can result in indications of hypothyroidism (drowsiness, depression, weight gain, edema, bradycardia, anorexia, cold intolerance, dry skin, menorrhagia).

NURSING ACTIONS
- Reduced dosages and temporary administration of thyroid supplements can be needed.
- Monitor thyroid function labs.

CLIENT EDUCATION: Report signs of overmedication to the provider.

Agranulocytosis

NURSING ACTIONS
- Monitor for early indications of agranulocytosis (sore throat, fever, fatigue), and instruct clients to report them promptly to provider.
- Monitor blood counts at baseline and periodically.
- If agranulocytosis occurs, stop treatment and monitor the client for reversal of agranulocytosis.
- Filgrastim can be indicated to treat agranulocytosis.

Liver injury, hepatitis (propylthiouracil)

NURSING ACTIONS: Monitor for jaundice, dark urine, light-colored stools, and elevated liver function tests during treatment.

CONTRAINDICATIONS/PRECAUTIONS

- Use is contraindicated in pregnancy (Pregnancy Risk Category D) and during lactation due to the risk of neonatal hypothyroidism. Propylthiouracil is safer than methimazole during the first trimester of pregnancy and is considered safer during lactation if an antithyroid medication is necessary. Qs
- Use cautiously in clients who have bone marrow depression and immunosuppression, and in clients at risk for liver failure.

INTERACTIONS

Concurrent use of antithyroid medications and anticoagulants can increase anticoagulation.
NURSING ACTIONS: Monitor PT, INR, and activated partial thromboplastin time (aPTT). Adjust dosages of anticoagulants accordingly.

Concurrent use of antithyroid medications and digoxin can increase glycoside level.
NURSING ACTIONS: Monitor digoxin level, and reduce digoxin dose as needed.

NURSING ADMINISTRATION

- Advise clients that therapeutic effects can take 1 to 2 weeks to be evident, while full benefit can take 3 to 12 weeks. Qpcc
- Propylthiouracil does not destroy the thyroid hormone that is present, but rather prevents continued synthesis of TH.
- Monitor thyroid function labs, vital signs, weight, and I&O at baseline and periodically.
- Instruct clients to take medication at consistent times each day and with meals to maintain a consistent therapeutic level and decrease gastric distress.
- Instruct clients not to discontinue the medication abruptly (risk of thyroid crisis due to stress response).
- Monitor for signs of hyperthyroidism (indicating inadequate medication).
- Clients who have hyperthyroidism may receive a beta adrenergic antagonist, such as propranolol, to decrease tremors and tachycardia.
- Monitor for indications of hypothyroidism (drowsiness, depression, weight gain, edema, bradycardia, anorexia, cold intolerance, dry skin) indicating overmedication.
- Monitor CBC for leukopenia or thrombocytopenia.
- Instruct clients to not take any OTC medications without consent of provider.
- Advise clients to avoid consumption of seafood, which contains iodine, and other iodine products.

NURSING EVALUATION OF MEDICATION EFFECTIVENESS

Depending on therapeutic intent, evidence of effectiveness can include the following.
- Weight gain
- Vital signs within expected reference range
- Decreased TSH and T_4 levels
- Absence of signs of hyperthyroidism (anxiety, tachycardia, palpitations, increased appetite, abdominal cramping, heat intolerance, fever, diaphoresis, weight loss, menstrual irregularities)

Radiopharmaceuticals

SELECT PROTOTYPE MEDICATION: Radioactive iodine (^{131}I)

PURPOSE

EXPECTED PHARMACOLOGICAL ACTION

The thyroid absorbs radioactive iodine, destroying some of the thyroid producing cells. At high doses, thyroid–radioactive iodine destroys thyroid cells.

THERAPEUTIC USES

At high doses
- Hyperthyroidism
- Thyroid cancer
- Clients who have not responded to other antithyroid treatments

At low doses: Thyroid function studies (Visualization of the degree of iodine uptake by the thyroid gland is helpful in the diagnosis of thyroid disorders.)

ROUTE OF ADMINISTRATION: Oral

COMPLICATIONS

Radiation sickness

NURSING ACTIONS
- Monitor for manifestations of radiation sickness (hematemesis, epistaxis, intense nausea, vomiting).
- Stop treatment and notify the provider.

Bone marrow depression

NURSING ACTIONS: Monitor for anemia, leukopenia, and thrombocytopenia.

Hypothyroidism

Intolerance to cold, edema, bradycardia, weight gain, depression

CLIENT EDUCATION: Report indications of hypothyroidism to the provider.

CONTRAINDICATIONS/PRECAUTIONS

- Pregnancy, childbearing age/intent, and lactation are contraindications to use due to irradiating effects. (Pregnancy Risk Category X) Qs
- Radioactive iodine use is not advisable for use in young children.

INTERACTIONS

Concurrent use of other antithyroid medications reduces uptake of radioactive iodine.
NURSING ACTIONS: Discontinue use of other antithyroid medications for a week prior to therapy.

NURSING ADMINISTRATION

- Instruct clients regarding radioactivity precautions.
- Limit contact with clients to 30 min/day/person.

CLIENT EDUCATION
- Increase fluid intake, usually 2 to 3 L/day.
- Dispose of body wastes per protocol.
- Avoid coughing and expectoration (source of radioactive iodine).
- Therapeutic effects can take 2 to 3 months.
- Maintain a distance of 6 feet from others. Do not prepare food for others or share utensils. Qpcc

Iodine products

SELECT PROTOTYPE MEDICATION: Strong iodine solution: nonradioactive iodine

PURPOSE

EXPECTED PHARMACOLOGICAL ACTION

Nonradioactive iodine creates high levels of iodide that will reduce iodine uptake (by the thyroid gland), inhibit thyroid hormone production, and block the release of thyroid hormones into the bloodstream.

THERAPEUTIC USES

- Nonradioactive iodine is used for the development of euthyroid state and reduction of thyroid gland size prior to thyroid removal surgery.
- Nonradioactive iodine is used for the emergency treatment of thyrotoxicosis.

ROUTE OF ADMINISTRATION: Oral

COMPLICATIONS

Iodism

- Repeated use can cause metallic taste, stomatitis, sore teeth and gums, nasal inflammation and sneezing, frontal headache, and skin rash.
- Iodism (early toxicity) can progress to overdose (severe GI distress, swelling of the glottis).

NURSING ACTIONS: Prepare to administer sodium thiosulfate (to reverse effects of iodine). Assist with gastric lavage as needed.

CLIENT EDUCATION: Notify the provider for any manifestations of overdose.

CONTRAINDICATIONS/PRECAUTIONS

Use in pregnancy is contraindicated (Pregnancy Risk Category D). Qs

INTERACTIONS

Concurrent intake of foods high in iodine (iodized salt, seafood containing iodine) increases risk for iodism.
NURSING ACTIONS
- Monitor for signs of iodism (brassy taste in mouth, burning sensation in mouth, sore teeth).
- Instruct clients regarding foods high in iodine.

Concurrent use of potassium-sparing diuretics, potassium supplements, and ACE inhibitors increases the risk of hyperkalemia.
NURSING ACTIONS: Do not use medications together.

NURSING ADMINISTRATION

- Nonradioactive iodine can be used in conjunction with other therapy because effects are not usually complete or permanent. Qpcc
- Obtain baseline vital signs, weight, and I&O, and monitor periodically.
- Instruct clients to dilute strong iodine solution with juice to improve taste.
- Instruct clients to take at the same time each day to maintain therapeutic levels.
- Encourage clients to increase fluid intake, unless contraindicated.
- Instruct clients to not take any OTC medications that contain iodine.
- Instruct clients not to discontinue medication abruptly.

NURSING EVALUATION OF MEDICATION EFFECTIVENESS

Depending on therapeutic intent, effectiveness can be evidenced by the following.
- Weight gain
- Vital signs within expected reference range
- Decreased T_4 levels
- Reduction in size of thyroid gland
- Client can get adequate sleep, achieve and maintain appropriate weight, maintain blood pressure and heart rate within expected reference range, and be free of complications of hyperthyroidism.

Anterior pituitary hormones/growth hormones

SELECT PROTOTYPE MEDICATION: Somatropin

PURPOSE

EXPECTED PHARMACOLOGICAL ACTION: Anterior pituitary hormones/growth hormones stimulate overall growth and the production of protein, and decrease the use of glucose.

THERAPEUTIC USES
- Anterior pituitary hormones/growth hormones are used to treat growth hormone deficiencies (pediatric and adult growth hormone deficiencies, Turner's syndrome, Prader–Willi syndrome).
- AIDS wasting syndrome

ROUTES OF ADMINISTRATION: Subcutaneous (preferred route) or IM

COMPLICATIONS

Hyperglycemia

NURSING ACTIONS
- Observe for indications of hyperglycemia (polyphagia, polydipsia, polyuria).
- Monitor glucose levels in clients who have diabetes. Insulin doses can need to be adjusted.

Hypercalciuria and renal calculi

CLIENT EDUCATION: Monitor for flank pain, fever, and dysuria, and report these to the provider.

CONTRAINDICATIONS/PRECAUTIONS

- These medications are Pregnancy Risk Category B or C (depending on the brand prescribed). Qs
- Use is contraindicated in clients who are severely obese or have serious respiratory impairment (sleep apnea) due to higher risk of mortality.
- Use cautiously in clients who have diabetes due to the risk of hyperglycemia.
- Use cautiously in clients who have hypothyroidism, as thyroid function can be suppressed. Evaluate thyroid function prior to administering and periodically.
- Treatment should not occur during or after epiphyseal closure.

INTERACTIONS

Concurrent use of glucocorticoids can counteract growth-promoting effects.
NURSING ACTIONS: Avoid concurrent use of glucocorticoids and somatrem.

NURSING ADMINISTRATION

- Obtain baseline height and weight.
- Therapy continues until a satisfactory adult height occurs or response can no longer be elicited.
- Monitor growth patterns during medication administration, usually monthly. Qpcc
- Reconstitute medication per directions. Mix gently, and do not shake prior to administration. Do not administer if medication contains particulates or is discolored.
- Rotate injection sites. Abdomen (subcutaneous) and thighs (subcutaneous, IM) are preferred.

NURSING EVALUATION OF MEDICATION EFFECTIVENESS

Depending on therapeutic intent, effectiveness can be evidenced by the client increasing height and weight.

Antidiuretic hormone

SELECT PROTOTYPE MEDICATION: Vasopressin

OTHER MEDICATION: Desmopressin

PURPOSE

EXPECTED PHARMACOLOGICAL ACTION

- Antidiuretic hormone (ADH), produced by the hypothalamus and stored in the posterior pituitary, promotes reabsorption of water within the kidney.
- Natural ADH causes vasoconstriction due to the contraction of vascular smooth muscle. Vasopressin simulates the potent action of ADH, while desmopressin causes much less vasoconstriction.

THERAPEUTIC USES

- These hormones are used to treat diabetes insipidus (DI). Desmopressin is the agent of choice for DI.
- Antidiuretic hormone (vasopressin) is sometimes used during CPR to temporarily decrease blood flow to the periphery and increase flow to the brain and heart.

ROUTE OF ADMINISTRATION
- Desmopressin: Oral, intranasal, subcutaneous, IV
- Vasopressin: Subcutaneous, IM, IV

COMPLICATIONS

Reabsorption of too much water

In general, clients should reduce fluid intake during therapy.

NURSING ACTIONS: Monitor for indications of overhydration (sleepiness, pounding headache).

CLIENT EDUCATION
- Monitor and record daily I&O and notify the provider of manifestations of overhydration.
- Use the smallest effective dose of desmopressin.

Myocardial ischemia

From excessive vasoconstriction (vasopressin)

NURSING ACTIONS: Monitor ECG and blood pressure.

CLIENT EDUCATION: Notify the provider of chest pain, tightness, or diaphoresis.

CONTRAINDICATIONS/PRECAUTIONS

- Use of vasopressin is contraindicated in clients who have coronary artery disease (risk for angina, MI), decreased peripheral circulation (risk for gangrene), or chronic nephritis. Qs
- Vasopressin is Pregnancy Risk Category C, and desmopressin is Pregnancy Risk Category B.
- Use caution in clients who have renal impairment, as risk of water intoxication is increased. ADH should not be administered to clients who have creatinine clearance less than 50 mL/min.

INTERACTIONS

Carbamazepine and tricyclic antidepressants can increase the antidiuretic action.
NURSING ACTIONS: Use cautiously together.

Concurrent use of alcohol, heparin, lithium, and phenytoin can decrease antidiuretic effects.
NURSING ACTIONS: Establish baseline I&O and weight, and monitor frequently.

NURSING ADMINISTRATION

- Monitor vital signs, I&O, specific gravity, and laboratory studies (potassium, sodium, BUN, creatinine, creatinine clearance, specific gravity, osmolality).
- Monitor blood pressure and heart rate.
- Monitor for headache, confusion, or other indications of water intoxication.
- With IV administration of vasopressin, monitor the IV site carefully because extravasation can lead to gangrene.
- Intranasal desmopressin starts with a bedtime dose. I&O is monitored. When nocturia is controlled, doses are given twice daily.

NURSING EVALUATION OF MEDICATION EFFECTIVENESS

Depending on therapeutic intent, evidence of effectiveness can include the following.
- Reduction in the large volumes of urine output associated with diabetes insipidus to normal levels of urine output (1.5 to 2 L/24 hr)
- Cardiac arrest survival

Adrenal hormone replacement

SELECT PROTOTYPE MEDICATION: Hydrocortisone

OTHER MEDICATIONS
- Glucocorticoids
  - Prednisone
  - Dexamethasone
- Mineralocorticoid: Fludrocortisone

PURPOSE

EXPECTED PHARMACOLOGICAL ACTION: Mimic effect of natural steroid hormones

THERAPEUTIC USES
- Acute and chronic replacement therapy for adrenocortical insufficiency (Addison's disease, adrenal crisis)
- Nonendocrine disorders (cancer, inflammation, allergic reactions)

ROUTE OF ADMINISTRATION: Oral, IV

COMPLICATIONS

Glucocorticoids

Osteoporosis
CLIENT EDUCATION: Take calcium supplements, vitamin D, and/or bisphosphonate. Get regular exercise.

Adrenal suppression
- NURSING ACTIONS: Increase dose with stress. Do not stop the medication suddenly. Taper dose to discontinue.
- CLIENT EDUCATION: Observe for manifestations (fatigue, muscle weakness, weight loss, hypotension), and notify the provider if they occur.

Peptic ulcer, GI discomfort
- NURSING ACTIONS: Administer prophylactic H$_2$ receptor antagonists.
- CLIENT EDUCATION: Observe for manifestations (coffee-ground emesis, bloody or tarry stools, abdominal pain), and notify the provider if they occur.

Infection
- NURSING ACTIONS: Monitor for any indications of infection, such as fever.
- CLIENT EDUCATION: Avoid contact with people who have a communicable disease.

Cushing's syndrome
- Risks are associated with long-term use of glucocorticoids and excessive doses.
- CLIENT EDUCATION: Observe for manifestations (muscle weakness, moon face, buffalo hump, cutaneous striations), and notify the provider if they occur.

Mineralocorticoids

Retention of sodium and water
- Can lead to hypertension, edema, heart failure and hypokalemia
- NURSING ACTIONS
  - Monitor weight, blood pressure, and electrolyte levels. Monitor breath sounds and urine output.
  - Educate clients on manifestations of sodium and water retention (weight gain, peripheral edema) and hypokalemia (muscle weakness, irregular pulse), and to notify provider if they occur.

CONTRAINDICATIONS/PRECAUTIONS

- Hydrocortisone and fludrocortisone are Pregnancy Risk Category C. **Qs**
- Use is contraindicated in clients who have a viral, bacterial, or fungal infection not controlled by antibiotics.
- Use with caution in clients who have had a recent MI, gastric ulcer, hypertension, kidney disorder, osteoporosis, diabetes mellitus, hypothyroidism, myasthenia gravis, glaucoma, or seizure disorder.

INTERACTIONS

Glucocorticoids: hydrocortisone

NSAIDs, acetaminophen, or alcohol use can cause increased gastric distress or bleed.
NURSING ACTIONS: Use together with caution.

Concurrent use with oral anticoagulants can increase or decrease anticoagulation.
NURSING ACTIONS: Monitor coagulation studies and medication levels.

Concurrent use with potassium depleting agents can cause increased potassium loss.
NURSING ACTIONS: Monitor serum potassium and ECG.

Concurrent use with vaccines and toxoids can reduce the antibody response.
NURSING ACTIONS: Do not use together.

Mineralocorticoid: fludrocortisone

Barbiturates and phenytoin can reduce effects of fludrocortisone.
NURSING ACTIONS: Monitor for reduced medication effects.

Antidiabetic effects of insulin and sulfonylureas decrease with concurrent use of fludrocortisone.
NURSING ACTIONS: Closely monitor blood glucose levels in clients who have diabetes mellitus.

NURSING ADMINISTRATION

- Monitor weight, blood pressure, glucocorticoid levels, and electrolytes at baseline and periodically.
- Give with food to reduce gastric distress.
- Advise clients to observe for indications of peptic ulcer (coffee-ground emesis, bloody or tarry stools, abdominal pain) and to notify the provider if they occur.
- Do not stop the medication suddenly. Taper dosage if discontinuing.
- Instruct clients to notify the provider of indications of acute adrenal insufficiency (fever, muscle and joint pain, weakness, fatigue).
- Instruct clients that dosages need to be increased during times of stress (infection, surgery, trauma).
- Advise clients that replacement therapy for Addison's disease must continue for life.
- Instruct clients to carry an extra supply of glucocorticoids for emergencies and to wear medical identification at all times.

NURSING EVALUATION OF MEDICATION EFFECTIVENESS

Depending on therapeutic intent, evidence of effectiveness can include relief of effects of adrenocortical deficiency (weakness, hypoglycemia, hyperkalemia, fatigue) with minimal adverse effects.

Hyperpituitarism medications

SELECT PROTOTYPE MEDICATION: Octreotide

OTHER MEDICATIONS
- Lanreotide
- Pegvisomant

PURPOSE

EXPECTED PHARMACOLOGICAL ACTION: Suppress growth hormone release in clients who do not respond to surgical excision or irradiation of the pituitary or adjunct therapy to surgery and/or radiation

THERAPEUTIC USES
- Gigantism in children
- Acromegaly in adults

ROUTE OF ADMINISTRATION
- Octreotide (IM, subcutaneous)
- Lanreotide (subcutaneous)
- Pegvisomant (subcutaneous)

COMPLICATIONS

Octreotide

Gastrointestinal disturbances
- Nausea, cramps, diarrhea, flatulence
- NURSING ACTIONS: Give injections without food or at bedtime to minimize symptoms.
- CLIENT EDUCATION: Symptoms usually subside in 1 to 2 weeks.

Hypo/hyperglycemia
NURSING ACTIONS: Monitor glucose levels regularly.

Lanreotide

Gastrointestinal disturbances
- Abdominal pain, diarrhea, nausea, vomiting, flatulence, cholelithiasis
- CLIENT EDUCATION: Notify the provider of symptoms.

Hypo/hyperglycemia
NURSING ACTIONS: Monitor glucose levels regularly.

Pegvisomant

Nausea, diarrhea
CLIENT EDUCATION: Notify the provider of symptoms.

Hypoglycemia
NURSING ACTIONS: Monitor glucose levels regularly.

Liver injury
NURSING ACTIONS
- Advise clients to discontinue the medication and notify the provider if jaundice appears.
- Monitor liver function studies.

Chest pain
CLIENT EDUCATION: Notify the provider of symptoms promptly.

Flu-like symptoms
CLIENT EDUCATION: Notify the provider of signs of infection.

CONTRAINDICATIONS/PRECAUTIONS

Octreotide
- Pregnancy Risk Category B Qs
- Use cautiously in clients who have diabetes, hypothyroidism, and kidney disease, and in older adult clients.

Lanreotide
- Pregnancy Risk Category C
- Use cautiously in clients who have gallbladder, liver, or renal disease; diabetes; hypothyroidism; and cardiac disease.

Pegvisomant
- Pregnancy Risk Category B
- Use cautiously in clients who have liver or kidney disease, diabetes, pituitary tumors, or neoplastic disease.

INTERACTIONS

Octreotide

Conduction delays can occur if used with antidysrhythmics.
NURSING ACTIONS: Monitor cardiac status.

Lanreotide

Bradycardia can occur with concurrent use of medications that affect heart rate.
NURSING ACTIONS: Monitor cardiac status.

Pegvisomant

Concurrent use with opioids can reduce the effect of pegvisomant.
NURSING ACTIONS: Dosage can need to be increased.

NURSING ADMINISTRATION

- Inform clients of proper technique for subcutaneous injection. Qs
- Minimize injection site pain by rotating sites. The abdomen, hip, and thigh are the preferred sites.
- IM injection of octreotide should be to a large muscle. Reinforce to clients to minimize injection site pain by administering slowly, after the medication reaches room temperature.

NURSING EVALUATION OF MEDICATION EFFECTIVENESS

Depending on therapeutic intent, evidence of effectiveness can include the suppression of excess growth hormone for the management of acromegaly when surgery or radiation has failed.

Application Exercises

1. A nurse is caring for a client who is taking methimazole. For which of the following adverse effects of this medication should the nurse monitor?
   - A. Bradycardia
   - B. Insomnia
   - C. Heat intolerance
   - D. Weight loss

2. A nurse is reinforcing teaching to a client who has Graves' disease about her prescribed medications. Which of the following statements by the client indicates an understanding of the use of propranolol in the treatment of Graves' disease?
   - A. "Propranolol helps increase blood flow to my thyroid gland."
   - B. "Propranolol is used to prevent excess glucose in my blood."
   - C. "Propranolol will decrease my tremors and fast heart beat."
   - D. "Propranolol promotes a decrease of thyroid hormone in my body."

3. A nurse is caring for an older adult client in a long-term care facility who has hypothyroidism and a new prescription for levothyroxine. Which of the following dosage schedules should the nurse expect for this client?
   - A. The client will start at a high dose, with dose adjustments as needed.
   - B. The client will remain on the initial dosage during the course of treatment.
   - C. The client's dosage will be adjusted daily based on blood levels.
   - D. The client will start on a low dose, with gradual increases in dosage.

4. A nurse is caring for a client who is taking somatropin to stimulate growth. The nurse should plan to monitor the client's urine for which of the following?
   - A. Bilirubin
   - B. Protein
   - C. Potassium
   - D. Calcium

5. A nurse is collecting data for a client who takes desmopressin for diabetes insipidus. For which of the following adverse effects should the nurse monitor?
   - A. Hypovolemia
   - B. Hypercalcemia
   - C. Agitation
   - D. Headache

Application Exercises Key

1. A. **CORRECT:** The nurse should monitor for bradycardia which is an adverse effect of methimazole.

   B. Drowsiness, rather than insomnia, is an adverse effect of methimazole.

   C. Cold intolerance rather than heat intolerance is an adverse effect of methimazole.

   D. Weight gain, rather than weight loss, is an adverse effect of methimazole.

   Ⓝ *NCLEX® Connection: Pharmacological Therapies, Adverse Effects/ Contraindications/Side Effects/Interactions*

2. A. Propranolol lowers blood pressure, but does not increase blood flow to the thyroid gland.

   B. Propranolol does not help prevent hyperglycemia.

   C. **CORRECT:** Propranolol is a beta adrenergic antagonist that decreases heart rate and controls tremors.

   D. Propranolol does not promote a decrease of thyroid hormone.

   Ⓝ *NCLEX® Connection: Pharmacological Therapies, Expected Actions/Outcomes*

3. A. The nurse should not expect that the levothyroxine will be started at a high dose.

   B. The nurse should not expect that the client's dosage will remain the same throughout treatment.

   C. The nurse should not expect that the client's dosage will be adjusted daily based on blood levels.

   D. **CORRECT:** The nurse should expect that levothyroxine will be started at a low dose and gradually increased over several weeks. This is especially important in older adult clients to prevent toxicity.

   Ⓝ *NCLEX® Connection: Pharmacological Therapies, Medication Administration*

4. A. Bilirubin can be present in the urine with liver or biliary disorders, but is not during somatropin therapy.

   B. Protein can be present in the urine during stress, infection, or glomerular disorders, but not during somatropin therapy.

   C. Somatropin therapy does not cause urinary excretion of potassium.

   D. **CORRECT:** A large amount of calcium can be present in the urine of a client who takes somatropin. This puts the client at risk for renal calculi.

   Ⓝ *NCLEX® Connection: Pharmacological Therapies, Adverse Effects/ Contraindications/Side Effects/Interactions*

5. A. Edema and hypervolemia, rather than hypovolemia, are adverse effects of desmopressin.

   B. Calcium imbalance is not an adverse effect of desmopressin.

   C. Sleepiness, rather than agitation, is an adverse effect of desmopressin, which can indicate water intoxication.

   D. **CORRECT:** Headache during desmopressin therapy is an indication of water intoxication.

   Ⓝ *NCLEX® Connection: Pharmacological Therapies, Adverse Effects/ Contraindications/Side Effects/Interactions*

PRACTICE Answer

Using the ATI Active Learning Template: Medication

THERAPEUTIC USES: Levothyroxine replaces T_4 for thyroid hormone replacement therapy. Replacement of T_4 also raises T_3 levels, because some T_4 converts into T_3.

COMPLICATIONS: Adverse effects are essentially the same as manifestations of hyperthyroidism: cardiac symptoms (hypertension, angina pectoris), insomnia, anxiety, weight loss, heat intolerance, increased body temperature, tremors, and menstrual irregularities.

NURSING INTERVENTIONS: The nurse should monitor thyroid function tests: T_3, T_4, and TSH.

CLIENT EDUCATION
- Take levothyroxine on an empty stomach, usually 1 hr before breakfast.
- Thyroid replacement therapy is usually for life
- Monitor for adverse effects that indicate that the dosage needs adjusting.
- Adverse effects include cardiac effects, chest pain, hypertension, and palpitations, especially in older adults.

Ⓝ *NCLEX® Connection: Pharmacological and Parenteral Therapies, Medication Administration*

Ⓝ *NCLEX® Connections*

When reviewing the following chapters, keep in mind the relevant topics and tasks of the NCLEX outline, in particular:

Health Promotion and Maintenance

HEALTH PROMOTION/DISEASE PREVENTION
Identify clients in need of immunizations (required and voluntary).

Identify precautions and contraindications to immunizations.

Pharmacological Therapies

EXPECTED ACTIONS/OUTCOMES: Use resources to check
on purposes and actions of pharmacological agents.

MEDICATION ADMINISTRATION: Administer a
subcutaneous, intradermal, or intramuscular medication.

UNIT 11   MEDICATIONS AFFECTING THE IMMUNE SYSTEM

CHAPTER 36 *Immunizations*

Administration of a vaccine causes the immune system to produce antibodies that target a specific microbe. Vaccines are made from inactivated toxins, killed viruses, or live attenuated (weakened) viruses.

IMMUNITY

Active immunity develops when the immune system produces antibodies in response to the entry of antigens into the body.

- **Artificial active immunity** develops when a vaccine is administered and the body produces antibodies in response to exposure to a killed or attenuated virus.
- **Natural active immunity** develops when an antigen enters the body naturally, without human assistance, stimulating the immune system to produce antibodies to the antigen.

Passive immunity is temporary, and develops when antibodies are created by another human or animal and then transferred to the client.

- **Natural passive immunity** develops when antibodies are passed from a client to the fetus through the placenta, and then to the newborn/infant via the colostrum and breast milk.
- **Artificial passive immunity** develops after antibodies in the form of immune globulins are administered to an individual who requires immediate protection against a disease after exposure has occurred.

RECOMMENDED CHILDHOOD IMMUNIZATIONS

Check the CDC website, www.cdc.gov, for current recommendations. Q EBP

Diphtheria and tetanus toxoids and acellular pertussis vaccine (DTaP): Administer doses at 2, 4, 6, and 15 to 18 months, and 4 to 6 years.

Tetanus and diphtheria toxoids and pertussis vaccine (Tdap): Administer one dose at 11 to 12 years.

Tetanus and diphtheria (Td) booster: Administer one dose every 10 years following Tdap.

Haemophilus influenzae **type B (Hib):** Administer doses at 2, 4, 6 (if a four-dose series), and 12 to 15 months.

Rotavirus (RV) oral vaccine
- Two formulations are available. The infant may receive either formulation. The first dose of either form should not be initiated for infants 15 weeks, 0 days or older.
  - RV-5 vaccine should be administered as a three-dose series at ages 2, 4, and 6 months.
  - RV-1 vaccine should be administered as two-dose series at 2 and 4 months.
- Maximum age for the final dose of RV vaccine is 8 months, 0 days.

Inactivated poliovirus vaccine (IPV): Administer doses at 2, 4, and 6 to 18 months, and 4 to 6 years.

Measles, mumps, and rubella vaccine (MMR): Administer doses at 12 to 15 months and 4 to 6 years.

Varicella vaccine: Administer one dose at 12 to 15 months and 4 to 6 years, or two doses a minimum of 4 weeks apart if administered after age 13 years.

Pneumococcal conjugate vaccine (PCV13): Administer doses at 2, 4, 6, and 12 to 15 months.

Hepatitis A: Administer the first dose between 12 and 23 months. Administer the second dose 6 to 18 months after the first.

Hepatitis B: Administer within 12 hr after birth with additional doses at age 1 to 2 months and 6 to 18 months. Do not give the third dose prior to 24 weeks of age.

Seasonal influenza vaccine
- Annually, beginning at age 6 months, administer inactivated influenza vaccine (IIV).
- Influenza immunization recommendations change periodically, check the CDC for current recommendations. The vaccine is typically available beginning in early fall.

Meningococcal vaccine (MenACWY): Administer first dose at age 11 to 12 years (earlier if specific risk factors are present). Administer a booster dose at age 16 years.

Human papillomavirus (HPV2, HPV4, or HPV9): Administer three doses over a 6-month period for males and females 11 to 12 years of age (minimum age of 9 years). Administer males only HPV4 or HPV9; administer females HPV2, HPV4, or HPV9. The second dose is administered 1 to 2 months after the first dose, and the third dose is administered 16 weeks after the second dose.

RECOMMENDED ADULT IMMUNIZATIONS

- For adults age 19 and older.
- Immunization recommendations change periodically.

Td/Tdap: Administer one dose of Tdap instead of Td, and then give Td booster every 10 years. Give one dose of Tdap to clients who are pregnant (with each pregnancy) between 27 and 36 weeks gestation.

MMR: Follow recommendations for administering one or two doses to clients between the ages of 19 and 49 who lack documentation of immunization or prior infection, or laboratory proof of immunity.

Varicella vaccine: Administer two doses to adults who do not have evidence of immunity. Administer a second dose to adults who had only one previous dose and lack evidence of immunity. Pregnant clients needing protection against varicella should wait until the postpartum period for immunization.

Pneumococcal polysaccharide vaccine (PPSV23) and pneumococcal conjugate vaccine (PCV13): Follow recommendations for administration to adults who are immunocompromised, have specific chronic diseases, smoke cigarettes, or live in a long-term care facility. For adults 65 years and older who have not been immunized with PCV13 or PPSV23, administer PCV13 first and then give PPSV23 in 6 to 12 months; do not administer both during the same visit. For adults who received a dose of PPSV23 at age 65 or older, an additional dose is not indicated. Ⓒ

Hepatitis A: Administer single-antigen vaccines as two doses spaced 6 to 12 months, or 6 to 18 months apart to high-risk individuals.

Hepatitis B: Administer three doses to high-risk individuals who lack completion of the series. There must be at least 1 month between doses one and two, and at least 2 months between doses two and three. A minimum of 4 months are required between doses one and three.

Influenza vaccine
- One dose annually is recommended for all adults.
- IIV is approved for individuals 6 months of age or older, including those who are pregnant.
- Recombinant influenza vaccine (RIV) is approved for adults 18 years of age and older.
- LAIV is available as a nasal spray.
- Influenza immunization recommendations change periodically. Check the CDC for current recommendations.

Meningococcal polysaccharide vaccine (MPSV4) and meningococcal ACWY (MenACWY) vaccine: Administer a dose of MenACWY to students up to age 21 years entering college and living in dormitories if a dose was not received on or after the 16th birthday. Two doses of MenACWY at least 2 months apart are recommended for individuals who have anatomical or functional asplenia. One dose is recommended for military recruits and those traveling to or living in areas of hyperendemic or epidemic rates of meningococcal disease. MPSV4 is preferred for adults who are 56 years of age or older, require a single dose, and have not had MenACWY previously. Reimmunization with MenACWY is recommended every 5 years for adults who remain at high risk for infection and were previously immunized with MenACWY or MPSV4.

HPV2, HPV4, or HPV9: Three doses are recommended for females up to age 26 years who were not immunized prior to age 18. Females can receive HPV2, HPV4, or HPV9. If not immunized as children, HPV4 or HPV9 is recommended for males age 19 to 21 years, and for males age 22 to 26 years who have a high risk for HPV.

Zoster vaccine: A one-time dose is recommended for all adults 60 years or older.

PURPOSE

EXPECTED PHARMACOLOGICAL ACTION

Vaccines cause the immune system to produce antibodies that provide passive active immunity. Immunizations can take months to have an effect but confer long-lasting protection against infectious diseases.

THERAPEUTIC USES

- Eradication of infectious diseases (polio, smallpox)
- Prevention of childhood and adult infectious diseases (measles, diphtheria, mumps, rubella, tetanus, *H. influenzae*) and their complications

COMPLICATIONS, CONTRAINDICATIONS, AND PRECAUTIONS

- Anaphylactic reaction to a vaccine is a contraindication for further doses of that vaccine. Qs
- Anaphylactic reaction to any component of a vaccine is a contraindication to use of subsequent vaccines containing that substance.
- Do not administer live virus vaccines (varicella, MMR) to a client who is severely immunocompromised. Severe febrile illness is a contraindication to all immunizations.
- Precautions to immunizations require the provider to analyze data and weigh the risks that come with immunizing or not immunizing. Qᴾᶜᶜ
- Moderate or severe illnesses with or without fever are precautions to receiving immunizations.
- The common cold and other minor illnesses are not contraindications or precautions for receiving immunizations.

DTaP

ADVERSE EFFECTS
- **Mild**
  - Redness, swelling, and tenderness at the injection site
  - Low fever
  - Behavioral changes (drowsiness, irritability, anorexia)
- **Moderate**
  - Inconsolable crying for 3 hr or more
  - Fever 40.6° C (105° F) or greater
  - Seizures (with or without fever)
  - Shock-like state
- **Severe:** Acute encephalopathy (rare)

CONTRAINDICATIONS
- Occurrence of encephalopathy within 7 days following prior dose of the vaccine
- Immediate anaphylactic reaction with a prior DTaP vaccine

PRECAUTIONS
- Guillain-Barré syndrome within 6 weeks of prior dose of tetanus toxoid
- Progressive neurologic disorders; uncontrolled seizures
- Fever 40.6° C (105° F) or greater within 48 hr of prior dose

- Shock-like state within 48 hr of prior dose
- Seizures within 3 days of prior dose
- Inconsolable crying for 3 hr or more within 48 hr of prior dose

Haemophilus influenzae type B

ADVERSE EFFECTS
- Redness, swelling, warmth, and tenderness at the injection site
- Fever greater than 38.3° C (101° F), vomiting, diarrhea, crying

CONTRAINDICATION: Age less than 6 weeks

Rotavirus

ADVERSE EFFECTS
- Irritability
- Mild, temporary diarrhea or vomiting
- Intussusception

CONTRAINDICATIONS
- History of intussusception
- Severe combined immunodeficiency (SCID), which is a rare disorder that is inherited
- Unresolved moderate to severe diarrhea or vomiting

PRECAUTIONS
- Unresolved inherited abnormalities of the GI tract
- Immunocompromised (other than SCID)

Inactivated poliovirus vaccine

ADVERSE EFFECTS: Tenderness at the injection site

PRECAUTION
- Pregnancy
- Allergy to neomycin, streptomycin, or bacitracin

Measles, mumps, and rubella

ADVERSE EFFECTS
- **Mild:** Local reactions (rash; fever; swollen glands in cheeks or neck)
- **Moderate**
  - Joint pain and stiffness lasting for days to weeks
  - Febrile seizure
  - Low platelet count
- **Severe**
  - Transient thrombocytopenia
  - Deafness
  - Long-term seizures
  - Brain damage

CONTRAINDICATION: Pregnancy

PRECAUTIONS
- History of thrombocytopenia or thrombocytopenic purpura
- Anaphylactic reaction to eggs, gelatin, or neomycin
- Transfusion with blood product containing antibodies within the prior 11 months
- Simultaneous tuberculin skin testing

Varicella

ADVERSE EFFECTS
- **Mild**
  - Tenderness and swelling at injection site
  - Fever
  - Rash (mild) for up to 1 month after immunization
- **Moderate:** Seizures
- **Severe**
  - Pneumonia
  - Low blood count (extremely rare)
  - Severe brain reactions (extremely rare)

CONTRAINDICATIONS
- Pregnancy
- Anaphylactic reaction to gelatin or neomycin
- Cancer (leukemia or lymphoma)
- Immunodeficiency

PRECAUTIONS
- Transfusion with blood product containing antibodies within the prior 11 months
- Treatment with antiviral medication within 24 hr prior to immunization (Avoid taking antivirals for 14 days following immunization.)
- Extended use (2 weeks or longer) of corticosteroids or other medications that affect the immune system
- Vaccinated patients should temporarily avoid close contact with susceptible, high-risk individuals such as neonates, pregnant clients and those immunocompromised.
- To avoid the risk of developing Reye's Syndrome, children receiving the vaccine should avoid aspirin and other salicylates for 6 weeks following vaccination.

Pneumococcal conjugate vaccine (PCV13)

ADVERSE EFFECTS
- Swelling, redness and tenderness at site of injection
- Fever
- Irritability
- Drowsiness
- Anorexia

CONTRAINDICATION: Anaphylactic reaction to any vaccine containing diphtheria toxoid

Pneumococcal polysaccharide vaccine (PPSV23)

ADVERSE EFFECTS
- Redness and tenderness at site of injection
- Fever
- Myalgia

CONTRAINDICATION: Age less than 2 years

PRECAUTION
- Pregnancy
- Moderate or severe acute illness

Hepatitis A

ADVERSE EFFECTS
- Tenderness at the injection site
- Headache
- Anorexia
- Malaise

CONTRAINDICATION: Severe allergy to previous vaccine

PRECAUTION: Moderate or severe acute illness, with or without fever

Hepatitis B

ADVERSE EFFECTS
- Tenderness at the injection site
- Temperature of 37.7° C (99.9° F) or greater

CONTRAINDICATION: Anaphylactic allergy to yeast or previous vaccine

PRECAUTION
- Infant weight less than 2 kg (4 lb, 6.5 oz)
- Moderate or severe acute illness, with or without fever

Inactivated influenza vaccine; influenza recombinant vaccine

ADVERSE EFFECTS
- Swelling, redness, and tenderness at the injection site
- Hoarseness
- Fever
- Malaise
- Headache
- Cough
- Aches
- Increased risk for Guillain-Barré syndrome
- Increased risk of seizures in children receiving PCV13 or DTaP simultaneously
- Influenza immunization recommendations change periodically. Check the CDC for current recommendations.

CONTRAINDICATIONS: Anaphylactic reaction to previous dose or vaccine with an egg protein

PRECAUTIONS
- Guillain-Barré syndrome within 6 weeks of prior influenza vaccine
- Moderate or severe acute illness with or without fever

Live attenuated influenza vaccine

ADVERSE EFFECTS
- Vomiting, diarrhea
- Cough
- Fever
- Headache
- Myalgia
- Nasal congestion/runny nose
- Influenza immunization recommendations change periodically. Check the CDC for current recommendations.

CONTRAINDICATIONS
- Age less than 2 years
- Age 50 years or older
- Pregnancy

PRECAUTIONS
- Guillain-Barré syndrome within 6 weeks of prior influenza vaccine
- Treatment with antiviral medication within 48 hr prior to immunization (avoid taking antivirals for 14 days following immunization)
- Some chronic conditions

Meningococcal ACWY

ADVERSE EFFECTS
- Redness and tenderness at the injection site
- Fever

CONTRAINDICATION: Anaphylaxis after a previous dose or to a vaccine component

PRECAUTION: Moderate or severe acute illness with or without fever

HPV4 and HPV9

ADVERSE EFFECTS
- Redness, swelling and tenderness at the injection site
- Mild to moderate fever
- Headache
- Fainting shortly after receiving the vaccine

CONTRAINDICATIONS
- Pregnancy
- Severe allergy to yeast

HPV2

ADVERSE EFFECTS
- Redness, swelling, and tenderness at the injection site
- Temperature 37.7° C (99.9° F) or greater
- Headache
- Fatigue
- Nausea, vomiting, abdominal pain
- Myalgia
- Fainting (shortly after receiving the vaccine)

CONTRAINDICATIONS
- Pregnancy
- Severe allergy to latex

Zoster

ADVERSE EFFECTS
- Redness, edema, itching, and tenderness at the injection site
- Headache

CONTRAINDICATIONS
- Immunosuppression
- Pregnancy (Pregnancy should be avoided for 4 weeks following zoster vaccination.)
- Treatment with medications that alter the immune system
- Anaphylaxis to neomycin, gelatin, or other vaccine component

PRECAUTIONS
- Moderate or severe illness with or without fever
- Receiving antiviral medication 24 hr prior to vaccine
- Receiving antiviral medication within 14 days after receiving vaccination

NURSING ADMINISTRATION

FOR INFANTS AND CHILDREN

- Obtain informed consent from the legal guardian prior to administration.
- Administer IM immunizations in the vastus lateralis or ventrogluteal muscle in infants and young children, and in the deltoid muscle for older children and adolescents.
- Administer subcutaneous injections in the outer aspect of the upper arm or anterolateral thigh.
- Use the appropriate size needle for route, site, age, and amount of medication. Adequate needle length reduces the incidence of swelling and tenderness at the injection site. Qpcc
- Use strategies to minimize discomfort.
  - Provide distraction.
  - Apply a topical anesthetic prior to injection.
  - Give infants a concentrated oral sucrose solution 2 min prior to, during, and 3 min after immunization administration.
- Analgesic-antipyretic medications can suppress the immune response and should not be given prophylactically prior to administration of vaccines.
- Do not allow the child to delay the procedure.
- Encourage caregivers to use comforting measures (cuddling, pacifiers) during procedure and measures such as application of cool compresses to injection site or gentle movement of the involved extremity after the procedure.
- Provide praise afterward.
- Apply a colorful bandage if appropriate.
- Instruct parents to avoid administration of aspirin to children to treat fever or local reaction following administration of a live virus vaccine due to the risk of developing Reye syndrome.

FOR ADULTS

- Administer subcutaneous immunizations in the outer aspect of the upper arm or anterolateral thigh.
- Administer IM immunizations into the deltoid muscle.

FOR CLIENTS OF ALL AGES

- Have emergency medications and equipment on standby in case the client experiences an allergic response such as anaphylaxis.
- Provide written vaccine information sheets (VIS) and review the content with legal guardians or clients. Include the publication date of each VIS given in documentation.
- Instruct parents and clients to observe for complications and to notify the provider if adverse effects occur.
- Document the administration of the vaccine.
  - Date, route, and site of immunization
  - Type, manufacturer, lot number, and expiration date of the vaccine
  - Evidence of informed consent from the legal guardian
  - Name, address and title of the administering nurse. Ql

NURSING EVALUATION OF MEDICATION EFFECTIVENESS

Depending on therapeutic intent, effectiveness can be evidenced by the following.

- Improvement of local reaction to immunization with absence of pain, fever, and swelling at the site of injection
- Development of immunity

Application Exercises

1. A nurse in a public health clinic is caring for several clients who request seasonal influenza immunization. Which of the following clients has a contraindication to receiving the influenza immunization?

   A. 2-month-old who has no health problems

   B. 17-year-old who has a hypersensitivity to penicillin

   C. 25-year-old who is pregnant

   D. 52-year-old who takes a statin for hyperlipidemia

2. A nurse is speaking to a group of new parents about immunizations. CDC recommendations call for completion of which of the following vaccines by the first birthday?

   A. Pneumococcal conjugate

   B. Meningococcal conjugate

   C. Varicella

   D. Rotavirus

3. A nurse at a provider's office is preparing to administer RV, DTaP, Hib, PCV13, and IPV immunizations to a 4-month-old infant. Which of the following actions should the nurse plan to take? (Select all that apply.)

   A. Administer IPV orally.

   B. Administer subcutaneous injections in the anterolateral thigh.

   C. Administer IM injections in the deltoid muscle.

   D. Give the infant his pacifier during vaccine injections.

   E. Tell the parents to give aspirin on a schedule for 24 hr after immunization.

4. A 12-month-old child just received the first measles, mumps, and rubella (MMR) vaccine. For which of the following possible reactions to this vaccine should the nurse inform the parents to monitor? (Select all that apply.)

   A. Rash

   B. Swollen glands

   C. Bruising

   D. Headache

   E. Inconsolable crying

5. A nurse is caring for a group of clients who do not have protection against varicella. The nurse should prepare to administer the varicella vaccine at this time to which of the following clients?

   A. 24-year-old client in the third trimester of pregnancy

   B. 12-year-old child who has a severe allergy to neomycin

   C. 2-month-old infant who has no health problems

   D. 32-year-old man who has essential hypertension

PRACTICE Active Learning Scenario

A nurse at a community health clinic is planning to administer the human papilloma virus (HPV4) vaccine to an 11-year-old female client. Use the ATI Active Learning Template: Medication to complete this item.

COMPLICATIONS: Identify two adverse effects the client should monitor for.

CONTRAINDICATIONS/PRECAUTIONS: Identify contraindications to receiving the HPV vaccine.

CLIENT EDUCATION: Describe two teaching points for a client who receives a first dose of the HPV vaccine.

Application Exercises Key

1. A. **CORRECT:** Children younger than 3 months of age are not eligible to receive the influenza immunization.

   B. A hypersensitivity to penicillin is not a contraindication for an influenza immunization.

   C. Pregnancy is not a contraindication for an influenza immunization.

   D. Taking statin medications is not a contraindication for an influenza immunization.

   Ⓝ *NCLEX® Connection: Health Promotion and Maintenance, Health Promotion/Disease Prevention*

2. A. Pneumococcal conjugate vaccine (PCV13) is a four-dose series with the final dose given between the ages of 12 to 15 months. A one-time dose of PCV13 followed by a dose of pneumococcal polysaccharide vaccine (PPSV23) in 6 to 12 months is also recommended for adults 65 years or older.

   B. Recommendations for meningococcal conjugate vaccine include a dose for children at age 11 to 12 years, followed by a booster dose at 16 to 18 years. Recommendations also include that adults at high risk for meningococcal disease receive the vaccine.

   C. Recommendations for varicella vaccine include a two-dose series at the age of 12 to 15 months, and 4 to 6 years. Recommendations also include that adults who have no evidence of immunity receive the vaccine.

   D. **CORRECT:** Rotavirus vaccine is administered only to infants less than 8 months, 0 days of age.

   Ⓝ *NCLEX® Connection: Health Promotion and Maintenance, Health Promotion/Disease Prevention*

3. A. The nurse should administer IPV subcutaneously. An oral polio vaccine is no longer available in the U.S.

   B. **CORRECT:** Subcutaneous immunizations may be administered in either the anterolateral thigh or the outer aspect of the upper arm to infants and children.

   C. The deltoid muscle of infants should not be used for IM injections until the approximate age of 18 months. The nurse should use the vastus lateralis muscle for immunizations in the infant.

   D. **CORRECT:** Giving the infant a pacifier during injections is a comfort measure that the nurse should encourage.

   E. The parents should not give aspirin to the infant on a schedule because this can increase the risk of developing Reye syndrome.

   Ⓝ *NCLEX® Connection: Pharmacological Therapies, Medication Administration*

4. A. **CORRECT:** A rash and fever can develop in children 1 to 2 weeks following MMR immunization.

   B. **CORRECT:** Swollen glands can develop in children 1 to 2 weeks following MMR immunization.

   C. **CORRECT:** A temporary low platelet count, causing bruising or bleeding, can occur occasionally following MMR immunization.

   D. Headache is an adverse reaction that can occur following immunization with the IIV or LAIV influenza vaccine.

   E. Inconsolable crying can occur in some infants following the DTaP immunization.

   Ⓝ *NCLEX® Connection: Pharmacological Therapies, Adverse Effects/ Contraindications/Side Effects/Interactions*

5. A. A client in the third trimester of pregnancy should wait until the postpartum period for varicella immunization. This live vaccine is not safe during pregnancy.

   B. A severe allergy to neomycin is a contraindication to receiving the varicella vaccine.

   C. A 2-month-old infant is too young to receive the varicella vaccine, which is a two-dose series recommended at age 12 to 15 months and 4 to 6 years.

   D. **CORRECT:** A 32-year-old man who has essential hypertension and did not receive two doses of varicella vaccine earlier in life should be immunized. Essential hypertension is not a contraindication for this vaccine.

   Ⓝ *NCLEX® Connection: Health Promotion and Maintenance, Health Promotion/Disease Prevention*

PRACTICE Answer

Using the ATI Active Learning Template: Medication

COMPLICATIONS
- The HPV4 vaccine can cause redness, tenderness, and swelling at the injection site.
- The vaccine can cause fainting shortly after administration.
- Headache and mild to moderate fever are also possible adverse effects.

CONTRAINDICATIONS/PRECAUTIONS:
Contraindications to receiving HPV include pregnancy and a severe allergy to yeast.

CLIENT EDUCATION
- Common adverse effects are mild and temporary.
- Recommendations for HPV4 call for three doses of the vaccine within 6 months. The schedule of administration includes receiving the second dose 1 to 2 months after the first dose, and the third dose 16 weeks after the second dose.

Ⓝ *NCLEX® Connection: Pharmacological and Parenteral Therapies, Medication Administration*

NCLEX® Connections

When reviewing the following chapters, keep in mind the relevant topics and tasks of the NCLEX outline, in particular:

Safety and Infection Control

ACCIDENT/ERROR/INJURY PREVENTION: Evaluate the appropriateness of a health care provider's order for the client.

Pharmacological Therapies

ADVERSE EFFECTS/CONTRAINDICATIONS/ SIDE EFFECTS/INTERACTIONS: Identify symptoms of an allergic reaction (to medication).

MEDICATION ADMINISTRATION: Maintain medication safety practices (storage, checking for expiration dates or compatibility).

CHAPTER 37

CHAPTER 37 *Principles of Antimicrobial Therapy*

Antimicrobial therapy is the use of medications to treat infections due to bacteria, viruses, or fungi. Antimicrobials (natural or synthetic) must use selective toxicity to kill or otherwise control microbes without destroying host cells.

Changes in the DNA of micro-organisms (conjugation), which produces resistance to multiple existing medications, mandates the continual creation of new antimicrobials.

Superinfection is a type of resistance that results when an antibiotic kills normal flora, thus favoring the emergence of a new infection that is difficult to eliminate.

METHODS OF ANTIMICROBIAL ACTIONS

- Destroying the cell wall that is present in bacteria but not in mammals
- Inhibiting the conversion of an enzyme unique for a particular bacterium's survival
- Impairing protein synthesis in the bacteria's ribosomes, which are never identical to mammalian cells

CLASSIFICATION OF ANTIMICROBIAL MEDICATIONS

- Requires defining which microbes are susceptible to each medication
  - **Narrow-spectrum antibiotics,** to which only a few types of bacteria are sensitive
  - **Broad-spectrum antibiotics,** to which a wide variety of bacteria are sensitive
- Requires identifying the mechanism of action of each antibacterial medication
  - **Bactericidal medications** are directly lethal to the micro-organism.
  - **Bacteriostatic medications** slow the growth of the micro-organism, but the immune-system response of phagocytic cells (macrophages, neutrophils) actually destroys the bacteria.
- Multiple factors determine which medication providers prescribe (antibacterial, antifungal, antiviral).

SELECTION OF ANTIMICROBIALS

IDENTIFICATION OF CAUSATIVE AGENT

Laboratory testing of body fluids, such as blood, urine, sputum, and wound drainage, identifies the micro-organism causing the infection.

Gram stain

Technicians examine an aspirate of the body fluid under a microscope to identify the micro-organisms directly.

Culture

Technicians apply the aspirate to a culture medium, where colonies of the micro-organism grow over several days. A culture is preferable when a Gram stain does not yield a positive identification.
- Nurses should obtain specimens for culture prior to treatment with antimicrobials. Q EBP
- Nurses must collect fluid for culture carefully to prevent contamination.

SENSITIVITY OF A MICRO-ORGANISM TO AN ANTIMICROBIAL

For organisms commonly resistant, technicians test the sensitivity of the organism to various antimicrobials.
- **The disk diffusion test** (Kirby-Bauer test) is most common. The size of the bacteria-free on the antibiotic-containing zone on the disk determines the degree of medication sensitivity.
- **Serial dilution** is a quantitative method using several test tubes with varying amounts of the antimicrobial that helps determine the amount necessary to treat a specific infection.
  - **Minimum inhibitory concentration (MIC):** The amount of antibiotic that inhibits bacterial growth completely but does not kill the bacteria
  - **Minimum bactericidal concentration:** The lowest concentration of the antibiotic that kills 99.9% of the bacteria
  - Providers should adjust the antibiotic dosage to produce the concentration equal to or greater than the MIC.
- **Gradient diffusion** uses a disk and strips with varying concentrations of antibiotic. No further growth of bacteria identifies the essential antibiotic concentration.

HOST FACTORS

Immune system

- In people who have an intact immune system, an antimicrobial works with host defense systems to suppress micro-organisms. Providers prescribe either bactericidal or bacteriostatic antibiotics.
- People with immune-system compromise need strong bactericidal antibiotics, not bacteriostatic medication.

Site of infection

Some sites are difficult for antimicrobials to reach and achieve the MIC.
- Infections in cerebrospinal fluid, where the antimicrobials have to cross the blood-brain barrier (meningitis)
- Bacterial infiltration within the heart (endocarditis)
  - Infectious micro-organisms vegetate on the thrombus that develops on the injured endocardium.
  - New thrombus formation covers and conceals the micro-organisms, making it difficult for defense mechanisms and antibiotics to kill them.
- Purulent abscesses anywhere within the body due to poor blood supply
- Surgical removal of drainage increases the effect of antimicrobials.
- Phagocytes that attack foreign objects (pacemaker, joint prosthesis, vascular grafts, heart valves, surgical mesh) and become less able to destroy micro-organisms that colonize around the foreign object

Age

- Infants are at increased risk for antimicrobial toxicity due to undeveloped kidney and liver function, causing slow excretion of the medication.
- Older adult clients easily develop toxicity due to the reduction in medication metabolism and excretion. Ⓖ

Pregnancy

- Antimicrobials can harm a developing fetus by crossing over to the placenta. Ⓠs
  - **Sulfonamides** can produce kernicterus (a severe neurologic disorder) in newborns.
  - **Gentamicin** causes hearing loss in infants.
  - **Tetracyclines** cause discoloratio n of developing teeth. Toxicity to these antibiotics is more likely during pregnancy.
- Lactation is usually a contraindication for antimicrobials because of possible danger to breastfeeding infants.

Presence of a previous allergic reaction

- Especially with penicillin
- Clients should not receive penicillin after an allergic reaction, narrowing the antibiotic choices for those clients.

Combination therapy

Combining more than one antimicrobial can cause additive, potentiating, or antagonistic effects.
- To treat severe infections
- To treat infections from more than one micro-organism
- Prevents bacterial resistance from causing an infection, such as tuberculosis
- Decreases the risk of toxicity by reducing the dosage of each medication
- Produces more effective treatment than using only one antimicrobial medication

Combining antimicrobials can cause adverse effects.
- Increased resistance to antimicrobials
- Increased cost of therapy
- More adverse or toxic reactions
- Antagonistic effects among the various antimicrobials
- Increased risk for a superinfection (a new infection that develops while treating another infection)

PROPHYLAXIS

- Indications for prophylactic use include prevention of the following.
  - Infections for clients undergoing gastrointestinal, cardiac, peripheral vascular, orthopedic, or gynecologic surgery
  - Sexually transmitted infections following sexual exposure
- Use antimicrobials for individuals who have the following.
  - Prosthetic heart valves prior to dental or other procedures because of the danger of bacterial endocarditis
  - Recurring urinary tract infections

PREVENTIVE MEASURES

- Perform hand hygiene before and after each client contact to prevent the spread of infection.
- Recognize invasive procedures that increase the risk of infection (indwelling urinary catheter, IV catheter, cardiac catheterization).
- Encourage prevention by having clients maintain an up-to-date immunization status.
- Reinforce with the client to take the full course of prescribed antimicrobials to prevent medication resistance and recurrence of infection.
- Use infection-control procedures to prevent transmission of resistant micro-organisms. Practice infection-control principles (aseptic technique, standard and transmission-based precautions, careful assignment of rooms within facilities).
- Monitor the effectiveness of treatment.
  - Check post-treatment cultures to confirm that they are negative for micro-organisms.
  - Monitor clients for improvement (clear breath sounds, resolution of fever).

Application Exercises

1. A nurse is implementing a plan of care for a client who has a wound infection. Which of the following actions should the nurse perform first?

    A. Administer antibiotic medication.

    B. Obtain a wound specimen for culture.

    C. Review WBC laboratory findings.

    D. Apply a dressing to the wound.

2. A nurse is caring for a client who has a urinary tract infection and a history of recurrence of this type of infection. The nurse should expect the provider to wait for the results of which of the following laboratory tests to identify which antibiotic to prescribe?

    A. Gram stain

    B. Culture

    C. Sensitivity

    D. Specific gravity

3. A nurse is assisting in preparing an in-service about the effectiveness of antimicrobial therapy for clients who have bacterial infections. Which of the following host factors are conditions that affect antimicrobial effectiveness? (Select all that apply.)

    A. Meningitis

    B. Pacemaker

    C. Endocarditis

    D. Pneumonia

    E. Pyelonephritis

4. A nurse is caring for a group of clients who are receiving antimicrobial therapy. Which of the following clients should the nurse plan to monitor for manifestations of antibiotic toxicity?

    A. An adolescent client who has a sinus infection

    B. An older adult client who has prostatitis

    C. A client who is postpartum and has mastitis

    D. A middle adult client who has a urinary tract infection

5. A nurse is reviewing the records of a group of clients. Which of the following clients should the nurse expect a prescription for prophylactic antimicrobial therapy? (Select all that apply.)

    A. A client who reports exposure to a sexually transmitted infection

    B. A client who is having orthopedic surgery

    C. A client who has a prosthetic heart valve and is planning to have dental work

    D. A client who has recurrent urinary tract infections

    E. A client who has an upper respiratory infection

PRACTICE Active Learning Scenario

A nurse is assisting a staff educator in providing information to a group of nurses about ways to prevent the spread of micro-organisms. What information should the nurse recommend? Use the ATI Active Learning Template: Basic Concept to complete this item.

RELATED CONTENT: Determine one related concept.

UNDERLYING PRINCIPLES: Describe one related to the concept.

NURSING INTERVENTIONS: Identify five related to the concept.

Application Exercises Key

1. A. The nurse should plan to administer antibiotics. However, according to evidence-based practice another action is the priority.

   B. **CORRECT:** According to evidence-based practice, the nurse should first obtain a culture of the wound before initiating antibiotic therapy.

   C. The nurse should review the WBC laboratory findings to identify any values outside the expected reference range. However, according to evidence-based practice another action is the priority.

   D. The nurse should apply dressings to the wound to absorb drainage and prevent the spread of infection. However, according to evidence-based practice another action is the priority.

   Ⓝ NCLEX® Connection: Pharmacological Therapies, Expected Actions/Outcomes

2. A. A Gram stain helps identify the micro-organism that is causing the infection.

   B. A culture determines the type of micro-organism causing the infection.

   C. **CORRECT:** A sensitivity test identifies the most effective antibiotic to prescribe to treat a specific micro-organism.

   D. A specific gravity test determines the dilution of fluid (typically urine) and does not provide information on the type of micro-organism or antibiotic to prescribe to treat the infection.

   Ⓝ NCLEX® Connection: Pharmacological Therapies, Medication Administration

3. A. **CORRECT:** The client who has meningitis might not respond to antimicrobial therapy because it is difficult for the medication to cross the blood-brain barrier to reach the infecting micro-organisms.

   B. **CORRECT:** The client who has a pacemaker might not respond to antimicrobial therapy due to colonization of micro-organisms around the pacemaker and the inability of phagocytic cells to destroy those micro-organisms.

   C. **CORRECT:** The client who has endocarditis can have difficulty responding to antimicrobial therapy because the medication cannot penetrate the vegetative thrombus that develops on the injured endocardium.

   D. The client who has pneumonia should respond effectively to antimicrobial therapy due to the vascularity of pulmonary tissue.

   E. The client who has pyelonephritis should respond to antimicrobial therapy effectively because of the vascularity of kidney tissue and the filtration system.

   Ⓝ NCLEX® Connection: Pharmacological Therapies, Expected Actions/Outcomes

4. A. An adolescent client who has a sinus infection should metabolize and excrete the medication without developing antibiotic toxicity.

   B. **CORRECT:** An older adult client who has prostatitis and is receiving antibiotics is at risk for toxicity due to the age-related reduction in medication metabolism and excretion.

   C. The client who is postpartum and has mastitis should metabolize and excrete the medication without developing antibiotic toxicity.

   D. A middle adult client who has a urinary tract infection should metabolize and excrete the medication without developing antibiotic toxicity.

   Ⓝ NCLEX® Connection: Pharmacological Therapies, Adverse Effects/Contraindications/Side Effects/Interactions

5. A. **CORRECT:** The client who suspects exposure to a sexually transmitted infection requires prophylactic antimicrobial therapy to prevent an infection.

   B. **CORRECT:** The client who is having orthopedic surgery requires prophylactic antimicrobial therapy to prevent an infection.

   C. **CORRECT:** The client who has prosthetic heart valve and is having dental work should receive prophylactic antimicrobial therapy to prevent an infection.

   D. **CORRECT:** The client who has recurrent urinary tract infections should receive prophylactic antimicrobial therapy to prevent an infection.

   E. The client who has an upper respiratory infection can develop resistance to antimicrobial therapy if taken for a viral infection or prophylactically.

   Ⓝ NCLEX® Connection: Pharmacological Therapies, Expected Actions/Outcomes

PRACTICE Answer

Using ATI Active Learning Template: Basic Concept

RELATED CONTENT: Preventive nursing measures

UNDERLYING PRINCIPLES: Controlling the spread of infection to staff and clients in a health care setting

NURSING INTERVENTIONS
- Perform hand hygiene before and after each client contact to prevent the spread of infection.
- Recognize invasive procedures that increase the risk of infection (indwelling urinary catheter, IV catheter, cardiac catheterization).
- Encourage prevention by having clients maintain an up-to-date immunization status.
- Reinforce with the client to take the full course of prescribed antimicrobials to prevent medication resistance and recurrence of infection.
- Use infection-control procedures to prevent transmission of resistant micro-organisms.
- Monitor the effectiveness of treatment.

Ⓝ NCLEX® Connection: Pharmacological and Parenteral Therapies, Medication Administration

UNIT 12   MEDICATIONS FOR INFECTION

CHAPTER 38 *Antibiotics Affecting the Bacterial Cell Wall*

Antibiotics that affect the cell wall are bactericidal. This group of antibiotics includes penicillins, cephalosporins, carbapenems, and monobactams.

Penicillins

SELECT PROTOTYPE MEDICATION: Penicillin G potassium, a narrow-spectrum medication for IM or IV use

OTHER MEDICATIONS
- **Narrow-spectrum**
  - Penicillin G for IM use
  - Penicillin V for PO use
- **Broad-spectrum**
  - Amoxicillin for PO use
  - Amoxicillin-clavulanate for PO use
  - Ampicillin for PO or IV use
- **Antistaphylococcal:**
  - Nafcillin for IM (rare) or IV use
  - Oxacillin for IV use
- **Antipseudomonal**
  - Ticarcillin-clavulanate for IV use
  - Piperacillin-tazobactam for IV use

PURPOSE

EXPECTED PHARMACOLOGICAL ACTION

Penicillins destroy bacteria by weakening the bacterial cell wall.

THERAPEUTIC USES

- Penicillins treat infections due to gram-positive cocci such as *Streptococcus pneumoniae* (pneumonia and meningitis), *Streptococcus viridans* (infectious endocarditis), and *Streptococcus pyogenes* (pharyngitis).
- Penicillins treat meningitis due to gram-negative cocci such as *Neisseria meningitides*.
- Penicillins kill spirochetes, such as *Treponema pallidum*, which causes syphilis.
- Extended-spectrum penicillins (piperacillin, ticarcillin) are effective against organisms such as *Pseudomonas aeruginosa*, *Enterobacter* species, *Proteus*, *Bacteroides fragilis*, and *Klebsiella*. Ticarcillin by itself is no longer available in the U.S., but ticarcillin in combination with clavulanic acid is available.
- Penicillins provide prophylaxis against bacterial endocarditis in at-risk clients prior to dental and other procedures.

COMPLICATIONS

Allergies, anaphylaxis

NURSING ACTIONS
- Interview clients for prior allergy.
- Advise clients to wear an allergy identification bracelet.
- Observe for allergic reactions for 30 min following parenteral administration of penicillin.
- Have epinephrine and equipment for respiratory support available for immediate use.

Kidney impairment

NURSING ACTIONS: Monitor kidney function and I&O.

Hyperkalemia, dysrhythmias, hypernatremia

Hyperkalemia, dysrhythmias: High doses of penicillin G potassium

Hypernatremia: IV ticarcillin-clavulanate

NURSING ACTIONS: Monitor cardiac status and electrolyte levels.

CONTRAINDICATIONS/PRECAUTIONS

- A history of severe allergic reactions to penicillin, cephalosporins, or imipenem is a contraindication for penicillins. Qs
- Use cautiously for clients who have or are at risk for kidney dysfunction (clients who are acutely ill, older adults, young children). Ⓖ
- Clients who are allergic to one penicillin are cross-allergic to other penicillins and are at risk for cross-sensitivity to cephalosporins.

INTERACTIONS

Penicillin in the same IV solution as aminoglycosides inactivates the aminoglycoside.
NURSING ACTIONS: Do not mix penicillin and aminoglycosides in the same IV solution.

Probenecid delays the excretion of penicillin.
Providers sometimes add probenecid to prolong the action of penicillin therapy.

NURSING ADMINISTRATION

- Instruct clients to take penicillin V, amoxicillin, and amoxicillin-clavulanate with meals. Tell them to take all others with 8 oz of water 1 hr before or 2 hr after meals. QEBP
- Instruct clients to report any manifestations of an allergic response (dyspnea, skin rash, itching, hives).
- Give IM injections cautiously to avoid injecting into a nerve or an artery.
- Advise clients to complete the entire course of therapy, even if manifestations of infection resolve.
- Advise clients to use an additional contraceptive method when taking penicillins.

Cephalosporins

SELECT PROTOTYPE MEDICATION: Cephalexin, first generation

OTHER MEDICATIONS
- **First generation:** Cefazolin for IM or IV use
- **Second generation:** Cefaclor for PO use, cefotetan for IM or IV use
- **Third generation:** Ceftriaxone, cefotaxime for IM or IV use
- **Fourth generation:** Cefepime for IM or IV use
- **Fifth generation:** Ceftaroline for IV use

PURPOSE

EXPECTED PHARMACOLOGICAL ACTION

- Cephalosporins are beta-lactam antibiotics, similar to penicillins, that destroy bacterial cell walls causing destruction of micro-organisms.
- Cephalosporins comprise five generations. Each subsequent generation is
  - More likely to reach cerebrospinal fluid.
  - Less susceptible to destruction by beta-lactamase.
  - More effective against gram-negative organisms and anaerobes.

THERAPEUTIC USES

Cephalosporins are broad-spectrum bactericidal medications with a high therapeutic index that treat urinary tract infections, postoperative infections, pelvic infections, and meningitis.

COMPLICATIONS

Allergy, hypersensitivity, anaphylaxis, possible cross-sensitivity to penicillin

NURSING ACTIONS
- If indications of allergy appear (urticaria, rash, hypotension, dyspnea), stop the cephalosporin immediately and notify the provider.
- Question clients carefully about a history of allergy to a penicillin or another cephalosporin, and notify the provider if present.
- Have epinephrine and equipment for respiratory support available for immediate use.

Bleeding tendencies from cefotetan and ceftriaxone

NURSING ACTIONS
- Avoid use for clients who have bleeding disorders and for clients taking anticoagulants.
- Observe clients for bleeding.
- Monitor prothrombin and bleeding times. Delays in clotting can require discontinuation of the medication.
- Administer parenteral vitamin K.

Thrombophlebitis with IV infusion

NURSING ACTIONS
- Rotate injection sites.
- Administer as a dilute intermittent infusion or slowly over 3 to 5 min and in a dilute solution for bolus dosing.

Kidney insufficiency

NURSING ACTIONS: Give a lower dosage of most cephalosporins to prevent accumulation to toxic levels.

Pain with IM injection

NURSING ACTIONS: Administer IM injections deep into a large muscle mass such as into the ventrogluteal site.

Antibiotic-associated pseudomembranous colitis

NURSING ACTIONS
- Observe for diarrhea, and notify the provider if present.
- Stop the medication.

CONTRAINDICATIONS/PRECAUTIONS

NURSING ACTIONS
- Do not give cephalosporins to clients who have a history of severe allergic reactions to penicillins. **Qs**
- Use cautiously with clients who have kidney impairment or bleeding tendencies.

INTERACTIONS

Disulfiram reaction (intolerance to alcohol) occurs with simultaneous use of alcohol and either cefotetan or cefazolin.
CLIENT EDUCATION: Do not consume alcohol while taking these cephalosporins.

Probenecid delays kidney excretion.
NURSING ACTIONS: Monitor I&O.

NURSING ADMINISTRATION

- Instruct clients to complete the entire course of therapy, even if manifestations of infection resolve. **Qebp**
- Advise clients to take oral cephalosporins with food.
- Instruct clients to store oral cephalosporin suspensions in a refrigerator.

Carbapenems

SELECT PROTOTYPE MEDICATION: Imipenem-cilastatin for IM or IV use

OTHER MEDICATIONS: Meropenem for IV use

PURPOSE

EXPECTED PHARMACOLOGICAL ACTION

Carbapenems are beta-lactam antibiotics that destroy bacterial cell walls, causing destruction of micro-organisms.

THERAPEUTIC USES

- Their broad antimicrobial spectrum is effective for serious infections such as pneumonia, peritonitis, and urinary tract infections due to gram-positive cocci, gram-negative cocci, and anaerobic bacteria.
- Resistance develops from using imipenem alone to treat *Pseudomonas aeruginosa* infections. This pathogen requires a combination of antipseudomonal medications.

COMPLICATIONS

Allergy, hypersensitivity, possible cross-sensitivity to penicillin or cephalosporins

NURSING ACTIONS
- Monitor for indications of allergic reactions (dyspnea, rash, pruritus).
- Question clients carefully about their history of allergy to a penicillin or cephalosporin, and notify the provider if present.

Gastrointestinal upset (nausea, vomiting, diarrhea)

NURSING ACTIONS
- Observe for manifestations, and notify the provider if they occur.
- Monitor I&O.

Superinfection

NURSING ACTIONS: Monitor for indications of colitis (diarrhea), oral thrush, and vaginal yeast infection.

CONTRAINDICATIONS/PRECAUTIONS

- Imipenem cilastatin is a Pregnancy Risk Category C medication. Qs
- Use cautiously in clients who have kidney impairment.

INTERACTIONS

Imipenem cilastatin can reduce blood levels of valproic acid. Breakthrough seizures are possible.
NURSING ACTIONS: Avoid using together. If concurrent use is unavoidable, monitor for increased seizure activity.

NURSING ADMINISTRATION

Advise clients to complete the entire course of therapy, even if manifestations of infection resolve.

Other inhibitors of cell wall synthesis

SELECT PROTOTYPE MEDICATIONS
- Vancomycin for PO or IV use
- Telavancin
- Aztreonam, a monobactam, for IM or IV use
- Fosfomycin for PO use

PURPOSE

EXPECTED PHARMACOLOGICAL ACTION

This group of antibiotics destroys bacterial cell walls, causing destruction of micro-organisms.

THERAPEUTIC USES

- Treat serious infections due to methicillin-resistant *Staphylococcus aureus*, *Staphylococcus epidermidis*, and streptococcal infections
- Treat antibiotic-associated pseudomembranous colitis due to *Clostridium difficile*

COMPLICATIONS

Ototoxicity (rare and reversible)

NURSING ACTIONS
- Monitor for indications of hearing loss.
- Monitor vancomycin levels.

CLIENT EDUCATION: Notify the provider if changes in hearing acuity develop.

Infusion reactions

Red man syndrome (rashes, flushing, tachycardia, hypotension)

NURSING ACTIONS: Administer vancomycin slowly over 60 min.

IM and IV injection-site pain, thrombophlebitis

NURSING ACTIONS
- Rotate injection sites.
- Monitor the infusion site for redness, swelling, and inflammation.

Kidney toxicity

NURSING ACTIONS
- Monitor I&O and kidney function tests.
- Monitor vancomycin trough levels.

CONTRAINDICATIONS/PRECAUTIONS

- An allergy to corn or corn products and previous allergy to vancomycin are contraindications. ⓠs
- Use cautiously for older adults and with clients who have kidney impairment or hearing loss. ⓒ

INTERACTIONS

Increased risk for ototoxicity when taking vancomycin concurrently with another medication that causes ototoxicity (loop diuretics, aminoglycoside antibiotics).
NURSING ACTIONS: Monitor for hearing loss.

NURSING ADMINISTRATION

- Monitor vancomycin trough levels routinely after blood levels have reached a steady state.
- For clients who have kidney insufficiency, creatinine clearance levels indicate IV dosage adjustments.

NURSING EVALUATION OF MEDICATION EFFECTIVENESS

Indications of effectiveness include the following.
- Reduction of manifestations such as fever, pain, inflammation, and adventitious breath sounds
- Resolution of infection

Application Exercises

1. A nurse in an outpatient facility is preparing to administer nafcillin IM to an adult client who has an infection. Which of the following actions should the nurse plan to take? (Select all that apply.)

   A. Select a 25-gauge, ½-inch needle for the injection.

   B. Administer the medication deeply into the ventrogluteal muscle.

   C. Ask the client about an allergy to penicillin before administering the medication.

   D. Monitor the client for 30 min following the injection.

   E. Tell the client to expect a temporary rash to develop following the injection.

2. A nurse is collecting data from a client who has been receiving cefotaxime IV for the past week. Which of the following findings indicates a potentially serious adverse reaction to this medication that the nurse should report to the provider?

   A. Diaphoresis

   B. Epistaxis

   C. Diarrhea

   D. Alopecia

3. A nurse is obtaining a medication history from a client who is to receive imipenem-cilastatin IV to treat an infection. Which of the following medications puts the client at risk for a medication interaction?

   A. Regular insulin

   B. Furosemide

   C. Valproic acid

   D. Ferrous sulfate

4. A nurse is reviewing prescriptions for a client who has a cerebrospinal fluid infection with gram-negative bacteria. Which of the following cephalosporin antibiotics should the nurse expect the provider to prescribe IV to treat this infection?

   A. Cefaclor

   B. Cefazolin

   C. Cefepime

   D. Cephalexin

5. A nurse is preparing to administer penicillin V to a client who has a streptococcal infection. The client tells the nurse that she has difficulty swallowing tablets and doesn't tolerate liquid or chewable medications because the taste gags her, even when mixed with food. The nurse should request a prescription for which of the following medications?

   A. Fosfomycin

   B. Amoxicillin

   C. Nafcillin

   D. Cefaclor

PRACTICE Active Learning Scenario

A nurse in an acute care facility is caring for a client who has a new prescription for vancomycin IV. What information should the nurse know about this medication? Use the ATI Active Learning Template: Medication to complete this item.

THERAPEUTIC USES: Identify for vancomycin for this client.

COMPLICATIONS: Identify two adverse effects the client should watch for.

NURSING INTERVENTIONS: Describe two nursing actions for clients receiving vancomycin.

Application Exercises Key

1. A. A 25-gauge, ½-inch needle is too small and short for an IM injection of nafcillin to an adult client. For this medication, a needle for an adult client's IM injection should be 19- to 22-gauge and 1½ inches long.

    B. **CORRECT:** It is important to administer nafcillin IM into a deep muscle mass, such as the ventrogluteal site.

    C. **CORRECT:** It is important to ask the client about an allergy to penicillin or other antibiotics before administering nafcillin. An allergy to another penicillin or to a cephalosporin is a contraindication for administering nafcillin.

    D. **CORRECT:** When administering a penicillin or other antibiotic parenterally, it is important to monitor the client for 30 min for an allergic reaction.

    E. A rash is not an expected reaction after nafcillin administration. A rash can be a manifestation of an allergy to the medication.

    Ⓝ *NCLEX® Connection: Pharmacological Therapies, Adverse Effects/ Contraindications/Side Effects/Interactions*

2. A. Diaphoresis is not an adverse effect of cefotaxime. Common adverse effects include rashes, nausea, headache, dizziness, and weakness.

    B. Epistaxis is not an adverse effect of cefotaxime. Two other cephalosporins, ceftriaxone and cefotetan, can cause bleeding.

    C. **CORRECT:** Diarrhea is an adverse effect of cefotaxime and other cephalosporins that the nurse should report to the provider. Severe diarrhea can indicate that the client has developed antibiotic-associated pseudomembranous colitis, a superinfection that could be life-threatening.

    D. Alopecia is not an adverse effect of cefotaxime.

    Ⓝ *NCLEX® Connection: Pharmacological Therapies, Expected Actions/Outcomes*

3. A. Regular insulin, an antidiabetes medication, does not interact with imipenem-cilastatin. Medications that interact with imipenem-cilastatin include probenecid, aminophylline, theophylline, ganciclovir, and cyclosporine.

    B. Furosemide, a loop diuretic, does not interact with imipenem-cilastatin.

    C. **CORRECT:** Imipenem-cilastatin decreases the blood levels of valproic acid (an antiseizure medication), putting the client at risk for increased seizure activity. If the client must take these two medications concurrently, the nurse should monitor for seizures.

    D. Ferrous sulfate does not interact with imipenem-cilastatin.

    Ⓝ *NCLEX® Connection: Pharmacological Therapies, Adverse Effects/ Contraindications/Side Effects/Interactions*

4. A. Cefaclor, a second-generation cephalosporin, is unlikely to be effective against gram-negative bacteria in cerebrospinal fluid.

    B. Cefazolin, a first-generation cephalosporin, is unlikely to be effective against gram-negative bacteria in cerebrospinal fluid.

    C. **CORRECT:** Cefepime, a fourth-generation cephalosporin, is more likely to be effective against this infection than the other medications, which are from the first or second generation. Medications from each progressive generation of cephalosporins are more effective against gram-negative bacteria, more resistant to destruction by beta-lactamase, and more able to reach cerebrospinal fluid.

    D. Cephalexin, a first-generation cephalosporin, is unlikely to be effective against gram-negative bacteria in cerebrospinal fluid.

    Ⓝ *NCLEX® Connection: Pharmacological Therapies, Expected Actions/Outcomes*

5. A. Fosfomycin is available only in a PO formulation. Acceptable alternatives to penicillin V within the penicillin classification include penicillin G, ampicillin, ticarcillin-clavulanate, and piperacillin tazobactam.

    B. Amoxicillin is available only in a PO formulation.

    C. **CORRECT:** Nafcillin is an acceptable alternative within the penicillin classification because it is available for IM or IV use.

    D. Cefaclor is available only in a PO formulation and is not a penicillin.

    Ⓝ *NCLEX® Connection: Pharmacological Therapies, Medication Administration*

PRACTICE Answer

Using the ATI Active Learning Template: Medication

THERAPEUTIC USES: Vancomycin is an antibiotic that kills bacteria by disrupting their cell wall. The IV form treats serious infections due to methicillin-resistant *Staphylococcus aureus*, *Staphylococcus epidermidis*, and streptococci.

COMPLICATIONS
- Infusion reactions (red man syndrome: rashes, flushing, tachycardia, and hypotension)
- Ototoxicity (rare and reversible)
- Kidney toxicity
- Thrombophlebitis at the IV site
- IM and IV injection-site pain

NURSING INTERVENTIONS
- Ensure vancomycin infuses over at least 60 min/dose to prevent an infusion reaction.
- Observe the IV site for redness, pain, or other manifestations of thrombophlebitis.
- Calculate I&O, and notify the provider for oliguria or other signs of acute kidney injury.
- Monitor for hearing loss.
- Ask the client about allergy to antibiotics before administering the medication. Watch for allergic manifestations during and after the infusion.

Ⓝ *NCLEX® Connection: Pharmacological and Parenteral Therapies, Medication Administration*

CHAPTER 39

CHAPTER 39 *Antibiotics Affecting Protein Synthesis*

Antibiotics affecting protein synthesis are bacteriostatic (tetracyclines, macrolides) or bactericidal (aminoglycosides). These medications treat respiratory, gastrointestinal (GI), urinary, and reproductive tract infections.

Tetracyclines

SELECT PROTOTYPE MEDICATION: Tetracycline

OTHER MEDICATIONS
- Doxycycline
- Minocycline
- Demeclocycline

PURPOSE

EXPECTED PHARMACOLOGICAL ACTION

Tetracycline medications are broad-spectrum antibiotics that inhibit micro-organism growth by preventing protein synthesis (bacteriostatic).

THERAPEUTIC USES

Treat the following
- Acne vulgaris (topically and orally)
- Periodontal disease (topically)
- Rickettsial infections (typhus fever, Rocky Mountain spotted fever)
- Infections of the urethra or cervix due to *Chlamydia trachomatis*
- Brucellosis
- Pneumonia due to *Mycoplasma pneumonia*
- Lyme disease
- Cholera
- Anthrax
- GI infections due to *Helicobacter pylori*

ADVERSE EFFECTS

GI discomfort

Cramping, nausea, vomiting, diarrhea, and esophageal ulceration

NURSING ACTIONS
- Monitor for nausea, vomiting, and diarrhea.
- Monitor I&O.
- Suggest taking doxycycline and minocycline with meals, although food can reduce absorption.

CLIENT EDUCATION: Avoid taking at bedtime to reduce the risk of esophageal ulceration.

Yellow or brown tooth discoloration, hypoplasia of tooth enamel

NURSING ACTIONS: Avoid administration to children younger than 8 years old and to clients who are pregnant.

Hepatotoxicity (lethargy, jaundice)

NURSING ACTIONS: Avoid administration of high daily doses IV.

Photosensitivity (intense sunburn)

CLIENT EDUCATION: Wear protective clothing and use sunscreen while outdoors in sunlight.

Superinfection

Pseudomembranous colitis (diarrhea) caused from an overgrowth of staphylococci or *Clostridium difficile*, yeast infections of the mouth, pharynx, vagina, bowels

CLIENT EDUCATION: Notify the provider of diarrhea or manifestations of a yeast infection.

Dizziness, lightheadedness (minocycline)

Parenteral administration can cause pain at IM injection site.

NURSING ACTIONS: Monitor IV infusion sites for manifestations of thrombophlebitis.

CLIENT EDUCATION: Take care with ambulation and report these findings to the provider.

CONTRAINDICATIONS/PRECAUTIONS

- Tetracycline medications are Pregnancy Risk Category D. Qs
- Taking tetracycline medications after the fourth month of pregnancy can stain the deciduous teeth of the infant, but does not affect the infant's permanent teeth. However, the medication can stain the permanent teeth of children when taken between the ages of 4 months and 8 years.
- Use cautiously with liver and kidney disease. Tetracycline and demeclocycline are filtered through the kidneys and can cause a toxic level in the client who has kidney disease.
- Doxycycline and minocycline are generally safe for clients who have kidney disease because the liver, not the kidneys, eliminates these two tetracycline medications.

INTERACTIONS

Interaction with milk products, calcium and iron supplements, laxatives containing magnesium, and antacids causes formation of nonabsorbable chelates, thus reducing the absorption of tetracycline medications.
CLIENT EDUCATION
- Take tetracyclines on an empty stomach with 8 oz water (1 hr before or 2 hr after meals). Take tetracycline medications with food if gastric distress occurs, but this will decrease absorption. Minocycline can be taken with food without causing a decrease in the absorption of the medication.
- Avoid milk products and antacids, or separate by 2 hr.

Tetracycline medications decrease the efficacy of oral contraceptives.
CLIENT EDUCATION: Use an alternative form of birth control.

Both minocycline and doxycycline increase the risk of digoxin toxicity and alter warfarin levels.
NURSING ACTIONS: Monitor digoxin and warfarin levels carefully if administered concurrently with tetracycline medications.

NURSING ADMINISTRATION

- Instruct clients to take tetracycline medications (except for minocycline) on an empty stomach with 8 oz water. It may be taken with food if gastric distress occurs. QEBP
- Tell clients not to take tetracycline medications just before lying down because it increases the risk of esophageal ulceration.
- Reinforce with the client to maintain a 2-hr interval between ingestion of chelating agents and tetracycline medications.
- Reinforce with the client to complete the entire course of therapy, even though manifestations may resolve sooner.
- Advise using additional contraception.

NURSING EVALUATION OF MEDICATION EFFECTIVENESS

Indications of effectiveness include the following.
- Decrease in the manifestations of infection (fever, pain, inflammation, adventitious breath sounds)
- Resolution of yeast infections of the mouth, vagina, and bowels
- Resolution of acne vulgaris

Macrolides

SELECT PROTOTYPE MEDICATION: Erythromycin

OTHER MEDICATION: Azithromycin, clarithromycin

PURPOSE

EXPECTED PHARMACOLOGICAL ACTION

Erythromycin slows the growth of micro-organisms by inhibiting protein synthesis (bacteriostatic), but it is bactericidal at high doses.

THERAPEUTIC USES

- Treat infections in the client who has a penicillin allergy, such as for prophylaxis against rheumatic fever and bacterial endocarditis
- Treat Legionnaires' disease, pertussis (whooping cough), and acute diphtheria (also eliminating the carrier state of diphtheria)
- Treat chlamydial infections (urethritis, cervicitis), pneumonia due to *Mycoplasma pneumoniae*, and streptococcal infections

ADVERSE EFFECTS

GI discomfort (nausea, vomiting, epigastric pain, diarrhea)

NURSING ACTIONS
- Administer erythromycin with meals.
- Monitor for and report adverse GI effects.

Prolonged QT intervals

Causing dysrhythmias and possible sudden cardiac death

NURSING ACTIONS: Avoid use in clients who have prolonged QT intervals.

Ototoxicity with high-dose therapy

NURSING ACTIONS: Monitor for and report hearing loss, vertigo, and tinnitus.

Superinfection of the bowel

NURSING ACTIONS: Monitor for diarrhea.

Thrombophlebitis

NURSING ACTIONS
- Administer the medication slowly in a dilute solution.
- Monitor IV site for manifestations of thrombophlebitis.

CONTRAINDICATIONS/PRECAUTIONS

Liver disease and QT prolongation are contraindications. Qs

INTERACTIONS

Erythromycin inhibits the metabolism of antihistamines, theophylline, carbamazepine, warfarin, and digoxin, which can lead to toxicity.
NURSING ACTIONS
- To minimize toxicity, avoid using erythromycin with medications that affect hepatic medication-metabolizing enzymes. If unavoidable, monitor liver function tests carefully for indications of toxicity.
- Avoid concurrent use of verapamil, diltiazem, HIV protease inhibitors, antifungal medications, and nefazodone, which inhibit the metabolism of erythromycin, lead to toxicity, and can cause tachydysrhythmias and possible cardiac arrest.

NURSING ADMINISTRATION

- Except for azithromycin, administer oral preparations on an empty stomach (1 hr before meals or 2 hr after) with 8 oz of water, unless GI upset occurs. QEBP
- Instruct the client to complete the entire course of antimicrobial therapy, even if manifestations resolve sooner.
- Carefully monitor the PT or INR of clients who take warfarin concurrently with erythromycin.
- Monitor liver function tests for therapy lasting longer than 2 weeks.

NURSING EVALUATION OF MEDICATION EFFECTIVENESS

Indications of effectiveness include the following.
- A decrease in the manifestations of infection (fever, sore throat, cough, inflammation, adventitious breath sounds)
- Resolution of urinary tract manifestations
- Resolution of bacterial endocarditis (negative blood cultures, WBC counts within the expected reference range)

Aminoglycosides

SELECT PROTOTYPE MEDICATION: Gentamicin

OTHER MEDICATIONS
- Tobramycin
- Neomycin
- Streptomycin
- Paromomycin

PURPOSE

EXPECTED PHARMACOLOGICAL ACTION

Aminoglycosides are bactericidal antibiotics that destroy micro-organisms by disrupting protein synthesis.

THERAPEUTIC USES

- Treat aerobic gram-negative bacilli (*Escherichia coli, Klebsiella pneumoniae, Proteus mirabilis, Pseudomonas aeruginosa*).
- Paromomycin (an oral aminoglycoside) treats intestinal amebiasis and tapeworm infections.
- Oral neomycin suppresses the normal flora of the GI tract preoperatively in preparation for colorectal surgery; topically, it treats infections of the eye, ear, and skin.
- Streptomycin can treat tuberculosis in combination with other medications, but newer and safer ones (ethambutol, rifampin, isoniazid) are preferable. Streptomycin also treats severe, uncommon infections (tularemia, plague, and brucellosis).

ADVERSE EFFECTS

Ototoxicity

- Cochlear damage due to the sensory hair cell injury, causing hearing loss
- Vestibular damage due to injury to sensory hair cells, causing loss of balance

NURSING ACTIONS
- Monitor for high-pitch tinnitus, headache caused from vestibular damage, hearing loss, nausea, dizziness, and vertigo.
- Do baseline audiometric studies (hearing tests).
- Stop aminoglycoside if manifestations occur.
- Monitor trough levels of the medication.
- Administer for no more than 10 days.

CLIENT EDUCATION: Notify the provider if tinnitus, hearing loss, or headaches occur.

Nephrotoxicity

Due to high total cumulative doses resulting in acute tubular necrosis (proteinuria, casts in the urine, dilute urine, elevated BUN, elevated creatinine)

NURSING ACTIONS
- Monitor I&O, BUN, and creatinine.
- Report hematuria and cloudy urine.
- Older adult clients and clients who have kidney disease have an increased risk for developing nephrotoxicity.

Intense neuromuscular blockade

Resulting in respiratory depression, muscle weakness, paralysis

NURSING ACTIONS: Closely monitor use in the client who has myasthenia gravis, is taking skeletal muscle relaxants, or is receiving general anesthetics.

Hypersensitivity

Rash, pruritus, paresthesia of hands and feet, urticaria

NURSING ACTIONS: Monitor for allergic effects.

STREPTOMYCIN

Neurologic disorder

Peripheral neuritis, optic nerve dysfunction, tingling/numbness of the hands and feet

CLIENT EDUCATION: Report any manifestations to the provider promptly.

CONTRAINDICATIONS/PRECAUTIONS

- Use cautiously with clients who have kidney impairment, hearing loss, and myasthenia gravis. Qs
- Use cautiously for clients taking ethacrynic acid (increases the risk for ototoxicity), amphotericin B, cephalosporins, vancomycin (increases the risk for nephrotoxicity), and neuromuscular blocking agents such as tubocurarine.
- The client who has a kidney impairment should receive lower doses of aminoglycosides.

INTERACTIONS

Penicillin inactivates aminoglycosides when in the same IV solution.
NURSING ACTIONS: Do not mix aminoglycosides and penicillins in the same IV solution.

Concurrent administration with other ototoxic medications, such as loop diuretics, increases the risk for ototoxicity.
NURSING ACTIONS: Check frequently for hearing loss with concurrent medication use.

NURSING ADMINISTRATION

- Most aminoglycosides, such as gentamicin and streptomycin (IM only), are parenteral. Neomycin also has oral and topical formulations; tobramycin also has an inhalation formulation.
- Base acquisition of aminoglycoside levels on dosing schedules. QEBP
  - With ONCE-A-DAY DOSING, it is only necessary to obtain a blood sample for measuring trough levels.
  - DIVIDED DOSES
    - **Peak:** 30 min after administration of aminoglycoside IM or 30 min after completion of an IV infusion
    - **Trough:** Right before the next dose

NURSING EVALUATION OF MEDICATION EFFECTIVENESS

Indications of effectiveness include the following.
- Decrease in the manifestations of infection (fever, inflammation, adventitious breath sounds)
- Resolution of urinary tract manifestations
- Wound healing

Application Exercises

1. A nurse is reinforcing teaching with a client about taking tetracycline to treat a GI infection due to *Helicobacter pylori*. Which of the following statements indicates understanding?

    A. "I will take this medication with 8 ounces of milk."

    B. "I will let my doctor know if I start having diarrhea."

    C. "I can stop taking this medication when I feel completely well."

    D. "I can take this medication just before bedtime."

2. A nurse is monitoring the administration of gentamicin by IV infusion at 0900. The medication will take 1 hr to infuse. Which of the following times should the nurse plan to obtain a blood sample for a peak serum level of gentamicin?

    A. 1000

    B. 1030

    C. 1100

    D. 1130

3. A nurse is caring for a client who is starting a course of gentamicin IV for a serious respiratory infection. For which of the following manifestations should the nurse monitor as an adverse effect of this medication? (Select all that apply.)

    A. Pruritus

    B. Hematuria

    C. Muscle weakness

    D. Nystagmus

    E. Vertigo

4. A nurse is caring for a client who has subacute bacterial endocarditis and is receiving several antibiotics, including streptomycin IM. For which of the following manifestations should the nurse monitor as an adverse effect of this medication?

    A. Extremity paresthesias

    B. Urinary retention

    C. Severe constipation

    D. Complex partial seizures

5. A nurse is caring for a client who is undergoing preparation for extensive colorectal surgery. Which of the following oral antibiotics should the nurse expect to administer specifically to suppress normal flora in the GI tract?

    A. Kanamycin

    B. Gentamicin

    C. Neomycin

    D. Tobramycin

PRACTICE Active Learning Scenario

A nurse is reinforcing teaching with a client who has a new prescription for oral erythromycin every 6 hr to treat pneumonia. What should the nurse reinforce with the client about this medication? Use the ATI Active Learning Template: Medication to complete this item.

THERAPEUTIC USES: Describe the therapeutic use for erythromycin in this client.

COMPLICATIONS: Identify two adverse effects the client should monitor for.

NURSING INTERVENTIONS: Describe two diagnostic tests to monitor for clients taking erythromycin.

CLIENT EDUCATION: Include two teaching points for clients taking erythromycin.

Application Exercises Key

1. A. Tetracycline can form a nonabsorbable chelate if clients take it with dairy products. They should take it with water on an empty stomach.

    B. **CORRECT:** Diarrhea can indicate that the client is developing a superinfection, which can be very serious. The client should notify the provider if diarrhea occurs.

    C. Client should take the full prescription of tetracycline and not stop the medication when they begin to feel well.

    D. Taking tetracycline in the morning helps prevent esophageal ulceration, which can occur if the client takes the medication just before lying down.

    Ⓝ *NCLEX® Connection: Pharmacological Therapies, Expected Actions/Outcomes*

2. A. The IV infusion should end at 1000, but that is not the time for the nurse to collect a blood specimen for the peak serum level.

    B. **CORRECT:** The nurse should obtain the blood specimen for the peak serum level at 1030, 30 min after the end of the IV infusion. For the trough level, the nurse should collect the blood sample just before starting the infusion.

    C. Collecting the specimen for the peak serum level 1 hr following the end of the IV infusion would yield an inaccurate peak level.

    D. Collecting the specimen for the peak serum level 1.5 hr following the end of the IV infusion would yield an inaccurate peak level.

    Ⓝ *NCLEX® Connection: Pharmacological Therapies, Expected Actions/Outcomes*

3. A. **CORRECT:** Paresthesias of the hands and feet, urticaria, rash, and pruritus are indications of a hypersensitivity reaction that can occur in clients taking gentamicin.

    B. **CORRECT:** Hematuria is an indication of acute kidney toxicity due to gentamicin.

    C. **CORRECT:** Muscle weakness and respiratory depression can occur in clients taking gentamicin as a result of neuromuscular blockade.

    D. Nystagmus is not an adverse effect of gentamicin.

    E. **CORRECT:** Vertigo, ataxia, and hearing loss are indications of ototoxicity that can occur in clients taking gentamicin.

    Ⓝ *NCLEX® Connection: Pharmacological Therapies, Adverse Effects/ Contraindications/Side Effects/Interactions*

4. A. **CORRECT:** Paresthesias of the hands and feet are a common adverse effect of streptomycin. This medication treats infections in combination with other antibiotics or to treat severe infections when other antibiotics failed.

    B. Urinary retention is not an adverse effect of streptomycin, but this medication can cause nephrotoxicity.

    C. Severe constipation is not an adverse effect of streptomycin. Common adverse effects include headache, ototoxicity, angioedema, muscle weakness, stomatitis, and optic nerve toxicity.

    D. Complex partial seizures are not an adverse effect of streptomycin.

    Ⓝ *NCLEX® Connection: Pharmacological Therapies, Adverse Effects/ Contraindications/Side Effects/Interactions*

5. A. To rid the large intestine of normal flora, the nurse should administer an antibiotic the client can take orally, so that it passes through the GI tract. Kanamycin, an aminoglycoside, is only available in parenteral formulations.

    B. To rid the large intestine of normal flora, the nurse should administer an antibiotic the client can take orally, so that it passes through the GI tract. Gentamicin, an aminoglycoside, is only available in parenteral formulations.

    C. **CORRECT:** The nurse should expect to administer neomycin, an aminoglycoside antibiotic, orally prior to GI surgery to rid the large intestine of normal flora.

    D. To rid the large intestine of normal flora, the nurse should administer an antibiotic the client can take orally, so that it passes through the GI tract. Tobramycin, an aminoglycoside, is only available in parenteral and inhalation formulations.

    Ⓝ *NCLEX® Connection: Pharmacological Therapies, Expected Actions/Outcomes*

PRACTICE Answer

Using the ATI Active Learning Template: Medication

THERAPEUTIC USES: Erythromycin inhibits protein synthesis in the cells of susceptible micro-organisms, usually gram-positive bacteria. Erythromycin can be either bacteriostatic or bactericidal, depending on the organism and on the medication's dosage. It also treats infections for clients who are allergic to penicillin.

COMPLICATIONS
- The most common adverse effects of erythromycin are GI manifestations (abdominal pain, nausea, vomiting, diarrhea).
- Hepatotoxicity with abdominal pain, anorexia, fatigue, and possibly jaundice can occur after 1 to 2 weeks of erythromycin therapy.
- Erythromycin can cause a prolonged QT interval on ECG, which can lead to potentially fatal tachydysrhythmias.
- Ototoxicity can occur with high doses, especially after prolonged periods.

NURSING INTERVENTIONS
- Monitor liver function tests for clients who take erythromycin over a period of several weeks.
- If the client is concurrently taking warfarin or digoxin with erythromycin, carefully monitor PT and INR or digoxin levels.
- Monitor WBC counts for effectiveness of erythromycin treatment.

CLIENT EDUCATION
- Take erythromycin on an empty stomach, 1 hr before or 2 hr after meals, with 8 oz of water.
- Monitor for adverse effects, and call the provider for severe GI distress, manifestations of liver toxicity, and ototoxicity.
- Take the entire course of the medication and do not stop when feeling better.

Ⓝ *NCLEX® Connection: Pharmacological and Parenteral Therapies, Medication Administration*

CHAPTER 40 *Urinary Tract Infections*

Sulfonamides, trimethoprim, and urinary tract antiseptics are medications that treat urinary tract infections (UTIs). Others include penicillins, aminoglycosides, cephalosporins, fluoroquinolones, and a phosphoric acid derivative. These medications treat active infections and prevent recurrent infections for susceptible individuals. Typical regimens are a single-dose; course of 3 days; traditional course of 7 days; or up to 14 days for severe infections.

Trimethoprim-sulfamethoxazole and nitrofurantoin treat uncomplicated cystitis. Fluoroquinolones treat UTIs resistant to trimethoprim-sulfamethoxazole and nitrofurantoin. Fosfomycin, which requires one dose, is a good alternative for clients who have difficulty with adherence. Qᴘᴄᴄ

Sulfonamides and trimethoprim

SELECT PROTOTYPE MEDICATIONS
- Trimethoprim-sulfamethoxazole
- Sulfadiazine
- Trimethoprim

PURPOSE

EXPECTED PHARMACOLOGICAL ACTION

Sulfonamides and trimethoprim inhibit bacterial growth by preventing the synthesis of a folic acid derivative for the replication bacteria.

THERAPEUTIC USES

Trimethoprim-sulfamethoxazole treats the following.
- UTIs, which are most often due to infection with *Escherichia coli*
- Otitis media, chancroid, pertussis, shigellosis, and *Pneumocystis jirovecii* pneumonia

COMPLICATIONS

Hypersensitivity

Including Stevens-Johnson syndrome

NURSING ACTIONS
- Do not administer trimethoprim-sulfamethoxazole to clients who have allergies to the following.
  - Sulfonamides (sulfa)
  - Thiazide diuretics (hydrochlorothiazide)
  - Sulfonylurea-type oral hypoglycemics (glipizide, glyburide)
  - Loop diuretics (furosemide)
- Stop trimethoprim-sulfamethoxazole at the first indication of hypersensitivity, such as rash.

Blood dyscrasias

Hemolytic anemia, agranulocytosis, leukopenia, thrombocytopenia, aplastic anemia

NURSING ACTIONS
- Obtain blood samples for baseline and periodic CBC counts to detect hematologic disorders.
- Observe for and instruct clients to report bleeding, sore throat, and pallor.

Crystalluria

Crystalline aggregates in the kidneys, ureters, and bladder, causing irritation and obstruction that causes acute kidney injury

NURSING ACTIONS
- Encourage adequate oral fluid intake (at least eight 8 oz glasses per day).
- Monitor urine output (should be at least 1,200 mL/day).

Kernicterus

Jaundice, increased bilirubin levels, neurotoxic for newborns

NURSING ACTIONS: Do not give trimethoprim-sulfamethoxazole to clients who are pregnant (during the first trimester or near term) or breastfeeding, or to infants younger than 2 months (due to the risk of kernicterus).

Hyperkalemia

NURSING ACTIONS: Monitor potassium levels.

CONTRAINDICATIONS/PRECAUTIONS

- Folate deficiency is a contraindication because it increases the risk of megaloblastic anemia.
- Use cautiously in clients who have impaired kidney function (give lower dosages).
- Administer with caution to adults older than 65 years who take ACE inhibitors or angiotensin II receptor blockers because of the risk for hyperkalemia. Ⓖ

INTERACTIONS

Increased effects of warfarin, phenytoin, and sulfonylurea oral hypoglycemics

NURSING ACTIONS
- Give lower dosages during trimethoprim-sulfamethoxazole therapy.
- Monitor laboratory levels (PT, INR, blood glucose, phenytoin levels).

NURSING ADMINISTRATION

- Instruct clients to take trimethoprim-sulfamethoxazole on an empty stomach with 8 oz water.
- Instruct clients to complete the entire course of therapy, even if manifestations resolve sooner.
- Advise female clients to use additional contraception to prevent pregnancy. Qs

NURSING EVALUATION OF MEDICATION EFFECTIVENESS

Indications of effectiveness include the following.
- Decrease in manifestations of UTI (frequency, burning, dysuria)
- Negative urine cultures and lower WBC counts

Urinary tract antiseptics

SELECT PROTOTYPE MEDICATION: Nitrofurantoin

OTHER MEDICATIONS: Methenamine

PURPOSE

EXPECTED PHARMACOLOGICAL ACTION

Nitrofurantoin is a broad-spectrum urinary antiseptic with bacteriostatic and bactericidal action. It injures bacteria by damaging DNA.

THERAPEUTIC USES

- Acute UTIs
- Prophylaxis for recurrent lower UTIs

COMPLICATIONS

Gastrointestinal (GI) discomfort

Anorexia, nausea, vomiting, diarrhea

NURSING ACTIONS
- Administer nitrofurantoin with milk or meals.
- Reduce dosages, and use macrocrystalline capsules.

Hypersensitivity reactions

With fever, chills, severe pulmonary manifestations (dyspnea, cough, chest pain, alveolar infiltrations)

CLIENT EDUCATION
- Stop taking the medication and report these reactions.
- Pulmonary manifestations should subside within several days after stopping nitrofurantoin.
- Do not take nitrofurantoin again.

Blood dyscrasias

Agranulocytosis, leukopenia, thrombocytopenia, megaloblastic anemia, hepatotoxicity

NURSING ACTIONS
- Obtain blood samples for a baseline CBC and periodic blood tests including liver function tests.
- Monitor for and report easy bruising and epistaxis (nose bleeding).

Peripheral neuropathy

Numbness, tingling of the hands and feet, muscle weakness

NURSING ACTIONS: Do not administer to clients who have chronic kidney disease (increased risk for peripheral neuropathy).

CLIENT EDUCATION
- Report neuropathy.
- Avoid chronic use of nitrofurantoin.

Headache, drowsiness, dizziness

CLIENT EDUCATION: Report these adverse effects.

CONTRAINDICATIONS/PRECAUTIONS

Impaired kidney function and a creatinine clearance less than 40 mL/min are contraindications. Impaired kidney function increases the risk of toxicity because of the inability to excrete nitrofurantoin.

NURSING ADMINISTRATION

- Inform clients that nitrofurantoin turns urine rust-yellow to brown and can stain teeth.
- Encourage clients to take nitrofurantoin with food if adverse GI effects occur.
- Instruct clients to complete the entire course of therapy, even if manifestations resolve sooner.
- Recommend that clients avoid crushing, chewing, or opening capsules due to the possibility of tooth staining.
- Instruct clients to avoid nitrofurantoin while pregnant (can cause birth defects).

NURSING EVALUATION OF MEDICATION EFFECTIVENESS

Indications of effectiveness include the following.
- Decrease in the manifestations of UTI (frequency, burning, dysuria)
- Negative urine cultures and lower WBC counts
- Resolution of GI disturbances (anorexia, diarrhea, nausea, vomiting)

Fluoroquinolones

SELECT PROTOTYPE MEDICATION: Ciprofloxacin

OTHER MEDICATIONS
- Ofloxacin
- Moxifloxacin
- Levofloxacin
- Norfloxacin

PURPOSE

EXPECTED PHARMACOLOGICAL ACTION

Fluoroquinolones are bactericidal due to inhibition of an enzyme necessary for DNA replication.

THERAPEUTIC USES

- Broad-spectrum antimicrobials treat a wide variety of micro-organisms—including some gram-positive bacteria (such as *Staphylococcus aureus*), and gram-negative bacteria (such as *Klebsiella* and *Escherichia coli*).
- Alternative to parenteral antibiotics for clients who have severe infections
- Urinary, respiratory, and GI tract infections
- Infections of bones, joints, skin, and soft tissues
- Prevention of anthrax for clients who have inhaled anthrax spores

COMPLICATIONS

GI discomfort (nausea, vomiting, diarrhea)

CLIENT EDUCATION: Take the medication with food (with the exception of dairy products) if GI discomfort occurs.

Achilles tendon rupture

CLIENT EDUCATION
- Observe for and report pain, swelling, and redness at the Achilles tendon site.
- Stop taking ciprofloxacin and avoid exercise until the inflammation subsides.

Superinfection (thrush, vaginal yeast infection, C. difficile infection [CDI])

NURSING ACTIONS: Observe for manifestations of CDI

CLIENT EDUCATION: Observe for and report manifestations of yeast infection (cottage-cheese or curd-like lesions on the mouth and genital area).

Phototoxicity (severe sunburn)

From direct and indirect sunlight and sun lamps, even with sunscreen use

CLIENT EDUCATION
- Avoid sun exposure. Wear protective clothing outdoors in sunlight.
- Stop taking the medication if phototoxicity occurs.

CONTRAINDICATIONS/PRECAUTIONS

- Do not administer ciprofloxacin to children younger than 18 years old (due to the risk of Achilles tendon rupture), unless the treatment is for *Escherichia coli* infections of the urinary tract or inhalational anthrax.
- Ciprofloxacin increases the risk for a *Clostridium difficile* infection because it destroys normal intestinal flora.
- Ciprofloxacin and several other fluoroquinolones can affect the CNS (dizziness, headache, restlessness, confusion). Use cautiously with older adults and clients who have cardiovascular disorders. ©

INTERACTIONS

Cationic compounds (aluminum-magnesium antacids, iron salts, sucralfate, dairy products) decrease the absorption of ciprofloxacin.
NURSING ACTIONS: Administer cationic compounds 6 hr before or 2 hr after ciprofloxacin.

Plasma levels of theophylline can increase with concurrent use of ciprofloxacin.
NURSING ACTIONS: Monitor levels, and adjust dosages.

Plasma levels of warfarin can increase with concurrent use of ciprofloxacin.
NURSING ACTIONS: Monitor prothrombin time and INR, and adjust dosages.

NURSING ADMINISTRATION

- Ciprofloxacin is available in oral and IV formulations. Discontinue other IV infusions or use another IV site when administering ciprofloxacin IV.
- Give lower dosages to clients who have impaired kidney function.
- Administer ciprofloxacin IV in a dilute solution slowly over 60 min in a large vein. ⓠEBP
- For inhalation anthrax infection, give ciprofloxacin every 12 hr for 60 days.
- Instruct clients to complete the entire course of therapy, even if manifestations resolve sooner.

NURSING EVALUATION OF MEDICATION EFFECTIVENESS

Indications of effectiveness include the following.
- Decrease in manifestations of UTI (frequency, burning, dysuria)
- Negative urine cultures and lower WBC counts
- No evidence of superinfection

Urinary tract analgesic

SELECT PROTOTYPE MEDICATION: Phenazopyridine

PURPOSE

EXPECTED PHARMACOLOGICAL ACTION: The medication is an azo dye that functions as a local anesthetic on the mucosa of the urinary tract.

THERAPEUTIC USES: Relieve manifestations of burning with urination, pain, frequency, and urgency

NURSING ADMINISTRATION

- Acute kidney injury and chronic kidney disease are contraindications.
- It changes urine to an orange-red color.
- Tell clients that the urine can stain clothes.
- Instruct clients to take it with or after meals to minimize GI discomfort.
- Instruct clients not to crush, break, or chew the tablets.

Application Exercises

1. A nurse is reviewing a client's medication history and notes an allergy to sulfonamides. This allergy is a contraindication for taking which of the following medications? (Select all that apply.)

   A. Hydrochlorothiazide

   B. Metoprolol

   C. Acetaminophen

   D. Glipizide

   E. Furosemide

2. A nurse is reinforcing teaching with a client who has a new prescription for nitrofurantoin. Which of the following information should the nurse include? (Select all that apply.)

   A. Observe for bruising on the skin.

   B. Take the medication with milk or meals.

   C. Expect brown discoloration of urine.

   D. Crush the medication if it is difficult to swallow.

   E. Expect insomnia when taking it.

3. A nurse is reviewing a medication information sheet about ciprofloxacin with a client. Which of the following information about adverse reactions should the nurse include? (Select all that apply.)

   A. Observe for pain and swelling of the Achilles tendon.

   B. Watch for a vaginal yeast infection.

   C. Expect excessive nighttime perspiration.

   D. Inspect the mouth for cottage cheese-like lesions.

   E. Take the medication with a dairy product.

4. A nurse is reviewing discharge teaching with a client who has a new prescription for trimethoprim-sulfamethoxazole. Which of the following information should the nurse include?

   A. Take the medication even if pregnant.

   B. Maintain a fluid restriction while taking it.

   C. Take it on an empty stomach.

   D. Stop taking it when manifestations subside.

5. A nurse is collecting data from a client who has been taking ofloxacin for an upper respiratory infection. Which of the following statements should the nurse report to the provider?

   A. "I have been limiting my time outdoors."

   B. "I have had foul-smelling diarrhea."

   C. "I kept taking the medication even though my symptoms stopped."

   D. "I have been taking loratadine for my allergies."

PRACTICE Active Learning Scenario

A nurse in a provider's office is talking with a client who has a UTI and a prescription for phenazopyridine. What information should the nurse review? Use the ATI Active Learning Template: Medication to complete this item.

EXPECTED PHARMACOLOGICAL ACTION

THERAPEUTIC USES: Describe four.

CLIENT EDUCATION: Include three teaching points.

Application Exercises Key

1. A. **CORRECT:** A sulfonamide allergy is a contraindication for taking hydrochlorothiazide. Hypersensitivity, including Stevens-Johnson syndrome, can result from taking hydrochlorothiazide and a sulfonamide concurrently.

   B. A sulfonamide allergy is not a contraindication for taking metoprolol. It is a contraindication for taking chlorpropamide, glimepiride, metolazone, and ethacrynic acid.

   C. A sulfonamide allergy is not a contraindication for taking acetaminophen. It is a contraindication for taking chlorpropamide, glimepiride, metolazone, and ethacrynic acid.

   D. **CORRECT:** A sulfonamide allergy is a contraindication for taking some oral antidiabetes medications, including glipizide and glyburide. Hypersensitivity, including Stevens-Johnson syndrome, can result from taking glipizide and a sulfonamide concurrently.

   E. **CORRECT:** A sulfonamide allergy is a contraindication for taking loop diuretics, such as furosemide. Hypersensitivity, including Stevens-Johnson syndrome, can result from taking furosemide and a sulfonamide concurrently.

   Ⓝ *NCLEX® Connection: Pharmacological Therapies, Adverse Effects/ Contraindications/Side Effects/Interactions*

2. A. **CORRECT:** Bruising can indicate a blood dyscrasia, and the client should notify the provider if this occurs.

   B. **CORRECT:** Taking the medication with milk or meals minimizes GI discomfort from nausea, vomiting, anorexia, and diarrhea.

   C. **CORRECT:** A brown discoloration of urine is a common adverse effect of nitrofurantoin.

   D. Crushing the medication can cause staining of the teeth.

   E. Nitrofurantoin is more likely to cause drowsiness than insomnia.

   Ⓝ *NCLEX® Connection: Pharmacological Therapies, Expected Actions/Outcomes*

3. A. **CORRECT:** Pain and swelling of the Achilles tendon indicate an adverse effect of ciprofloxacin to report to the provider.

   B. **CORRECT:** A vaginal yeast infection is an overgrowth of *Candida albicans*, which commonly occurs when taking ciprofloxacin.

   C. An alteration in perspiration is not an adverse effect of this medication. Common adverse effects include headache, tremors, dizziness, and dysphagia.

   D. **CORRECT:** Cottage cheese-like lesions in the mouth indicate an overgrowth of *Candida albicans*, a common adverse effect when taking ciprofloxacin.

   E. Milk and other dairy products contain calcium ions that reduce the effect of ciprofloxacin. The client should take the medication 6 hr before or 2 hr after ingesting dairy products.

   Ⓝ *NCLEX® Connection: Pharmacological Therapies, Adverse Effects/ Contraindications/Side Effects/Interactions*

4. A. Trimethoprim-sulfamethoxazole can cause birth defects and fetal kernicterus, especially when taking it during the first trimester or near term

   B. The client should take trimethoprim-sulfamethoxazole with at least eight 8 oz glasses of water each day to prevent crystalluria, which results in kidney damage.

   C. **CORRECT:** The nurse should inform the client that the medication can be taken with or without food.

   D. The client should take the entire prescribed course of medication to destroy all the bacteria and prevent a rebound infection.

   Ⓝ *NCLEX® Connection: Pharmacological Therapies, Expected Actions/Outcomes*

5. A. Fluoroquinolone medications can cause phototoxicity. The client should prevent exposure to sunlight.

   B. **CORRECT:** Foul-smelling diarrhea and abdominal cramping are possible manifestations of a superinfection caused by *C. difficile*. The nurse should report this statement to the provider so the client receives treatment for the secondary infection.

   C. It is appropriate and important to take a full dose of antibiotic therapy even after manifestations resolve.

   D. Loratadine and fluoroquinolones have no known interaction. Fluoroquinolone medications can increase the plasma levels of theophylline or warfarin, and medications containing calcium or magnesium can decrease fluoroquinolone absorption.

   Ⓝ *NCLEX® Connection: Pharmacological Therapies, Adverse Effects/ Contraindications/Side Effects/Interactions*

PRACTICE Answer

Using the ATI Active Learning Template: Medication

EXPECTED PHARMACOLOGICAL ACTION: Phenazopyridine is an azo dye, which acts as a local anesthetic on the mucosa of the urinary tract. It is not an antibiotic.

THERAPEUTIC USES: Relieves urinary burning, urgency, pain, and frequency

CLIENT EDUCATION
- Acute kidney injury and chronic kidney disease are contraindications.
- It changes urine to an orange-red color.
- Urine can stain clothes.
- Take medication with or after meals to minimize GI discomfort.

Ⓝ *NCLEX® Connection: Pharmacological and Parenteral Therapies, Expected Actions/Outcomes*

UNIT 12   MEDICATIONS FOR INFECTION

CHAPTER 41

Mycobacterial, Fungal, and Parasitic Infections

Mycobacterium tuberculosis is a slow-growing pathogen that necessitates long-term treatment. Long-term treatment increases the risk for toxicity, poor client adherence, and development of medication-resistant strains. Treatment for tuberculosis requires the use of at least two medications to which the pathogen is susceptible. Isoniazid and rifampin are two effective antituberculosis medications.

Metronidazole is the medication of choice for parasitic infections.

Antifungal medications belong to a variety of chemical families and can treat systemic and superficial mycoses.

Antimycobacterial (selective antituberculosis)

SELECT PROTOTYPE MEDICATION: Isoniazid

OTHER MEDICATIONS
- Pyrazinamide
- Ethambutol (bacteriostatic only to *M. tuberculosis*)
- Rifapentine

PURPOSE

EXPECTED PHARMACOLOGICAL ACTION

This medication is highly specific for mycobacteria. Isoniazid inhibits growth of mycobacteria by preventing synthesis of mycolic acid in the cell wall.

THERAPEUTIC USES

Indicated for active and latent tuberculosis

Latent: Isoniazid only daily for 9 months, or isoniazid with rifapentine once weekly for 3 months. (Contraindicated in children younger than 2 years old, clients who have HIV, pregnant clients, and clients resistant to either medication.)

Active: The client requires several antimycobacterial medications to treat active tuberculosis in order to decrease medication resistance. Treatment usually consists of a four-medication regimen, often including isoniazid and rifampin.

The initial phase (induction phase) focuses on eliminating the active tubercle bacilli, which will result in noninfectious sputum. **The second phase** (continuation phase) works toward eliminating any other pathogens in the body. Length of treatment varies and can be as short as 6 months for medication-sensitive tuberculosis (2 months for the initial phase and 4 to 7 months for the continuation phase) or as long as 24 months for medication-resistant infections.

COMPLICATIONS

Peripheral neuropathy

Tingling, numbness, burning, and pain resulting from deficiency of pyridoxine, vitamin B_6

NURSING ACTIONS: Administer 50 to 200 mg vitamin B_6 daily.

CLIENT EDUCATION: Observe for manifestations and notify the provider if they occur.

Hepatotoxicity

- Anorexia, malaise, fatigue, nausea, and yellowish discoloration of skin and eyes
- Elevated liver function test results can indicate the need to discontinue the medication.

NURSING ACTIONS: Monitor liver function tests.

CLIENT EDUCATION
- Observe for manifestations and notify the provider if they occur.
- Avoid consumption of alcohol.

CONTRAINDICATIONS/PRECAUTIONS

Clients who have liver disease should not take isoniazid.
NURSING ACTIONS: Use cautiously in older adult clients and clients who have diabetes mellitus or alcohol use disorder. Qs

INTERACTIONS

Isoniazid inhibits metabolism of phenytoin, leading to buildup of medication and toxicity. Ataxia and incoordination can indicate toxicity.
NURSING ACTIONS: Monitor levels of phenytoin. Adjust dosage of phenytoin based on phenytoin levels.

Concurrent use of tyramine foods (aged cheeses, cured meats), alcohol, rifampin, and pyrazinamide increases the risk for hepatotoxicity.
- NURSING ACTIONS: Monitor liver function.
- CLIENT EDUCATION
  ○ Avoid foods with high levels of tyramine.
  ○ Avoid alcohol consumption.

NURSING ADMINISTRATION

- The client usually takes isoniazid orally. When given IM, the medication should be at room temperature to ensure that the solution is free of crystals. Inject the medication deeply into a large muscle.
- For active tuberculosis, direct observation therapy can ensure adherence. Qᴾᶜᶜ
- Advise clients to take isoniazid 1 hr before or 2 hr after meals. If gastric discomfort occurs, the client can take isoniazid with meals.
- Instruct clients to complete the prescribed course of antimicrobial therapy, even though manifestations can resolve before the full course is completed.

Broad-spectrum antimycobacterial (antituberculosis)

SELECT PROTOTYPE MEDICATION: Rifampin

PURPOSE

EXPECTED PHARMACOLOGICAL ACTION

Rifampin is bactericidal as a result of inhibition of protein synthesis.

THERAPEUTIC USES

- Rifampin is a broad-spectrum antibiotic effective for gram-positive and gram-negative bacteria.
- Rifampin is part of combination medication therapy with at least one other antituberculosis medication to help prevent antibiotic resistance. Qᴱᴮᴾ

COMPLICATIONS

Discoloration of body fluids

NURSING ACTIONS: Inform clients of expected orange color of urine, saliva, sweat, and tears.

Hepatotoxicity (jaundice, anorexia, and fatigue)

NURSING ACTIONS: Monitor liver function.

CLIENT EDUCATION
- Manifestations include anorexia, fatigue, and malaise. Notify the provider if they occur.
- Avoid alcohol.

Mild GI discomfort

- Anorexia, nausea, and abdominal discomfort
- Abdominal discomfort is mild and usually does not require intervention.

Pseudomembranous colitis

CLIENT EDUCATION: Monitor and report fever, diarrhea, abdominal pain, or bloody stool.

CONTRAINDICATIONS/PRECAUTIONS

Use cautiously in clients who have liver dysfunction. Qₛ

INTERACTIONS

Rifampin accelerates metabolism of warfarin, oral contraceptives, protease inhibitors, and non–nucleoside reverse transcriptase inhibitors (NNRTIs) for HIV, resulting in diminished effectiveness.
- Increased dosages of HIV medications are often necessary.
- NURSING ACTIONS: Monitor PT and INR.
- CLIENT EDUCATION: Use a nonhormonal form of contraception.

Concurrent use with isoniazid and pyrazinamide increases risk of hepatotoxicity.
- NURSING ACTIONS: Monitor liver function.
- CLIENT EDUCATION: Avoid alcohol consumption.

NURSING ADMINISTRATION

- Administer orally or by IV route.
- Administer oral rifampin 1 hr before or 2 hr after meals. Food decreases medication absorption.

CLIENT EDUCATION

Use a nonhormonal form of contraception.

NURSING EVALUATION OF MEDICATION EFFECTIVENESS

Depending on therapeutic intent, the following findings indicate medication effectiveness.
- Improvement of tuberculosis manifestations (clear breath sounds, no night sweats, increased appetite, no afternoon rises of temperature)
- Three negative sputum cultures for tuberculosis, usually taking 3 to 6 months to achieve

Antiprotozoals

SELECT PROTOTYPE MEDICATION: Metronidazole

PURPOSE

EXPECTED PHARMACOLOGICAL ACTION

Metronidazole is a broad-spectrum antimicrobial with bactericidal activity against anaerobic micro-organisms.

THERAPEUTIC USES

- Treatment of protozoal infections (intestinal amebiasis, trichomoniasis) and obligate anaerobic bacteria
- Prophylaxis for clients who will have surgical procedures and are at high risk for anaerobic infection
- Treatment of *H. pylori* in combination with tetracycline and bismuth subsalicylate in clients who have peptic ulcer disease

COMPLICATIONS

GI discomfort

Nausea, vomiting, dry mouth, metallic taste

CLIENT EDUCATION: Take the medication with meals to reduce these effects.

Darkening of urine

CLIENT EDUCATION: This is a harmless effect of metronidazole.

Neurotoxicity, CNS effects

Numbness of extremities, ataxia, and seizures

NURSING ACTIONS: Stop metronidazole.

CLIENT EDUCATION: Notify the provider if manifestations occur.

Superinfection

CLIENT EDUCATION: Monitor for and report fever, vaginal itching blackened tongue, diarrhea, or bloody stool.

CONTRAINDICATIONS/PRECAUTIONS

- Contraindicated in the first trimester of pregnancy Qs
- Use cautiously in clients in second or third trimesters of pregnancy.

INTERACTIONS

Alcohol causes a disulfiram-like reaction (facial flushing, vomiting, dyspnea, tachycardia).
CLIENT EDUCATION: Avoid alcohol consumption.

Metronidazole inhibits inactivation of warfarin, phenytoin, and lithium.
NURSING ACTIONS: Monitor prothrombin time and INR, phenytoin and lithium levels. Adjust dosages accordingly.

NURSING ADMINISTRATION

Administer by oral or IV route.

CLIENT EDUCATION

- Complete the prescribed course of antimicrobial therapy, even though manifestations can resolve before the full course is completed. Qpcc
- Avoid sexual intercourse or use condoms if using this medication for treatment of trichomoniasis.

NURSING EVALUATION OF MEDICATION EFFECTIVENESS

Depending on therapeutic intent, the following findings can indicate medication effectiveness.
- Resolution of bloody mucoid diarrhea
- Formed stools
- Negative stool results for amoeba and giardia
- Decrease or absence of watery vaginal/urethral discharge
- Negative blood cultures for anaerobic organisms in the CNS, blood, bones and joints, and soft tissues

Antifungals

SELECT PROTOTYPE MEDICATIONS
- Amphotericin B (a polyene antibiotic for systemic mycoses)
- Ketoconazole (an azole for treating both superficial and systemic mycoses)

OTHER MEDICATIONS
- Flucytosine
- Nystatin
- Miconazole
- Clotrimazole
- Terbinafine
- Fluconazole
- Griseofulvin

PURPOSE

EXPECTED PHARMACOLOGICAL ACTION

Amphotericin B is an antifungal agent that acts on fungal cell membranes to cause cell death. Depending on concentration, these agents can be fungistatic (slows growth on the fungus) or fungicidal (destroys the fungus).

THERAPEUTIC USES

- Antifungals are the treatment of choice for systemic fungal infection (candidiasis, aspergillosis, cryptococcosis) and nonopportunistic mycoses.
- Some antifungals treat superficial fungal infections of the nails and skin (especially groin and feet) and the mucous membranes.

COMPLICATIONS

Infusion reactions

Fever, chills, rigors, and headache 1 to 3 hr after initiation
- A test dose of 1 mg amphotericin B, infused slowly IV, can test client reaction to the medication.
- The client can require meperidine, dantrolene, or hydrocortisone for rigors.

NURSING ACTIONS: Pretreat with diphenhydramine and acetaminophen prior to IV infusion. Qs

Thrombophlebitis

NURSING ACTIONS
- Observe infusion sites for of erythema, swelling, and pain.
- Rotate injection sites.
- Administer in a large vein.

Nephrotoxicity

NURSING ACTIONS
- Obtain baseline kidney function (BUN and creatinine) and monitor weekly kidney function tests.
- Monitor I&O.

Electrolyte imbalance

NURSING ACTIONS
- Monitor electrolyte levels, especially potassium.
- Administer supplements for deficiencies.

Bone marrow suppression

NURSING ACTIONS: Obtain baseline CBC and hematocrit, and monitor weekly.

KETOCONAZOLE

Hepatotoxicity

Anorexia, nausea, vomiting, jaundice, dark urine, and clay-colored stools

NURSING ACTIONS: Obtain baseline liver function studies, and monitor liver function monthly.

CLIENT EDUCATION: If manifestations occur, notify the provider and discontinue the medication.

Effects on sex hormones

Male clients: Gynecomastia (enlargement of breast), decreased libido, erectile dysfunction

Female clients: Irregular menstrual flow

CLIENT EDUCATION: Observe for these effects and notify the provider.

CONTRAINDICATIONS/PRECAUTIONS

- Clients who have impaired kidney function should not take antifungals due to the risk for nephrotoxicity. Qs
- Use antifungals with caution in clients who have anemia, electrolyte imbalance, and bone marrow suppression.
- Fluconazole is Pregnancy Risk Category D in high doses. The provider might permit use during breastfeeding because only trace amounts are present in human milk.

INTERACTIONS

Aminoglycosides (gentamicin, streptomycin, cyclosporine) have additive nephrotoxic risk when used concurrently with antifungal medications.
NURSING ACTIONS: Avoid use of these antimicrobials when clients are taking amphotericin B due to additive nephrotoxicity risk.

Antifungal effects of flucytosine are potentiated with concurrent use of amphotericin B.
NURSING ACTIONS: Potentiated flucytosine effects allow for a reduction in amphotericin B dosages.

Azole antibiotics increase levels of multiple medications (digoxin, warfarin, sulfonylurea antidiabetic medications).
NURSING ACTIONS: If concurrent administration is necessary, carefully monitor for toxicity.

NURSING ADMINISTRATION

- Amphotericin B is highly toxic and should be reserved for severe life-threatening fungal infections.
- Ensure amphotericin B IV infuses slowly over 2 to 6 hr.
- Observe infusion solutions for precipitation and discard or stop the infusion if precipitates are present. Use a filter to prevent infusion of undissolved crystals. Administering 1 L of 0.9% sodium chloride IV on the day of amphotericin B infusion lessens the risk of kidney injury. Qᴱᴮᴾ
- Instruct clients to complete the prescribed course of antimicrobial therapy, even though manifestations might resolve before the full course is completed.
- Apply antifungals for topical use to treat superficial vulvovaginal candidiasis as vaginal suppository or cream.

NURSING EVALUATION OF MEDICATION EFFECTIVENESS

Depending on therapeutic intent, the following findings can indicate medication effectiveness.
- Improvement of findings of systemic fungal infections
- Improvement of findings of superficial infections (clear mucus membranes, clear nails, intact skin)

> **PRACTICE** Active Learning Scenario
>
> A nurse in a public health department is reviewing medication information with a client who has latent tuberculosis (TB) and a new prescription for isoniazid twice weekly for 6 months. What should the nurse reinforce with the client about this medication? Use the ATI Active Learning Template: Medication to complete this item.
>
> **THERAPEUTIC USES:** Describe the therapeutic use for isoniazid in this client.
>
> **COMPLICATIONS:** List two adverse effects the client should watch for.
>
> **NURSING INTERVENTIONS:** Describe one test to monitor for clients taking isoniazid.
>
> **CLIENT EDUCATION:** Describe two teaching points for clients taking isoniazid.

Application Exercises

1. A nurse is caring for a client who has diabetes mellitus, pulmonary tuberculosis, and a new prescription for isoniazid. Which of the following supplements should the nurse expect to administer to prevent an adverse effect of INH?
   - A. Ascorbic acid
   - B. Pyridoxine
   - C. Folic acid
   - D. Cyanocobalamin

2. A nurse is assisting with monitoring a client receiving IV amphotericin B. The nurse should monitor the client for which of the following adverse effects of this medication?
   - A. Polyuria
   - B. Hypothermia
   - C. Rigors
   - D. Hyperkalemia

3. A nurse is caring for a client receiving an IV amphotericin B infusion. Which of the following serum laboratory values should the nurse plan to monitor? (Select all that apply.)
   - A. Albumin
   - B. Amylase
   - C. Magnesium
   - D. Hematocrit
   - E. Creatinine

4. A nurse is reinforcing teaching with a client who is beginning a course of metronidazole. The nurse should remind the client to stop taking the medication and notify the provider if which of the following manifestations occur?
   - A. Metallic taste
   - B. Nausea
   - C. Ataxia
   - D. Dark-colored urine

5. A nurse is reviewing discharge teaching with a client who has active tuberculosis. The client asks why he must take four different medications. Which of the following responses should the nurse make?
   - A. "Four medications decrease the risk for a severe allergic reaction."
   - B. "Four medications reduce the chance that the bacteria will become resistant."
   - C. "Four medications reduce the risk for adverse reactions"
   - D. "Four medications decrease the chance of having a positive tuberculin skin test."

Application Exercises Key

1. A. Clients who have a vitamin C deficiency require ascorbic acid supplementation. However, it will not prevent an adverse effect of INH.

   B. **CORRECT:** Clients often take pyridoxine (vitamin B₆) along with INH to prevent peripheral neuropathy. Clients who have diabetes mellitus or alcohol use disorder are at increased risk for this complication.

   C. Clients who have hepatic disease and folic acid deficiency can benefit from folic acid supplementation; however, it will not prevent an adverse effect of INH.

   D. Clients who have malabsorption syndrome can require cyanocobalamin supplementation; however, it will not prevent an adverse effect of INH.

   ⓝ *NCLEX® Connection: Pharmacological Therapies, Adverse Effects/ Contraindications/Side Effects/Interactions*

2. A. Amphotericin B can impair kidney function. The nurse should monitor for decreased urine output.

   B. Amphotericin B can cause an increased body temperature.

   C. **CORRECT:** Amphotericin B can cause fever, chills, and nausea during the infusion. Pretreatment with diphenhydramine and acetaminophen can reduce these effects.

   D. Amphotericin B can cause hypokalemia, a serious adverse effect.

   ⓝ *NCLEX® Connection: Pharmacological Therapies, Adverse Effects/ Contraindications/Side Effects/Interactions*

3. A. Amphotericin B does not affect serum protein levels.

   B. Amphotericin B does not cause pancreatitis.

   C. **CORRECT:** Amphotericin B can cause hypomagnesemia. The nurse should monitor serum magnesium values. The client is also at risk for potassium and calcium deficiency.

   D. **CORRECT:** Amphotericin B can cause bone marrow suppression. The nurse should monitor CBC and platelet count periodically.

   E. **CORRECT:** Amphotericin B can cause nephrotoxicity. The nurse should monitor kidney function (with serum creatinine, BUN, and creatinine clearance).

   ⓝ *NCLEX® Connection: Pharmacological Therapies, Adverse Effects/ Contraindications/Side Effects/Interactions*

4. A. A metallic taste in the mouth is an adverse effect of metronidazole, but it is not necessary to stop the medication or notify the provider.

   B. Nausea is an adverse effect of metronidazole, but it is not necessary to stop taking the medication or notify the provider.

   C. **CORRECT:** Ataxia, tremors, paresthesias of the extremities, and seizures are manifestations of CNS toxicity. The client should stop taking the medication and notify the provider if any of these effects occur.

   D. Dark-colored urine is a harmless effect. It is not necessary to stop taking the medication or notify the provider.

   ⓝ *NCLEX® Connection: Pharmacological Therapies, Adverse Effects/ Contraindications/Side Effects/Interactions*

5. A. Taking several antituberculosis medications concurrently does not decrease the chance of an allergic reaction to any of the individual medications.

   B. **CORRECT:** If the client took only one medication to treat active tuberculosis, resistance to the medication would occur quickly. Taking three or four medications decreases the possibility of resistance.

   C. Taking several antituberculosis medications concurrently does not minimize the chance of adverse effects to any of the medications. Risk for liver toxicity increases when the client takes more than one medication that causes liver toxicity (isoniazid, rifampin, pyrazinamide).

   D. Taking several antituberculosis medications concurrently does not change the fact that the client will have a positive tuberculin skin test indefinitely.

   ⓝ *NCLEX® Connection: Pharmacological Therapies, Expected Actions/Outcomes*

PRACTICE Answer

Using the ATI Active Learning Template: Medication

THERAPEUTIC USES

- A client who has latent tuberculosis has a *Mycobacterium tuberculosis* infection and is at risk for (but has not yet developed) active tuberculosis.
- Some clients who have latent tuberculosis, such as those who are immunocompromised or who have recently immigrated to the U.S. from a country where active TB is common, can require treatment with isoniazid, with or without rifapentine, in order to prevent the onset of active TB.
- The client who has latent TB has a positive tuberculin test but a negative sputum culture and negative chest x-ray for TB. The client cannot infect others with tuberculosis unless the infection becomes active.

COMPLICATIONS

- Paresthesias in the extremities caused by vitamin B₆ deficiency
- Hepatotoxicity

NURSING INTERVENTIONS: The client who starts isoniazid should have baseline liver function testing and be tested periodically throughout treatment.

CLIENT EDUCATION

- Watch for paresthesias, and ask the provider about taking pyridoxine to reverse the effects.
- Indications of hepatitis include anorexia, fatigue, nausea, and jaundice. Notify the provider if these occur.
- Take isoniazid as prescribed, and do not stop until the entire course of treatment is completed. The client who has latent tuberculosis does not feel ill.
- Avoid foods with high levels of tyramine such as aged cheese and meats.
- Avoid alcohol consumption.

ⓝ *NCLEX® Connection: Pharmacological and Parenteral Therapies, Medication Administration*

UNIT 12   MEDICATIONS FOR INFECTION

CHAPTER 42 *Viral Infections, HIV, and AIDS*

Most antiviral medications act by altering viral reproduction. Antiviral medications are only effective during viral replication. Therefore, they are ineffective when the virus is dormant.

The human immunodeficiency virus (HIV) is a retrovirus. A retrovirus must attach to a host cell in order to replicate. RNA converts to DNA using the enzyme reverse transcriptase.

Antiretroviral agents treat HIV infections. These medications do not cure HIV infection and do not decrease the risk of passing HIV infection to others. Antiretroviral agents act by preventing the virus from entering the cells (fusion/entry inhibitors and chemokine receptor 5 [CCR5] antagonists). Others act by inhibiting enzymes needed for HIV replication (nucleoside reverse transcriptase inhibitors [NRTIs], non-nucleoside reverse transcriptase inhibitors [NNRTIs], protease inhibitors [PIs], and an integrase inhibitor [INSTI]). Skipping doses or taking decreased dosages of antiretroviral medications causes medication resistance and possible treatment failure.

Highly active antiretroviral therapy

- Highly active antiretroviral therapy (HAART) involves using three to four HIV medications in combination with other antiretroviral medications to reduce medication resistance, adverse effects, and dosages.
- HAART is an aggressive treatment method to reduce the amount of virus and increase CD4 counts.
- In addition to HAART, clients who have HIV infection take additional medications to treat adverse effects of antiretrovirals and treat or prevent secondary infections, such as pneumocystis pneumonia.

Antivirals

SELECT PROTOTYPE MEDICATIONS
- Acyclovir (oral, topical, IV)
- Ganciclovir (oral, IV)

OTHER MEDICATIONS
- Interferon alfa-2b
- Lamivudine
- Oseltamivir
- Ribavirin
- Amantadine
- Boceprevir
- Telaprevir

PURPOSE

EXPECTED PHARMACOLOGICAL ACTION: Acyclovir and ganciclovir prevent the reproduction of viral DNA and thus interrupt cell replication.

THERAPEUTIC USES
- Acyclovir is used to treat herpes simplex and varicella-zoster viruses
- Ganciclovir can treat and prevent cytomegalovirus (CMV). Clients who have HIV/AIDS, organ transplants, and other immunocompromised states can take ganciclovir prophylactically.
- Interferon alfa-2b and lamivudine can treat hepatitis B and C.
- Oseltamivir can treat influenza A and B.
- Ribavirin can treat respiratory syncytial virus, hepatitis C, and influenza (unlabeled use).
- Boceprevir and telaprevir are protease inhibitors that treat hepatitis C virus.

COMPLICATIONS

Acyclovir

Phlebitis and inflammation at the site of infusion
NURSING ACTIONS
- Rotate IV injection sites.
- Monitor IV sites for swelling and redness.

Nephrotoxicity
NURSING ACTIONS
- Administer acyclovir infusion slowly over 1 hr.
- Ensure adequate hydration during infusion and 2 hr after to minimize nephrotoxicity by increasing oral fluid intake as prescribed. The client might require IV fluid replacement.
- Use with caution in clients who have kidney impairment or are dehydrated.
- Monitor BUN and creatinine levels.

Mild discomfort associated with oral therapy
- Nausea, headache, diarrhea
- NURSING ACTIONS: Observe for manifestations and notify the provider.

Ganciclovir

Bone marrow suppression (leukocytes, thrombocytes)
- NURSING ACTIONS
  - Obtain baseline CBC and platelet count.
  - Administer granulocyte colony-stimulating factors.
  - Monitor WBC, absolute neutrophil, and platelet counts frequently during treatment.
- CLIENT EDUCATION: Report manifestations of infection and bleeding, and avoid crowds or individuals who have any infections.

Fever, headache, nausea, diarrhea
- NURSING ACTIONS: Administer with food.
- CLIENT EDUCATION: Report indications of infection.

CONTRAINDICATIONS/PRECAUTIONS

- Use caution when administering acyclovir to clients who have kidney impairment or dehydration, and clients taking nephrotoxic medications. Qs
- Ganciclovir is Pregnancy Risk Category C. It can cause infertility. Advise clients to use barrier contraception during treatment and for 3 months following treatment. Clients who have a neutrophil count less than 500/mm³ or platelet counts less than 25,000/mm³ should not take ganciclovir. Use cautiously in older adults and clients who have dehydration or kidney insufficiency. ©

INTERACTIONS

Acyclovir

Probenecid can decrease elimination of acyclovir.
NURSING ACTIONS: Monitor for medication toxicity.

Concurrent use of zidovudine can cause drowsiness.
NURSING ACTIONS: Use with caution.

Ganciclovir

Cytotoxic medications can cause increased toxicity.
NURSING ACTIONS: Use together with caution.

NURSING ADMINISTRATION

Instruct clients to complete the prescribed course of antimicrobial therapy, even though manifestations can resolve before the full course is completed.

Acyclovir

- Ensure slow IV infusion, over 1 hr or longer.
- Clients who have healed herpetic lesions should continue to use condoms to prevent transmission of the virus.

CLIENT EDUCATION
- For topical administration, wear rubber gloves to avoid transfer of virus to other areas of the body. Qᴇʙᴘ
- Expect relief of manifestations, but not a cure.
- Wash affected area with soap and water three to four times per day and keep the lesions dry after washing.
- Refrain from sexual contact while lesions are present.

Ganciclovir

- Ensure IV infuses slowly, with an infusion pump, over at least 1 hr.
- Administer oral medication with food.
- Encourage extra fluid intake during therapy.
- Administer intraocular for CMV retinitis. Do not use contact lenses with medication.
- Avoid getting ganciclovir solution or powder on skin. Wash well if contact occurs.

CLIENT EDUCATION: Use barrier contraception if using this medication.

NURSING EVALUATION OF MEDICATION EFFECTIVENESS

Depending on therapeutic intent, findings of medication effectiveness can include healed genital lesions, decreased inflammation and pain, and improvement in vision

Antiretrovirals: Fusion/entry inhibitors

SELECT PROTOTYPE MEDICATION:
Enfuvirtide (subcutaneous; T-20)

PURPOSE

EXPECTED PHARMACOLOGICAL ACTION: Decreases and limits the spread of HIV by blocking HIV from attaching to and entering CD4 T cell

THERAPEUTIC USES: Treatment of HIV that is unresponsive to other antiretrovirals

COMPLICATIONS

Localized reaction at injection site
NURSING ACTIONS: Rotate injection sites. Monitor for swelling and redness. Avoid sites with an active reaction.

Bacterial pneumonia
NURSING ACTIONS
- Check breath sounds prior to start of therapy.
- Monitor for manifestations of pneumonia (fever, cough, shortness of breath).
- Use cautiously with clients who are at an increased risk for pneumonia.

Fever, chills, rash, hypotension
NURSING ACTIONS: Monitor for medication reaction. Discontinue and notify the provider.

CONTRAINDICATIONS/PRECAUTIONS

- Clients who have medication hypersensitivity and clients who are breastfeeding should not take enfuvirtide. Qs
- This medication is Pregnancy Risk Category B.

NURSING ADMINISTRATION

- Enfuvirtide is only available for subcutaneous administration. Rotate injection sites and avoid previous skin reaction areas. Q_{EBP}
- Bring the solution to room temperature before injection.
- Monitor for bacterial pneumonia.
- Monitor for systemic hypersensitivity reaction.
- Remind the client to take medication exactly as prescribed to minimize development of resistance.
- Advise the client to notify the provider of possible pregnancy.
- Inspect medication solution to ensure it is free of particles or bubbles prior to administration.

NURSING EVALUATION OF MEDICATION EFFECTIVENESS

Depending on therapeutic intent, a reduction of manifestations and absence of opportunistic infection indicate medication effectiveness.

Antiretrovirals: CCR5 antagonists

SELECT PROTOTYPE MEDICATION: Maraviroc (oral)

PURPOSE

EXPECTED PHARMACOLOGICAL ACTION: Prevent HIV from entering lymphocytes by binding to CCR5 on cell membranes

THERAPEUTIC USE: Treat HIV infection in conjunction with other antiretroviral medications

COMPLICATIONS

Cough and upper respiratory tract infections
CLIENT EDUCATION: Report respiratory findings.

CNS effects (dizziness, paresthesias), orthostatic hypotension
CLIENT EDUCATION: Move carefully from lying or sitting to standing, and prevent injury caused by dizziness.

Hepatotoxicity
- Jaundice, right upper quadrant pain, and nausea, often preceded by allergic reaction (hives, rash)
- CLIENT EDUCATION: Stop maraviroc and notify provider for these findings.

Cardiovascular effects (myocardial infarction, myocardial ischemia)
CLIENT EDUCATION: Report chest pain or discomfort.

CONTRAINDICATIONS/PRECAUTIONS

- Contraindicated in clients who have kidney impairment. Q_s
- Use caution in clients who have existing cardiovascular disorders, kidney or liver disease, dehydration, or orthostatic hypotension.
- Use caution in older adults and clients who are breastfeeding. Ⓖ
- Pregnancy Risk Category B

INTERACTIONS

Most protease inhibitors raise maraviroc levels.
NURSING ACTIONS: Adjust maraviroc dosage.

Rifampin, efavirenz, phenytoin, some other anticonvulsants, and St. John's wort decrease maraviroc levels.
NURSING ACTIONS: Adjust maraviroc dosage.

NURSING ADMINISTRATION

- Administer orally in conjunction with other antiretroviral medications.
- Monitor liver function tests, blood pressure, and CBC at baseline and periodically during treatment.
- Tell the client to notify the provider of possible pregnancy.
- Administer at regular intervals to maintain therapeutic blood levels.

NURSING EVALUATION OF MEDICATION EFFECTIVENESS

Decrease in manifestations of HIV infection and absent of opportunistic infections indicates therapeutic effectiveness.

Antiretrovirals: NRTIs

SELECT PROTOTYPE MEDICATION: Zidovudine

OTHER MEDICATIONS
- Didanosine
- Stavudine
- Lamivudine
- Abacavir

COMBINATION MEDICATIONS: Fixed medication dosages in one tablet or capsule
- Abacavir, lamivudine, zidovudine
- Abacavir, lamivudine
- Lamivudine, zidovudine
- Tenofovir/emtricitabine

ROUTE OF ADMINISTRATION: Oral, IV

PURPOSE

EXPECTED PHARMACOLOGICAL ACTION: Reduce HIV manifestations by inhibiting DNA synthesis and thus viral replication

THERAPEUTIC USE: First-line antiretrovirals to treat HIV infection

COMPLICATIONS

Bone marrow suppression
- Zidovudine can cause bone marrow suppression, resulting in anemia, agranulocytosis (neutropenia), and thrombocytopenia.
- NURSING ACTIONS: Monitor CBC and platelets.
- CLIENT EDUCATION: Monitor for bleeding, easy bruising, sore throat, and fatigue.

Lactic acidosis
NURSING ACTIONS
- Monitor for indications of lactic acidosis (hyperventilation, nausea, abdominal pain).
- Pregnancy increases the risk of lactic acidosis.

Nausea, vomiting, diarrhea
NURSING ACTIONS
- Provide food with medication to reduce gastric irritation.
- Monitor fluids and electrolytes.

Hepatomegaly/fatty liver
NURSING ACTIONS: Monitor liver enzymes.

CONTRAINDICATIONS/PRECAUTIONS

- These medications are Pregnancy Risk Category C. Pregnancy increases risk for lactic acidosis, liver enlargement, and fatty liver. Qs
- Clients who have medication hypersensitivity should not take these medications.
- Use with caution in clients who have liver disease and bone marrow suppression.

INTERACTIONS

Probenecid, valproic acid, and methadone can increase zidovudine serum levels.
NURSING ACTIONS: Reduce dosage. Monitor for medication toxicity.

Ganciclovir or medications that decrease bone marrow production can further suppress bone marrow.
NURSING ACTIONS: Use together with caution. Monitor blood counts, and report sore throat or fever.

Rifampin and ritonavir can reduce zidovudine levels.
NURSING ACTIONS: Adjust dosage if needed.

NURSING ADMINISTRATION

- Monitor for bone marrow suppression. Obtain baseline CBC and platelets at the start of therapy, and monitor periodically as needed. Q EBP
- Treat anemia with epoetin alfa or transfusions.
- Treat neutropenia with colony-stimulating factors.

CLIENT EDUCATION

- Take medications exactly as prescribed to minimize development of medication resistance.
- Notify the provider if pregnancy is suspected.

NURSING EVALUATION OF MEDICATION EFFECTIVENESS

Depending on therapeutic intent, effectiveness is evidenced by a reduction of manifestations and absent of opportunistic infection.

Antiretrovirals: NNRTIs

SELECT PROTOTYPE MEDICATIONS
- Delavirdine
- Efavirenz

OTHER MEDICATIONS
- Nevirapine
- Etravirine

ROUTE OF ADMINISTRATION: Oral

PURPOSE

EXPECTED PHARMACOLOGICAL ACTION: NNRTIs act directly on reverse transcriptase to stop HIV replication.

THERAPEUTIC USES
- Primary HIV-1 infection
- Often used in combination with other antiretroviral agents to prevent medication resistance

COMPLICATIONS

Rash
- Can become serious and lead to Stevens–Johnson syndrome
- NURSING ACTIONS
  - Monitor for rash. Treat with diphenhydramine.
  - Notify the provider for fever or blistering.

Flu-like manifestations, headache, fatigue
NURSING ACTIONS
- Monitor for adverse reactions.
- Encourage rest and adequate oral fluid intake.

CNS manifestations
- Dizziness, drowsiness, insomnia, nightmares (especially with efavirenz)
- CLIENT EDUCATION
  - These findings should decrease within the first month of therapy.
  - Do not perform activities that require alertness until able to predict the adverse effects.

Nausea, diarrhea
CLIENT EDUCATION: Take at night on an empty stomach.

CONTRAINDICATIONS/PRECAUTIONS

- Efavirenz is Pregnancy Risk Category D, including the first trimester. Delavirdine is Pregnancy Risk Category C. **Qs**
- Clients who have medication hypersensitivity or severe liver disease should not take these medications.
- Use with caution in clients who have liver or kidney disease.

INTERACTIONS

Antacids can decrease absorption of delavirdine.
NURSING ACTIONS: Allow 1 hr between medications.

Rifampin and phenytoin can cause decreased levels of delavirdine.
NURSING ACTIONS: Do not use together.

Didanosine can reduce absorption of both medications.
NURSING ACTIONS: Allow 1 hr between medications.

NNRTIs can cause increase in sildenafil level.
NURSING ACTIONS: Monitor for hypotension and changes in vision. Use together with caution.

Efavirenz and delavirdine can decrease the effects of hormonal contraceptives.
CLIENT EDUCATION: Use a barrier form of contraception, such as condoms, in addition to a hormonal contraceptive.

NURSING ADMINISTRATION

- Monitor for rash.
- Administering with a high-fat meal can increase absorption.

CLIENT EDUCATION

- Take exactly as prescribed and do not skip doses to minimize development of resistance. **Q**EBP
- Use a barrier form of contraception, such as condoms, in addition to a hormonal contraceptive.

NURSING EVALUATION OF MEDICATION EFFECTIVENESS

Depending on therapeutic intent, a reduction of manifestations and absent of opportunistic infection can indicate medication effectiveness.

Antiretrovirals: Protease inhibitors

SELECT PROTOTYPE MEDICATION: Ritonavir

OTHER MEDICATIONS
- Saquinavir
- Indinavir
- Fosamprenavir
- Nelfinavir
- Lopinavir/ritonavir combination

ROUTE OF ADMINISTRATION: Oral

PURPOSE

EXPECTED PHARMACOLOGICAL ACTION: Protease inhibitors act against HIV-1 and HIV-2 to alter and inactivate the virus by inhibiting enzymes needed for HIV replication.

THERAPEUTIC USES
- Treat HIV infections
- Usually combined with one or two reverse transcriptase inhibitors
- Ritonavir is usually given with other PIs to increase their effect.

COMPLICATIONS

Bone loss/osteoporosis
- The client can require treatment with medications such as raloxifene and alendronate to manage severe bone loss.
- CLIENT EDUCATION: Eat a diet high in calcium and vitamin D.

Diabetes mellitus/hyperglycemia
- NURSING ACTIONS: Monitor serum glucose. Adjust diet and administer antidiabetic medications.
- CLIENT EDUCATION: Monitor for increased thirst (polydipsia) and increased urine output (polyuria).

Hypersensitivity reaction
NURSING ACTIONS: Monitor for rash. Notify the provider if rash develops.

Elevated serum lipids
NURSING ACTIONS: Monitor for hyperlipidemia. Adjust diet.

Altered fat distribution
NURSING ACTIONS: Warn clients of these effects.

Rhabdomyolysis
NURSING ACTIONS: Monitor and report muscle pain and weakness.

CONTRAINDICATIONS/PRECAUTIONS

- Protease inhibitors are Pregnancy Risk Category B or C. **Qs**
- Use with caution in clients who have liver disease, diabetes mellitus, AV block, and hypercholesterolemia.
- Contraindications exist with many other medications. Advise the client to notify the provider before taking any new medications.

INTERACTIONS

All protease inhibitors (especially ritonavir) cause multiple medications (quinidine) to raise to toxic levels.
NURSING ACTIONS: Check any new medication with the list of medications to avoid in clients taking protease inhibitors.

Ritonavir can increase medication levels of sildenafil, tadalafil, and vardenafil.
NURSING ACTIONS: Use with caution. Reduce dosages as needed.

Ritonavir decreases levels of ethynyl estradiol in oral contraceptives.
CLIENT EDUCATION: Use an alternative form of birth control.

Phenobarbital, phenytoin, carbamazepine, and St. John's wort all significantly reduce level of protease inhibitors.
NURSING ACTIONS: Avoid concurrent use, or adjust dosages.

Grapefruit juice can decrease metabolism of PIs.
CLIENT EDUCATION: Avoid grapefruit juice.

NURSING ADMINISTRATION

- Except for indinavir, administer protease inhibitors with food to increase absorption.
- Administer with another antiretroviral to reduce the risk of medication resistance.

CLIENT EDUCATION

- Report all other medications, including over-the-counter and herbal medications, to the provider.
- Use a barrier form of contraception, such as condoms, in addition to a hormonal contraceptive.

NURSING EVALUATION OF MEDICATION EFFECTIVENESS

Depending on therapeutic intent, effectiveness can be evidenced reduction of HIV manifestations and freedom from opportunistic infections.

Antiretrovirals: Integrase inhibitors (INSTIs)

SELECT PROTOTYPE MEDICATION: Raltegravir (oral)

PURPOSE

EXPECTED PHARMACOLOGICAL ACTION: Interfere with the enzyme integrase to prevent HIV replication within the cell

THERAPEUTIC USE: A first-line treatment for HIV when combined with two or three other antiretroviral medications

COMPLICATIONS

Headache and difficulty sleeping
CLIENT EDUCATION: Notify the provider if these findings occur.

Skin rash
- Can indicate Stevens-Johnson syndrome or other serious disorder, such as allergy
- CLIENT EDUCATION: Notify the provider if a rash or other skin manifestations occur.

Liver injury
- Anorexia, nausea, right upper quadrant pain, jaundice
- NURSING ACTIONS
  - Monitor liver function tests.
  - Notify the provider for manifestations of liver injury (jaundice, anorexia).

Kidney failure, hematuria
NURSING ACTIONS: Monitor for hematuria and decreased urinary output.

Suicidal ideation
CLIENT EDUCATION: Notify the provider of suicidal thoughts.

CONTRAINDICATIONS/PRECAUTIONS

- Contraindicated during lactation **Qs**
- Pregnancy Risk Category C
- Use cautiously in older adult clients or clients who have existing liver disorders.

INTERACTIONS

Concurrent use of rifampin or tipranavir/ritonavir can decrease raltegravir levels.
NURSING ACTIONS: Increase raltegravir dosage if needed.

NURSING ADMINISTRATION

- Administer raltegravir with or without food.
- Monitor baseline and periodic liver function tests and CBC.

CLIENT EDUCATION

- Take the medication exactly as prescribed without skipping doses to prevent medication resistance.
- Notify the provider of possible pregnancy.

NURSING EVALUATION OF MEDICATION EFFECTIVENESS

Depending on therapeutic intent, a reduction of HIV manifestations and absence of opportunistic infections indicates medication effectiveness.

PRACTICE Active Learning Scenario

A nurse is caring for a client who is immunocompromised and has a new prescription for ganciclovir IV twice per day to prevent cytomegalovirus. What should the nurse instruct the client about this medication? Use the ATI Active Learning Template: Medication to complete this item.

THERAPEUTIC USES: Identify for ganciclovir in this client.

COMPLICATIONS: Identify two adverse effects.

NURSING INTERVENTIONS: Describe two for clients taking ganciclovir, and two tests the nurse should monitor.

Application Exercises

1. A nurse is reviewing discharge teaching with a client who has a new prescription for combination oral NRTIs (abacavir, lamivudine, and zidovudine) for treatment of HIV. Which of the following statements should the nurse include?

    A. "These medications work by blocking HIV entry into cells."

    B. "These medications work by weakening the cell wall of the HIV virus."

    C. "These medications work by inhibiting enzymes to prevent HIV replication."

    D. "These medications work by preventing protein synthesis within the HIV cell."

2. A nurse is caring for a client who takes several antiretroviral medications, including the NRTI zidovudine, to treat HIV infection. The nurse should monitor for which of the following adverse effects of zidovudine? (Select all that apply.)

    A. Fatigue

    B. Blurred vision

    C. Ataxia

    D. Hyperventilation

    E. Vomiting

3. A nurse is caring for a client who is taking ritonavir, a protease inhibitor, to treat HIV infection. The nurse should monitor for which of the following adverse effects of this medication?

    A. Increased TSH level

    B. Decreased ALT level

    C. Hypoglycemia

    D. Hyperlipidemia

4. A nurse is caring for a client who has a new prescription for enfuvirtide to treat HIV infection. The nurse should monitor the client for which of the adverse reactions of this medication? (Select all that apply.)

    A. Bleeding

    B. Pneumonia

    C. Cerebral edema

    D. Localized erythema

    E. Hypotension

5. A nurse is administering IV acyclovir to a client who has varicella. Which of the following actions should the nurse take?

    A. Administer a stool softener.

    B. Decrease fluid intake following infusion.

    C. Infuse acyclovir over 1 hr.

    D. Monitor for hypotension

6. A nurse is reinforcing teaching with a client about ways to prevent medication resistance when taking highly active antiretroviral therapy (HAART). Which of the following information should the nurse include?

    A. Taking low dosages of antiretroviral medication minimizes resistance.

    B. Taking one antiretroviral medication at a time minimizes resistance.

    C. Taking medication at the same times daily without missing doses minimizes resistance.

    D. Changing the medication regimen when adverse effects occur minimizes resistance.

Application Exercises Key

1. A. The fusion/entry inhibitor enfuvirtide and the CCR5 antagonist maraviroc are newer antiretroviral medications that work by blocking HIV entry into cells.

   B. Some bactericidal antibiotics, such as penicillin, work by weakening the cell walls of bacteria.

   C. **CORRECT:** The NRTI antiretroviral medications this client takes work by inhibiting the enzyme reverse transcriptase and preventing HIV replication.

   D. Some antibiotics, such as aminoglycosides, kill bacteria by preventing protein synthesis within the cell.

   Ⓝ *NCLEX® Connection: Pharmacological Therapies, Expected Actions/Outcomes*

2. A. **CORRECT:** Fatigue is a manifestation of anemia, an adverse effect of zidovudine. Neutropenia can also occur, causing a high risk for infection.

   B. Zidovudine can cause hearing loss and photophobia.

   C. Zidovudine can cause vertigo.

   D. **CORRECT:** Hyperventilation is a finding that can occur if the client develops lactic acidosis, a serious adverse effect of zidovudine.

   E. **CORRECT:** Vomiting and other GI effects are adverse effects of zidovudine.

   Ⓝ *NCLEX® Connection: Pharmacological Therapies, Adverse Effects/ Contraindications/Side Effects/Interactions*

3. A. Increased TSH and T4 levels indicate hyperthyroidism, which is not an adverse effect of ritonavir.

   B. An increase in liver function tests, including AST and ALT levels, can occur as an adverse effect of ritonavir.

   C. Hyperglycemia indicating a possible onset or worsening of diabetes mellitus can occur as an adverse effect of ritonavir.

   D. **CORRECT:** Hyperlipidemia with increased cholesterol and triglyceride levels can occur as an adverse effect of ritonavir.

   Ⓝ *NCLEX® Connection: Pharmacological Therapies, Adverse Effects/ Contraindications/Side Effects/Interactions*

4. A. Bleeding is not an adverse effect of enfuvirtide.

   B. **CORRECT:** Bacterial pneumonia with fever, cough, and difficulty breathing are manifestations of an adverse reaction to enfuvirtide. The nurse should check breath sounds regularly.

   C. Cerebral edema is not an adverse reaction to enfuvirtide.

   D. **CORRECT:** Enfuvirtide is administered subcutaneously. Injection-site reactions (pain, redness, itching, bruising) are common.

   E. **CORRECT:** A systemic allergic reaction can occur when taking enfuvirtide. Manifestations of hypersensitivity include rash, hypotension, fever, and chills.

   Ⓝ *NCLEX® Connection: Pharmacological Therapies, Adverse Effects/ Contraindications/Side Effects/Interactions*

5. A. Acyclovir can cause diarrhea.

   B. The nurse should increase fluids during and for 2 hr following acyclovir infusion to prevent nephrotoxicity.

   C. **CORRECT:** The nurse should administer IV acyclovir slowly, over at least 1 hr, to prevent nephrotoxicity.

   D. Acyclovir can cause thrombocytopenia in clients who are immunocompromised.

   Ⓝ *NCLEX® Connection: Pharmacological Therapies, Adverse Effects/ Contraindications/Side Effects/Interactions*

6. A. Taking low dosages of the medication can cause medication resistance.

   B. Taking a combination of antiretroviral medications helps prevent resistance to each medication. Taking only one medication can lead to quick resistance.

   C. **CORRECT:** The nurse should emphasize the importance of taking each dose of medication exactly as prescribed. Missing even a few doses of antiretroviral medication can promote medication resistance, which can cause treatment failure.

   D. Changing the medication regimen when adverse effects occur can promote medication resistance.

   Ⓝ *NCLEX® Connection: Pharmacological Therapies, Expected Actions/Outcomes*

PRACTICE Answer

Using the ATI Active Learning Template: Medication

THERAPEUTIC USES: Ganciclovir prevents reproduction of viral DNA and thus prevents viral cell replication. It is used is to prevent or treat cytomegalovirus in clients who are immunocompromised.

COMPLICATIONS
- Minor discomforts, such as fever, headache, and nausea
- Suppresses the bone marrow, causing a decrease in WBCs (especially granulocytes)
- Causes thrombocytopenia frequently
- The client should report any discomforts and be sure to report new onset of fatigue, easy bruising, or sore throat.
- The client should report manifestations of infection or bleeding, and avoid crowds or individuals who have respiratory infections.

NURSING INTERVENTIONS
- Monitor client blood counts, especially WBC, absolute neutrophil count, and thrombocyte count. The nurse should expect ganciclovir therapy to be interrupted for an absolute neutrophil count less than 500/mm^3 or a thrombocyte count less than 25,000/mm^3.
- Monitor blood counts.
- Prepare to administer granulocyte colony-stimulating factors for a low absolute neutrophil count.
- Monitor I&O, and encourage the client to increase fluid intake.
- Avoid direct contact with the powder from oral ganciclovir or the IV solution, and wash well if contact occurs.
- Advise clients to use barrier contraception, such as condoms, during treatment and for 3 months following treatment.

Ⓝ *NCLEX® Connection: Pharmacological and Parenteral Therapies, Medication Administration*

References

Berman, A., Snyder, S., & Frandsen, G. (2016). *Kozier & Erb's fundamentals of nursing: Concepts, process, and practice* (10th ed.). Upper Saddle River, NJ: Prentice-Hall.

Burchum, J. R., & Rosenthal, L. D. (2016). *Lehne's pharmacology for nursing care* (9th ed.). St. Louis, MO: Elsevier.

Centers for Disease Control and Prevention. (2017). *Vaccines and immunizations*. Retrieved from https://www.cdc.gov/vaccines/index.html

Dudek, S. G. (2014). *Nutrition essentials for nursing practice* (7th ed.). Philadelphia: Lippincott Williams & Wilkins.

Eliopoulos, C. (2014). *Gerontological nursing* (8th ed.). Philadelphia: Lippincott Williams & Wilkins.

Ford, S. M., & Roach, S. S. (2014). *Roach's introductory clinical pharmacology* (10th ed.). Philadelphia: Lippincott Williams & Wilkins.

Grodner, M., Escott-Stump, S., & Dorner, S. (2016). *Nutritional foundations and clinical applications of nutrition: A nursing approach* (6th ed.). St. Louis, MO: Mosby.

Halter, M. J. (2014). *Varcarolis' foundations of psychiatric mental health nursing: A clinical approach* (7th ed.). St. Louis, MO: Saunders.

Hinkle, J. L., & Cheever, K. H. (2014). *Brunner and Suddarth's textbook of medical-surgical nursing* (13th ed.). Philadelphia: Lippincott Williams & Wilkins.

Hockenberry, M. J., & Wilson, D. (2015) *Wong's nursing care of infants and children* (10th ed.). St. Louis, MO: Mosby.

Ignatavicius, D. D., & Workman, M. L. (2016). *Medical-surgical nursing* (8th ed.). St. Louis, MO: Elsevier.

Immunization Action Coalition. (2017). *Advisory Committee on Immunization Practice*. Retrieved from http://www.immunize.org/acip/

Lilley, L. L., Rainforth-Collins, S., & Snyder, J. S. (2017). *Pharmacology and the nursing process* (8th Ed.). St. Louis, MO: Elsevier.

Lowdermilk, D. L., Perry, S. E., Cashion, M. C., & Aldean, K. R. (2016). *Maternity & women's health care* (11th ed.). St. Louis, MO: Elsevier.

Pagana, K. D., & Pagana, T. J. (2014). *Mosby's manual of diagnostic and laboratory tests* (5th ed.). St. Louis, MO: Elsevier.

Potter, P. A., Perry, A. G., Stockert, P., & Hall, A. (2017). *Fundamentals of nursing* (9th ed.). St. Louis, MO: Elsevier

Taketomo, C. K., Hodding, J. H., & Kraus, D. M. (2016). *Lexi-Comp's Pediatric & Neonatal Dosage Handbook: A universal resource for clinicians treating pediatric and neonatal patients* (23rd ed.). Hudson, OH: Lexi-Comp.

Touhy, T.A., & Jett, K.F. (2016) *Ebersole & Hess' toward healthy aging: Human needs and nursing response* (9th ed.). St. Louis, MO: Elsevier.

Townsend, M. C. (2017). *Essentials of psychiatric mental health nursing: Concepts of care in evidence-based practice* (7th ed.). Philadelphia: F. A. Davis.

Vallerand, A.H., & Sanoski, C.A. (2017). *Davis's drug guide for nurses* (15th Ed.). Philadelphia: Elsevier.

STUDENT NAME _____

CONCEPT_____ REVIEW MODULE CHAPTER_____

Related Content

(E.G., DELEGATION,
LEVELS OF PREVENTION,
ADVANCE DIRECTIVES)

Underlying Principles

Nursing Interventions

WHO? WHEN? WHY? HOW?

STUDENT NAME _____

PROCEDURE NAME _____ REVIEW MODULE CHAPTER_____

Description of Procedure

Indications

CONSIDERATIONS

Nursing Interventions (pre, intra, post)

Interpretation of Findings

Client Education

Potential Complications

Nursing Interventions

Growth and Development

STUDENT NAME _____

DEVELOPMENTAL STAGE _____ REVIEW MODULE CHAPTER_____

EXPECTED GROWTH AND DEVELOPMENT

Physical Development	Cognitive Development	Psychosocial Development	Age-Appropriate Activities

Health Promotion

Immunizations	Health Screening	Nutrition	Injury Prevention

STUDENT NAME _____

MEDICATION _____ REVIEW MODULE CHAPTER_____

CATEGORY CLASS_____

PURPOSE OF MEDICATION

Expected Pharmacological Action

Therapeutic Use

Complications

Medication Administration

Contraindications/Precautions

Interactions

Nursing Interventions

Client Education

Evaluation of Medication Effectiveness

STUDENT NAME _____

SKILL NAME_____ REVIEW MODULE CHAPTER_____

Description of Skill

Indications

CONSIDERATIONS

Nursing Interventions (pre, intra, post)

Outcomes/Evaluation

Client Education

Potential Complications

Nursing Interventions

STUDENT NAME _____

DISORDER/DISEASE PROCESS _____ REVIEW MODULE CHAPTER_____

Alterations in Health (Diagnosis)	Pathophysiology Related to Client Problem	Health Promotion and Disease Prevention

ASSESSMENT

Risk Factors

Expected Findings

Laboratory Tests

Diagnostic Procedures

SAFETY CONSIDERATIONS

PATIENT-CENTERED CARE

Nursing Care

Medications

Client Education

Therapeutic Procedures

Interprofessional Care

Complications

STUDENT NAME _____

PROCEDURE NAME _____ REVIEW MODULE CHAPTER_____

Description of Procedure

Indications

Outcomes/Evaluation

Potential Complications

CONSIDERATIONS

Nursing Interventions (pre, intra, post)

Client Education

Nursing Interventions